Clinical implications of
laboratory tests

Clinical implications of laboratory tests

SARKO M. TILKIAN, M.D.

Director of Medical Education, Northridge Hospital; Staff Physician,
Northridge Hospital Foundation, Northridge, California,
and Tarzana Medical Center, Tarzana, California

MARY BOUDREAU CONOVER, R.N., B.S.

Instructor and Education Consultant, California Hospital Medical Center,
Los Angeles, California; Instructor of Intermediate and Advanced
Arrhythmia Workshops, West Hills Hospital, Canoga Park,
California; Education Consultant, Holy Cross Hospital
Cardiac Arrhythmia Center, Mission Hills, California

ARA G. TILKIAN, M.D., F.A.C.C.

Assistant Clinical Professor of Medicine, University of California,
Los Angeles; Associate Director of Cardiology, Holy Cross Hospital and
Valley Presbyterian Hospital, San Fernando Valley, California

THIRD EDITION

with **70** illustrations

The C. V. Mosby Company

ST. LOUIS • TORONTO • LONDON   1983

MOSBY

A TRADITION OF PUBLISHING EXCELLENCE

Editor: Michael R. Riley
Assistant editor: Sally Gaines
Manuscript editor: Stephen C. Hetager
Book design: Jeanne Bush
Cover design: Suzanne Oberholtzer
Production: Susan Trail

THIRD EDITION

The C.V. Mosby Company
11830 Westline Industrial Drive, St. Louis, Missouri 63141

Library of Congress Cataloging in Publication Data

Tilkian, Sarko M., 1936-
    Clinical implications of laboratory tests.

    Bibliography: p.
    Includes index.
    1. Diagnosis, Laboratory. I. Conover, Mary
Boudreau, 1931- . II. Tilkian, Ara G., 1944-
III. Title.
RB37.T54   1983   616.07′5   82-18829
ISBN 0-8016-4960-9

GW/VH/VH 9 8 7 6 5 4 3 2 1   03/D/310

Lovingly dedicated to
our parents
Garabed and Nevart Tilkian
Essel and Eleanor Boudreau

Preface

This book is designed for persons in the nursing and allied health professions who need a concise reference and comprehensive guide to the clinical significance of laboratory tests. In addition to the standard clinical laboratory tests, we have included various forms of organ imaging (roentgenography, ultrasound, nuclear medicine), graphic studies (electrocardiography, vascular studies, sleep studies), and invasive diagnostic tests (cardiac catheterization, bronchoscopy, various organ biopsies). Our intention is to bridge the gap between the voluminous clinical pathology textbooks and the handbooks that merely list the conditions associated with abnormal results of laboratory tests, while still giving the reader an understanding of the physiological basis for each test and of the physiology of the organ being tested.

Since the publication of the second edition of this book, advances in nuclear medicine, computerized tomography techniques, and ultrasound studies have brought about many changes in laboratory tests, necessitating that most of the chapters in Unit Two be almost completely rewritten. In addition, we have included chapters on diagnostic tests for vascular disorders, nutritional disorders, and sleep disorders, three important disciplines that have developed rapidly during the past five years. A fourth new chapter, on miscellaneous diseases and tests, discusses allergy, porphyrias, diabetes, and other conditions.

Two other important additions can be found in the appendices: "Recommended procedure for necessary contrast studies in patients with a history of reaction to contrast material" and "Critical limits (panic values) for laboratory tests and drug levels."

Unit One deals with the tests in the routine laboratory screening panels. The discussion of each test includes suggestions of disease entities that could be suspected when the results of a particular laboratory test, or combination of tests, are abnormal. The tables provided at the end of Unit One guide the reader to the page in Unit Two where further discussion of a suspected disease entity and additional diagnostic laboratory tests can be found. The tests described in Chapter 1, "Blood Chemistry," have been arranged alphabetically for easy reference.

Unit Two is divided into chapters according to organ systems. Each chapter includes sections on anatomy and physiology, laboratory tests, and the application of those tests to specific disease entities. The descriptions of the laboratory tests include discussions of clinical value, indications, contraindications, dangers, pitfalls, and, when appropriate, patient preparation. The sections on the clinical application of the tests include brief descriptions of the diseases in question and lists of the diagnostic laboratory tests in the usual order of performance, followed by differential diagnosis.

H. Steven Aharonian, M.D., Assistant Clinical Professor of Medicine, University of California, Los Angeles, has revised the chapter on diagnostic tests for gastrointestinal disorders. Harry W. Rein, M.D., Director of Neurology, Valley Presbyterian Hospital, Van Nuys, California, has completely rewritten the chapter on diagnostic tests in neurologic disorders. We are grateful to these people and to Jeff Aaronson, M.D., Associate Clinical Professor of Medicine, University of Southern California, Los Angeles, who reviewed the chapter on diagnostic tests for bronchopulmonary disease and made many valuable contributions; Myron T. Berdischewsky, M.D., Instructor, Departments of Medicine and Infectious Diseases, University of California, Los Angeles, for his review of the chapter on infectious diseases; and Ronald Tung, M.D., for his contribution to the allergy section of the chapter on miscellaneous tests.

Sarko M. Tilkian
Mary Conover
Ara G. Tilkian

Contents

11 Diagnostic tests for neurologic disorders, 280

12 Diagnostic tests for collagen vascular diseases, 302

Routine multisystem screening tests

An increase in the number, availability, and sophistication of laboratory tests has made them valuable tools in the study of clinical problems. In recent years multiphasic screening tests have been adopted widely to supplement the conventional history and physical examination. These tests are based on the fact that a group of laboratory determinations can now be carried out on a single specimen at a relatively low cost.

These helpful diagnostic procedures, however, do not release one from the careful study and observation of the patient, nor should they be ordered without an understanding and appreciation of their merits and limitations as well as their hazards and expense. When performed as part of the total physical examination they have the following advantages:

1. Biochemical aberrations that are usually undetectable by routine history and physical can be discovered more easily.
2. When the patient has a known disease, the screening panels serve as a gauge of the overall biochemical state relative to the existing malady.
3. When there is a diagnostic problem, the findings of the screening panels may help with the differential diagnosis.
4. The screening panels supply data concerning the biochemical parameters necessary for the safe administration of medications.

The most commonly used biochemical screening panels are blood chemistry, hematology, and urinalysis.

Blood chemistry usually includes determination of the levels of calcium, phosphorus, glucose, uric acid, cholesterol, total protein, albumin, alkaline phosphatase, bilirubin, lactic dehydrogenase (LDH), serum glutamic-oxaloacetic transaminase (SGOT), blood urea nitrogen (BUN), creatinine, and electrolytes.

Hematology consists of a white blood cell count and differential and a red blood cell count, and determinations of hematocrit, hemoglobin level, mean corpuscular volume, mean corpuscular hemoglobin concentration, and sedimentation rate.

Urinalysis consists of determinations of pH, specific gravity, and glucose level, tests for the presence of blood and protein, and a microscopic examination.

ONE Blood chemistry

The tests in this chapter are listed alphabetically, with the electrolytes and enzymes being grouped together under their general titles.

If an automated analyzer is used, a single specimen of blood may be used to determine levels of electrolytes and chemical constituents.

BILIRUBIN (total serum)

Bilirubin is formed by the reticuloendothelial system, from the hemoglobin of destroyed erythrocytes; it is the predominant pigment of the bile. Being a by-product of hemoglobin metabolism, bilirubin is a waste product and thus must be excreted.

Bilirubin exists in two forms in the body, soluble (conjugated or direct-reacting) and protein-bound (unconjugated or "indirect-reacting"). The routine test for bilirubin level does not differentiate between the two, and further tests are run if the total bilirubin level is elevated. These tests and normal bilirubin physiology are discussed in Chapter 8, on p. 213.

◗ Normal bilirubin (serum)

Total:	0.1-1.2 mg/dl
Newborn total:	1-12 mg/dl

A normal level of total bilirubin rules out any significant impairment of the excretory function of the liver. It also rules out hemolysis.

Greatly elevated total bilirubin level (>12 mg/dl)

A markedly elevated total bilirubin level along with a significant drop in hemoglobin level and significant reticulocytosis strongly suggests massive hemolysis. If massive hemolysis is indeed taking place, further tests will show the bilirubin to be of the indirect-reacting type (Chapter 8, p. 213).

Significant elevation of the level of direct-reacting bilirubin indicates obstructive jaundice, which may result from the obstructive phase of hepatitis, cholangiolitis, or lower bilary tree obstruction caused by either calculus or carcinoma.

CALCIUM (Ca)

More than 98% of the calcium in the body is in the skeleton and teeth. The calcium in the extracellular fluid is only a small fraction of the total; its level and the level of phosphorus in that fluid are regulated precisely by the parathyroid gland and by the total serum protein level. The level of calcium in extracellular fluid rarely varies more than 5% above or below normal.

Of the total plasma calcium, 50% is ionized, while most of the rest is protein bound. The ionized calcium is important in blood coagulation, in the function of the heart, muscles, and nerves, and in membrane permeability.

Parathyroid hormone raises the plasma ionized calcium concentration by acting directly on osteoclasts to release bone salts into the extracellular fluid, thus affecting both calcium and phosphorus (usually measured as phosphate [PO_4]) levels in the plasma. Parathyroid hormone also increases the rate of absorption of calcium from the intestines and acts on the renal tubular cells, causing calcium to be saved and phosphorus to be lost.

Two other factors important in calcium metabolism are vitamin D and the potent hypocalcemic hormone calcitonin. Vitamin D increases the efficiency of intestinal calcium absorption; the effects of calcitonin are the opposite of those of parathyroid hormone in that calcitonin increases renal calcium clearance.

♦ Normal serum calcium

Ionized: 4.2-5.2 mg/dl
2.1-2.6 mEq/L or 50% to 58% of total
Total: 9.0-10.6 mg/dl
4.5-5.3 mEq/L
Infants: 11-13 mg/dl

Generally, a normal serum calcium value along with a normal overall biochemical screening panel rules out any significant disease entity involving calcium metabolism. However, a normal calcium value along with an abnormal level of phosphorus may indicate significant disease. In serum, the product of Ca × P (mg/dl) is normally about 50 in children. This product may be below 30 in rickets.

A normal blood calcium level in association with an elevated blood urea nitrogen (BUN) level would be very suggestive of one of two things: (1) secondary hyperparathyroidism, in which case uremia and acidosis have initially lowered the serum calcium level, which in turn will stimulate the parathyroid, resulting in a normal serum calcium level or (2) primary hyperparathyroidism, which would initially elevate the serum calcium level. The development of secondary kidney disease and uremia would then lower the elevated calcium level to normal by phosphate retention.

A normal serum calcium value associated with a marked decrease in serum albumin level should be considered abnormal hypercalcemia. Since about 50% of the total serum calcium is protein bound, the blood level of calcium should be depressed in the presence of hypoproteinemia. Free calcium ions are not measured directly; therefore the concentration of serum proteins is an important factor in estimating the level of ionized calcium in the blood.

Hypercalcemia

If all other biochemical values are normal, an elevation in calcium level should raise the possibility of laboratory error, and a second determination of calcium and phosphorus levels should then be made.

Hypercalcemia associated with hypophosphatemia is characteristic of hyperparathyroidism.

Hypercalcemia associated with hypergammaglobulinemia indicates three main possibilities: (1) sarcoidosis, (2) multiple myeloma, or (3) malignancies.

Hypercalcemia associated with metabolic alkalosis should raise the possibility of milk-alkali syndrome, particularly if there is a history of peptic ulcer, in which case there may have been ingestion of large amounts of calcium (milk) and absorbable antacids.

Hypercalcemia with a significant elevation in alkaline phosphatase level may suggest Paget's disease of bone.

Other causes of hypercalcemia are severe thyrotoxicosis, malignant tumors with or without bone metastasis, and bone fractures, especially during bed rest. Hypercalcemia may also be found in acute bone atrophy, hypervitaminosis D, polycythemia vera, some cases of acromegaly, Cushing's syndrome with osteoporosis, and in patients taking thiazide diuretics. In addition, hypercalcemia may be idiopathic.

Hypocalcemia

Whenever hypocalcemia is encountered, it is advisable to perform serum protein electrophoresis. If there is significant diminution of the albumin fraction, the hypocalcemia may not be true hypocalcemia and may not be significant in terms of calcium metabolism. This condition is termed pseudohypocalcemia. In such a situation, a reduction of the albumin fraction would also cause the serum calcium level to be low.

The causes of hypocalcemia, after pseudohypocalcemia has been ruled out, are:

1. Hypoparathyroidism, especially if the patient has undergone thyroid or parathyroid surgery
2. Osteomalacia in adults and rickets in children, both of which result from vitamin D deficiency
3. Chronic steatorrhea, resulting from pancreatic insufficiency, sprue, celiac disease, or biliary obstruction, all of which cause decreased absorption of calcium from the gastrointestinal tract (malabsorption syndrome). In such a case, as well as in acute pancreatitis, fatty acids form calcium soaps, which precipitate, causing calcium to be lost in the feces.
4. Pregnancy
5. Diuretic intake, if there is a history of such intake—particularly "loop" diuretics such as furosemide or ethacrynic acid
6. Respiratory alkalosis and hyperventilation. Since alkalosis causes calcium ions to bind to protein, the ionized calcium fraction decreases.
7. Hypomagnesemia, possibly secondary to suppression of release of parathyroid hormone

Certain types of hypocalcemia in the newborn respond to magnesium administration, indicating a primary etiology of hypomagnesemia.

Effect of calcium on an electrocardiogram

The S-T segment changes of an electrocardiogram (ECG) may be very helpful in case of doubt as to laboratory error or in situations where a quick evaluation of the serum calcium level is desirable, particularly in the hyperventilation syndrome. Usually, hypocalcemia causes significant prolongation of the S-T segment of the Q-T interval. Hypercalcemia causes shortening of the Q-T interval and perhaps a widening and rounding of the T waves. (Refer to Table 4-1, p. 77.)

CHOLESTEROL (Chol)

Cholesterol exists in the body in both a free form and an esterified form (combined with a fatty acid). Most ingested cholesterol is esterified in the intestine and absorbed as such into the lymph. The liver synthesizes cholesterol from acetate. This synthesis is presumably inhibited by a high level of circulating cholesterol.

Cholesterol is used in the body to form cholic acid in the liver, which in turn forms bile salts, important for fat digestion. A small quantity of cholesterol is used in the formation of hormones by the adrenal glands, ovaries, and testes. A large amount is used to make the skin highly resistant to the absorption of water-soluble substances.

The concentration of cholesterol in the blood is influenced by thyroid hormones and estrogens, both of which cause a decrease. The plasma cholesterol level is elevated when biliary flow is obstructed, and also in hereditary hypercholesterolemia and untreated diabetes mellitus, in spite of a decrease in cholesterol synthesis in diabetes.

There is popular interest in cholesterol values because hypercholesterolemia is a much publicized risk factor for coronary artery disease. This is discussed in Chapter 4. It is important to keep in mind that normal values for cholesterol are arbitrarily defined and show much variation in different populations and age groups.

⧫ Normal serum cholesterol

150-250 mg/dl (varies with diet and age, and from country to country)

Marked hypercholesterolemia (>400 mg/dl)

Marked hypercholesterolemia is seen in:
1. Liver disease associated with biliary obstruction. In this condition elevated alkaline phosphatase and bilirubin levels accompany hypercholesterolemia.
2. Nephrotic stage of glomerulonephritis. Elevated BUN and creatinine levels may be present.
3. Familial hypercholesterolemia, a genetically transmitted disorder, more pronounced if homozygous

Other causes of hypercholesterolemia are hypothyroidism, pancreatectomy, and pancreatic dysfunction such as that in diabetes mellitus and chronic pancreatitis.

Significant hypocholesterolemia (<150 mg/dl)

A significantly low blood cholesterol concentration may reflect dietary habits, malnutrition, extensive liver disease, or possibly hyperthyroidism, which by itself causes a low-normal serum cholesterol level.

In liver disease it is advisable to fractionate the cholesterol to the esterified form, since esterification is affected by liver damage much more than is the total cholesterol level.

Other conditions that may be associated with hypocholesterolemia are severe sepsis, anemia (megaloblastic and hypochromic), serum α and β lipoprotein deficiency, and certain enzyme deficiencies associated with cholesterol metabolism.

CREATININE (Creat), SERUM

Creatinine is a waste product of creatine, which is present in skeletal muscle as creatine phosphate, a high-energy compound.

Determination of serum creatinine level is a test of renal function. The creatinine level reflects the balance between the production of creatinine (proportional to the body's muscle mass) and its filtration by the renal glomerulus.

♦ **Normal creatinine (serum)**

0.6-1.2 mg/dl

Elevated serum creatinine level

The serum creatinine concentration is elevated in all diseases of the kidney in which 50% or more of the nephrons are destroyed. Nonrenal causes of elevation or fluctuation in serum creatinine levels are few, making the creatinine test fairly specific for renal failure. People with large muscle mass or patients with acromegaly may have values slightly above the normal range and still have normal kidney function.

ELECTROLYTES

The serum electrolyte panel traditionally has included tests for sodium (Na^+), potassium (K^+), and chloride (Cl^-) levels and carbon dioxide (CO_2) content. Recently, however, there has been increased awareness that electrolyte disorders often involve abnormalities in the levels of magnesium (Mg^{++}) and, to a lesser degree, phosphorus (PO_4) and calcium (Ca^{++}). It is likely that in the near future a *complete* electrolyte panel will include all seven.

The levels of electrolytes in the blood result from the fine regulation of ionic charges and the osmotic balance of the extracellular fluid. This regulation is accomplished through the marvelous adaptation of the kidneys, the lungs, and the endocrine system to varying and multidirectional forces. The kidneys and the lungs are involved in acid-base balance, while osmotic balance is finely governed by the endocrine system, with the hypothalamus, the posterior pituitary gland, and the kidneys being intricately interrelated.

It is apparent, then, that the determination of the serum level of a single electrolyte is insufficient for an overall evaluation of a patient's metabolic state. When one wishes to determine the serum level of any electrolyte, the whole series should be ordered. This approach will have a profound bearing on the correct interpretation and evaluation of the patient's electrolyte status.

The following example is given to emphasize the importance of a complete electrolyte analysis. A serum potassium level of 4.5 mEq/L means one thing if the CO_2 content is 35 mEq/L and something altogether different if the CO_2 content is 10 mEq/L. In the first case, the patient probably has a metabolic alkalosis. This would cause the potassium to migrate into the cells and be excreted in the urine. A serum potassium level of 4.5 mEq/L does not, then, reflect a true potassium homeostasis, since when the alkalosis is corrected the potassium will return to its extracellular position, with a possible decrease in total body potassium.

In the second case (CO_2 content of 10 mEq/L), the patient probably has a metabolic acidosis. This would cause the potassium to leave the cells. A serum potassium level of 4.5 mEq/L would, then, reflect a much lower potassium level when acidosis is corrected, since the available potassium will migrate back into the cells when the acidosis is corrected.

In addition to electrolyte level determination, it is extremely important that the blood urea nitrogen (BUN) and creatinine levels be determined as well. These serve two purposes. First, serum electrolyte values have one implication in the presence of an elevated BUN level with the associated metabolic acidosis, but when the BUN level is normal the implication changes. In addition, the BUN level is a relatively good indication of a patient's overall water metabolism and hydration status, which has a pronounced effect on the levels of the various electrolytes. Second, if therapy must be instituted, particularly potassium replacement, it is essential to know kidney function. It is preferable that a creatinine clearance test be ordered. However, if this is not available, at least one BUN determination should be ordered so that the patient's condition may be managed safely.

It is preferable to measure the arterial pH, P_{O_2}, and P_{CO_2} directly, because the pH affects and is affected by the serum electrolyte levels. This is particularly true in complex metabolic and/or respiratory acid-base problems, in which it is extremely difficult to evaluate the patient's electrolyte levels without knowing the arterial blood gas levels and pH.

Serum electrolyte levels may vary from moment to moment; therefore they are only rough indicators of the total body content of the ions. For example, in the condition known as dilutional hyponatremia the serum sodium level is below normal, but the total body sodium content is increased.

There is no direct way of measuring intracellular levels of electrolytes. It is known, however, that an electrocardiogram reflects the ratio of intracellular electrolytes to extracellular electrolytes. Initial information about a patient's overall electrolyte and acid-base state, therefore, may be drawn from this source.

By keeping in mind the above principles and problems, one can evaluate electrolyte levels much more rationally and obtain a more significant insight into a patient's overall metabolic state. At the present time electrolyte level determinations are usually performed in critical care units and in hospital environments. However, the value of these determinations is being appreciated more and more in the daily office practice of physicians, particularly in view of the large number of medications that alter electrolyte levels and body water metabolism.

Collecting and handling the specimen

When blood is being drawn for electrolyte level determinations, the procedure should be as atraumatic as possible, and the blood obtained should be centrifuged quickly. If there is any hemolysis, this fact should be noted, because tissue breakdown or hemolysis will cause a false elevation of serum potassium levels.

Carbon dioxide (CO_2) content

Total CO_2 content determination is the usual laboratory test done for the detection of acid-base abnormalities. Since direct determination of the pH of the blood is not clinically practical in ordinary circumstances, the CO_2 content is used instead. This test measures the total carbonic acid (H_2CO_3) and bicarbonate (HCO_3) in the plasma.

♦ Normal CO_2 content

24-30 mM/L

Elevated CO_2 content

In the absence of chronic obstructive lung disease, elevated CO_2 content indicates serum alkalosis and intracellular acidosis, which are most frequently associated with hypokalemia and hypochloremia.

For practical and therapeutic consideration, metabolic alkalosis can be divided into two groups, chloride responsive and chloride nonresponsive. The chloride-responsive type constitutes 90% of all hypochloremic alkalosis and can easily be corrected with potassium chloride administration. The usual causes of this type of metabolic alkalosis are gastrointestinal losses and diuretics.

The chloride-nonresponsive type makes up the remaining 10% of all metabolic alkalosis and occurs with Cushing's syndrome (particularly resulting from the ectopic ACTH production syndrome), primary aldosteronism, Bartter's syndrome, and licorice ingestion.

The two groups of metabolic alkalosis can be differentiated from each other by a 24-hour urine chloride measurement. In chloride-responsive alkalosis, the urinary chloride excretion is less than 10 mEq/L.

Low CO_2 content

A low CO_2 content occurs in conditions associated with metabolic acidosis, such as uremic acidosis, diabetic ketoacidosis, lactic acidosis, and renal tubular acidosis. However, if the arterial blood pH is found to be elevated (alkalosis), a low CO_2 content would indicate respiratory alkalosis as seen in the hyperventilation syndrome.

Metabolic acidosis and the anion gap. In the serum the numbers of cations and anions should be more or less equal, producing a neutral pH. The measurable electrolytes contributing to this anion-cation electroneutrality are sodium, chloride, and bicarbonate. Potassium, being an intracellular ion, contributes minimally and is usually not considered. The term "anion gap" refers to the number of unmeasurable anions, which is calculated by subtracting chloride and bicarbonate from the sodium concentration. With normal electrolytes, there is usually an anion gap of approximately 12.

Metabolic acidosis is commonly divided into two groups, normal anion gap and increased anion gap.

Metabolic acidosis with a normal anion gap is usually caused by diarrhea (because of a loss of bicarbonate), chronic interstitial nephritis, mild renal failure, renal tubular acidosis with hyperchloremia, urethrosigmoidostomy, administration of therapeutic ammonium chloride, or administration of acetazolamide.

Metabolic acidosis with an increased anion gap is usually caused by diabetic ketoacidosis, lactic acidosis, azotemic renal failure, or ingestion of toxins such as salicylates, ethylene glycol, paraldehyde, and methyl alcohol.

Serum chloride (Cl)

Chloride, chiefly an extracellular ion, is present in large quantities in the serum, exerting an important influence on acid-base balance and osmotic pressure.

♦ Normal serum chloride

95-103 mEq/L

Hyperchloremia

Hyperchloremia is most frequently associated with renal tubular acidosis, decreased CO_2 content, and hypokalemia.

Hypochloremia

Most often, hypochloremia is associated with hypokalemia and alkalosis; this condition has been termed hypokalemic-chloremic alkalosis. In such a situation the electrolyte analysis reflects low potassium and chloride levels and elevated CO_2 content. Most of the conditions associated with hypokalemia and alkalosis are also associated with hypochloremia.

Hypochloremia may also be associated with a normal serum potassium level if the patient's potassium deficiency is being corrected with potassium preparations that do not contain chloride, or if the patient is receiving potassium-saving diuretics. These facts bring into focus two points of clinical importance: (1) potassium replacement therapy should be accompanied by a one-to-one ratio of potassium to chloride, and (2) when potassium-saving diuretics are used one should watch very closely for the possible development of hypochloremia and hypochloremic alkalosis.

The development of hypochloremic alkalosis may occur when chronic respiratory acidosis is very rapidly corrected, precipitating significant chloride attrition from the kidneys.

Serum magnesium (Mg)

The magnesium ion is an essential cation, the fourth most abundant in the human body (after Na^+, K^+, and Ca^{++}). Numerous enzymatic reactions, including oxidative phosphorylation, depend upon adequate supplies of Mg^{++}. DNA transcription, RNA aggregation, protein synthesis, and numerous cell membrane functions require an optimal concentration of Mg^{++}. Of the total body Mg^{++}, only 1%-2% is in the extracellular fluid and the plasma. The remainder is found in bone (60%) or in the intracellular compartments of muscle cells, red blood cells, and so on. Thus, one major limitation of the value of a serum Mg^{++} determination is that a total body Mg^{++} deficit with intracellular depletion can occur without lowering the serum content. Therefore, a determination of Mg^{++} content in red blood cells is sometimes used to obtain an accurate assessment of Mg^{++} deficiency. In addition, a determination of the amount of Mg^{++} excreted in the urine after an intravenous load can provide an accurate assessment. At least 80% of such a load should be excreted in 24 hours if a Mg^{++} deficit is not present. Although one third of Mg^{++} is protein bound, the *ionized* Mg concentration is not measured routinely.

The average daily intake of Mg^{++} is approximately 300 mg (25 mEq). Normally, gastrointestinal (GI) losses are small and the kidney regulates Mg^{++} hemostasis. Either decreased or increased Mg^{++} levels can exist, as a result of gastrointestinal, renal, or endocrine factors.

Hypomagnesemia

Nutritional Mg^{++} deficiency is rare; it is seen in severe malnutrition or when a patient is receiving parenteral alimentation. Most instances of clinical Mg^{++} deficiency result from excessive losses, either from the kidney or from the GI tract. Infrequently, endocrine or metabolic causes are also present.

Gastrointestinal diseases or procedures that cause Mg^{++} deficiency include:
1. Malabsorption syndromes
2. Bowel resection
3. Chronic diarrhea
4. Intestinal and biliary fistulae
5. Nasogastric suction
6. Pancreatitis
7. Protein-calorie malnutrition

Causes of increased *renal* Mg^{++} loss include:
1. Diuretics of various types
2. Diabetic ketoacidosis
3. Aldosteronism
4. Congestive heart failure
5. Hypercalcemia
6. Other drugs (cisplatin, gentamycin, digoxin)
7. Alcohol
8. Renal diseases, including pyelonephritis, glomerulonephritis, and tubular disorders

Endocrine and metabolic causes of Mg^{++} loss include:
1. Hypoparathyroidism
2. Hyperthyroidism
3. Hypothyroidism
4. Phosphate deficiency

Manifestations of Mg^{++} deficiency include:
1. Hypocalcemia—secondary to both impaired parathyroid hormone secretion and end-organ resistance to the action of parathyroid hormone
2. Hypokalemia. Intracellular K^+ depletion and renal K^+ wasting occur because of compromise of the Na-K pump. These deficiencies prove resistant to K^+ supplements unless Mg^{++} deficiencies are also corrected.
3. Life-threatening arrhythmias, including ventricular tachycardia and fibrillation, can occur secondary to severe Mg^{++} depletion. The role of accompanying intracellular K^+ in the genesis of these arrhythmias is difficult to discern.
4. Enhanced digitalis toxicity
5. Neuromuscular hyperexcitability is frequent; tremulousness, fasciculation, weakness, and tetany are seen, and seizures can occur.
6. Dysphagia and anemias (rarely)

Treatment of hypomagnesemia includes Mg^{++} supplementation, oral or parenteral, and attempts to control the reason for the losses.

♦ Normal serum magnesium

1.8-2.2 mEq/L (a tightly controlled and narrow range)

♦ Some degree of magnesium depletion

1.5-1.8 mEq/L

♦ Definite hypomagnesemia

<1.5 mEq/L

♦ Potentially life-threatening hypomagnesemia

<1.0 mEq/L

Hypermagnesemia

Mild hypermagnesemia (2.5-3.0 mEq/L) is seen in the setting of excess intake of Mg^{++}, usually in the form of antacids or cathartics. Also, decreased renal function will predispose a person to elevated levels of Mg^{++}.

Severe (symptomatic) hypermagnesemia (>4-5 mEq/L) is seen infrequently, usually in the setting of increased intake with poor renal function or the setting of parenteral administration of Mg^{++} with poor control.

Manifestations of hypermagnesemia include (in progressive order):

1. Loss of deep tendon reflexes
2. Somnolence, and ultimately neuromuscular paralysis with respiratory arrest
3. Hypotension secondary to vasodilation and vascular collapse
4. Complete heart block and cardiac arrest (with very toxic levels—15 mEq/L or more)

Treatment includes control of Mg^{++} intake, Ca^{++} infusions, and in some cases peritoneal dialysis or hemodialysis.

Serum potassium (K)

Potassium is the major cation of the intracellular fluid, functioning as sodium does in the extracellular fluid, by influencing acid-base balance, osmotic pressure, and cellular membrane potential.

Serum potassium levels are profoundly affected by momentary acid-base changes. A discussion of serum potassium can be divided into three major categories: hyperkalemia, normokalemia with normal or decreased total body potassium, and hypokalemia, which is usually associated with decreased total body potassium levels.

♦ Normal serum potassium

3.8-5.0 mEq/L

Hyperkalemia

Hyperkalemia is encountered most frequently in renal failure. Ingestion of potassium chloride by a person with normal kidneys and normal creatinine clearance rarely results in hyperkalemia.

Addison's disease, accompanied by hypovolemia and retention of blood urea nitrogen, is the second most common clinical condition associated with hyperkalemia.

Massive tissue destruction, particularly destruction of muscle tissue, will result in hyperkalemia because of cellular trauma and leakage of intracellular potassium into the serum. Also, any causes of significant metabolic acidosis, such as lactic acidosis and diabetic ketoacidosis, can produce initial hyperkalemia.

Pseudohyperkalemia, a relatively rare condition, should be suspected when one encounters hyperkalemia without electrocardiographic evidence. Once documented, pseudohyperkalemia should suggest a myeloproliferative disease such as thrombocytosis. In such cases, the plasma potassium level should be checked instead of the serum potassium level, in order to obtain a true potassium level.

Normokalemia with normal or decreased total body potassium

The most commonly encountered clinical cause of normal potassium serum levels with decreased total body potassium levels is chronic diuretic use with inadequate potassium chloride supplementation. Other causes will be discussed under hypokelamia.

The following are a few clues that may be helpful in recognizing total body potassium depletion with normokalemia:

1. Alkalosis. This can be verified either directly, by arterial blood pH measurement, or indirectly, by checking for an elevation of the CO_2 content in the absence of chronic obstructive lung disease.
2. In the presence of significant hypochloremia and alkalosis, significant total body potassium depletion, not reflected in the serum, may exist.
3. An aberration in the cellular level of Na-K dependent adenosinetriphosphatase (ATPase) and in the Na-K pump may cause gradual cellupotassium depletion and may be reflected by hyponatremia rather than by hypokalemia.
4. The presence of a U wave or an apparent Q-T prolongation on the ECG should suggest cellular potassium depletion.

Hypokalemia

Most often, significant hypokalemia reflects total body depletion of potassium, which may have profound metabolic consequences.

Causes of hypokalemia are as follows:

1. Iatrogenic causes
   a. Diuretic therapy that depletes the body stores of potassium and chloride
   b. Diuretic therapy with supplementation of potassium and not chloride, causing a continual alkalosis with only a partial correction of the hypokalemia
2. Hypomagnesemia is quite frequently associated with hypokalemia. In such a situation, there will be continuous renal loss of potassium until the hypomagnesemia is corrected.
3. Endocrine causes
   a. Cushing's syndrome
   b. Primary or secondary hyperaldosteronism

   c. Liver disease with ascites

   d. Excessive ingestion of licorice, which contains a chemical very similar to aldosterone. The symptoms are, therefore, those of primary aldosteronism.

   e. Antiinflammatory drugs, indomethacin, phenylbutazone, and steroids and sex hormones, particularly estrogens

   f. Conditions associated with hyperreninemia, in which an excessive amount of renin introduced into the system can cause a secondary aldosteronemia. Such conditions include malignant hypertension, hypertensive disease, and (occasionally) unilateral renal vascular hypertension.

4. Poor dietary habits and crash diets with inadequate intake of potassium

5. Chronic stress

6. Excessive loss of potassium without adequate replacement

   a. Gastrointestinal tract (chronic diarrhea, malabsorption syndrome)

   b. Perspiration and chronic fever

7. Renal losses of potassium associated with either potassium-losing nephropathy or other kinds of renal tubular acidosis, which typically involve hypokalemia in association with acidosis and hyperchloremia and which sometimes are also associated with aminoacidurias

Electrocardiographic recognition of hyperkalemia and hypokalemia

An electrocardiogram is a sensitive indicator of the ratio of intracellular potassium to extracellular potassium; it shows signs of hypokalemia even when the serum potassium level is still within normal limits. Hypokalemia and hyperkalemia can cause life-threatening arrhythmias. It is, therefore, important to know the changes that a potassium deficit or excess will initiate on the ECG. This is discussed in Chapter 4.

Serum sodium (Na)

Sodium is the major cation of the extracellular fluid. It plays an important part in regulating acid-base equilibrium, protecting the body against excessive fluid loss, and preserving the normal function of muscle tissue.

♦ Normal serum sodium

136-142 mEq/L

Hypernatremia

Hypernatremia in a normally functioning individual is very uncommon. The condition most frequently occurs in a critical care unit, when an excessive amount of intravenous sodium is given to an unconscious patient, whose thirst mechanism is absent. Serum sodium levels have a strong influence on the body's osmoreceptors, and in the healthy individual this initiates the thirst mechanism. The individual then drinks water until the serum sodium level is back to normal.

Hyperglycemia is associated with hypernatremia in some rare hypothalamic lesions, in head trauma, and in hyperosmolar states. Other causes of hypernatremia are dehydration and steroid (mineralocorticoid) administration or excess.

Hyponatremia

Hyponatremia is more frequently encountered clinically than is hypernatremia. In ambulatory patients and in those seen in a physician's office, hyponatremia may reflect or be associated with diminution of total body sodium, with normal body sodium, or with excess body sodium.

Hyponatremia associated with an absolute sodium loss. Hyponatremia is associated with absolute sodium loss in the following conditions:

1. Addison's disease. In the absence of adrenal steroids, sodium reabsorption is impaired and the clinical picture is that of hyponatremia, hyperkalemia, and mild dehydration, reflected by a slight BUN elevation.
2. Chronic sodium-losing nephropathy. This is probably a more frequent cause than Addison's disease, and may be a stage in chronic glomerulonephritis or pyelonephritis, either of which is manifested by abnormal results of renal function tests and by an elevated BUN level.
3. Loss of gastrointestinal secretions because of vomiting, diarrhea, or tube drainage, with replacement of fluid but not electrolytes
4. Loss of sodium from the skin through diaphoresis or burns, with replacement of fluids but not electrolytes
5. Loss of sodium from the kidneys as a result of the use of diuretics (mercurial, chlorothiazide) or as a result of chronic renal insufficiency with acidosis
6. Metabolic loss of sodium through starvation with acidosis and diabetic acidosis
7. Loss of sodium from serous cavities through paracentesis or thoracentesis

Dilutional hyponatremia. Hyponatremia resulting from excessive water is associated with either normal or even excess total body sodium concentrations and is found in the following conditions or situations: chronic diuretic use with sodium restriction, secondary hyperaldosteronemia, hepatic failure with ascites, congestive heart failure, excessive water administration, acute or chronic renal insufficiency (oliguria), and diabetic acidosis (therapy without adequate sodium replacement).

Hyponatremia associated with inappropriate antidiuretic hormone syndrome. In this condition the patient continues reabsorbing water from the distal tubules and excreting a concentrated urine in spite of serum hypoosmolarity. Inappropriate antidiuretic hormone syndrome has been described in association with various other diseases, such as bronchogenic carcinoma (releasing ADH-like chemicals), pulmonary infections, metabolic diseases such as porphyria, and diuretic-induced hypokalemia.

Hyponatremia associated with intracellular potassium depletion. An impairment of the sodium-potassium pump mechanism results in an excessive intracellular sodium influx and a potassium efflux. The potassium is then lost in the urine, leaving the patient with a normal serum potassium level and a low serum sodium level, a situation that reflects the degree of intracellular sodium influx and corresponding potassium loss.

ENZYMES

Enzymes are found in all tissues. They are complex, naturally occurring compounds that catalyze the biochemical reactions of the body; that is, they speed up reactions that might otherwise proceed very slowly. Each tissue has its own specific enzyme; however, one enzyme can be common to more than one type of tissue. For example, alkaline phosphatase is found mainly in bone and liver and in small amounts in kidneys and the gastrointestinal tract. Glutamic-oxaloacetic transaminase (GOT) is found mainly in heart and skeletal muscle but also in the liver, kidneys, and red blood cells.

One looks for elevation of the levels of these enzymes in a laboratory examination, the rationale being that if a particular tissue is damaged significantly, it will release significant quantities of an enzyme into the blood.

Alkaline phosphatase (alk phos)

Alkaline phosphatase is an enzyme that mediates some of the complex reactions of bone formation. When the osteoblasts are actively depositing bone matrix, they secrete large quantities of alkaline phosphatase.

The two main sources of alkaline phosphatase are bone and liver. Consequently, an elevation of alkaline phosphatase immediately directs attention to either liver problems or bone disease that will correlate with clinical findings, such as jaundice (indicating liver disease). The chemical composition of the enzyme varies slightly according to its source, so that if the enzyme is fractionated one of the fractions (isoenzymes) is specific to the particular organ or tissue from which it came. For clinical purposes, the isoenzymes are not separated, although in highly specialized laboratories the different isoenzymes can be isolated by the process of electrophoresis (p. 27).

♦ Normal alkaline phosphatase (total serum)

Adults: 1.5-4.5 U/dl (Bodansky)
         4-13 U/dl (King-Armstrong)
         0.8-2.3 U/ml (Bessey-Lowry)
         15-35 U/ml (Shinowara-Jones-Reinhart)
Children: 5.0-14.0 U/dl (Bodansky)
         3.4-9.0 U/ml (Bessey-Lowry)
         15-30 U/dl (King-Armstrong)

Extreme elevation of alkaline phosphatase level with liver disease

When an extremely high level of alkaline phosphatase (15 U/dl or more, Bodansky) is associated with liver disease (abnormal results of liver function tests), one or both of the following are indicated:

1. Early phases of obstructive jaundice, with obstruction at the level of the major biliary ducts (gallstone or carcinoma of the head of the pancreas). In such a case the patient initially has a slight bilirubinemia; it gradually increases and is accompanied by the extremely high alkaline phosphatase level.
2. Space-occupying lesions of the liver, either widespread metastatic liver disease or an obstructive tumor of the biliary ducts. In the case of an obstructive tumor of the biliary ducts, the alkaline phosphatase is presumed to come from the cells that line the ducts. The obstruction and the damage cause the enzyme to leak from the cells and appear in the bloodstream.

Extreme elevation of alkaline phosphatase level without liver disease

In the absence of any indication of liver disease (normal results of liver function tests), an extreme elevation in alkaline phosphatase level along with some indication of bone pathology suggests Paget's disease of bone, in which disorder the highest level of the enzyme is found, especially if osteogenic sarcoma develops.

Extreme elevations in alkaline phosphatase level can also be found in carcinomas metastatic to bone.

Moderate or slight elevation of alkaline phosphatase level with liver disease

In the presence of liver disease, moderate elevation (8-12 U/dl, Bodansky) in the alkaline phosphatase level is usually associated with cholangiolitis hepatitis.

A slight elevation in the presence of liver disease usually indicates cirrhosis of the liver with some active hepatitis.

Moderate or slight elevation of alkaline phosphatase level without liver disease

In the absence of liver involvement (normal liver function test results) and in the presence of hypercalcemia, an elevated alkaline phosphatase level indicates the possibility of hyperparathyroidism. In this situation there is a slight elevation of the enzyme level in the initial stage. At a later stage there may be significant elevations. In secondary and tertiary hyperparathyroidism, borderline elevations may be encountered.

If other indicators of bone pathology (bone scan revealing evidence of bone disease) are present, mild to moderate elevations in the alkaline phosphatase level suggest osteomalacia. Usually such elevation will supply the differential diagnosis between osteomalacia and osteoporosis. In the latter condition the alkaline phosphatase level is normal.

In addition, a slight elevation in the alkaline phosphatase level occurs in childhood and during the growth period, in pregnancy, and in rickets.

Low alkaline phosphatase level

A low alkaline phosphatase level is usually not of much clinical significance. However, if a low value for this enzyme persists, one should consider some extremely rare entities, such as hypophosphatasia, achondroplasia, cretinism, and vitamin C deficiency.

Glutamic-oxaloacetic transaminase (GOT)

The transaminase enzymes catalyze the conversion of one amino acid to the corresponding keto acid, with simultaneous conversion of another keto acid to an amino acid. Transamination reactions occur in many tissues.

Glutamic-oxaloacetic transaminase is found mainly in heart muscle and the liver and to a certain degree in skeletal muscle, kidney, and red blood cells. Normally, almost all of this enzyme is intracellular. Following the injury or death of physiologically active cells, the enzyme is released into the serum (SGOT). Elevated SGOT values may be found 8 hours after injury and should peak in 24 to 36 hours if the original episode is not repeated. The SGOT level usually falls to normal in 4 to 6 days. The amount of SGOT is directly proportional to the number of cells damaged and the interval of time between tissue injury and the SGOT test.

◗ Normal SGOT
8-33 U/ml

Extreme elevation of SGOT value (>1000 U/ml)

There are extremely high levels of SGOT in the acute stages of severe fulminating hepatitis, in which there is massive destruction of liver tissue; in severe liver necrosis; and in skeletal muscle damage.

High SGOT values also occur in acute myocardial infarction. The level found following infarction depends on the size of the infarct and the time that elapses between the onset of the infarct and the drawing of the blood.

Minor elevation of SGOT value (40-100 U/ml)

Minor elevations in the SGOT level can be seen in congestive heart failure, tachyarrhythmias in the presence of shock, pericarditis, pulmonary infarction, and dissecting aneurysm, as well as in cirrhosis, cholangiolitic jaundice, metastatic liver disease, skeletal muscle disease, posttraumatic states, and generalized infections such as infectious mononucleosis.

Glutamic-pyruvic transaminase (GPT)

Glutamic-pyruvic transaminase is found mainly in liver cells; thus an elevated serum level (SGPT) is a definite sign of acute hepatocellular injury. In the presence of elevated SGOT and lactic dehydrogenase (LDH) values, a normal SGPT value rules out hepatic origin of the enzymes. On the other hand, a markedly elevated SGPT value in the presence of a mild to moderate elevation in the SGOT value definitely suggests either hepatic disease or hepatic disease combined with other conditions.

♦ Normal SGPT

1-36 U/ml

Lactic dehydrogenase (LDH)

Lactic dehydrogenase is an enzyme that catalyzes the reversible oxidation of lactic acid to pyruvic acid. It is present in nearly all metabolizing cells, with highest concentrations in heart, liver, kidney, brain, skeletal muscle, and erythrocytes. Damage to nearly any tissue can cause this enzyme to be released into the bloodstream. The origin of the release cannot be determined by routine examination. However, LDH can be separated into five isoenzymes, thus sharpening its diagnostic value. Electrophoresis is used to separate the isoenzymes of LDH and thus to determine the source of an elevated level of this enzyme.

One should be aware of the possibility of falsely elevated LDH levels as a result of hemolyzed blood specimens. Thus when all other parameters are normal except the LDH level, the LDH test should be repeated before any further investigations are undertaken.

♦ Normal LDH (serum)

80-120 Wacker units
71-207 IU/L
150-450 Wroblewski units

Extreme elevation of LDH level (>1500 Wroblewski units)

The highest values for this enzyme are seen in patients with myocardial infarction, hemolytic disorders, and pernicious anemia.

Slight elevation of LDH level (500-700 Wroblewski units)

Slight elevations that are persistent should direct attention to the following disease entities: chronic viral hepatitis; malignancies of skeletal muscles, liver, kidney, brain, blood, and heart; destruction of pulmonary tissue (pneumonia and pulmonary emboli); generalized viral infection involving multiple organs (infectious mononucleosis); low-grade hemolytic disorders; cerebrovascular accidents with brain damage; and renal tissue destruction (renal infarcts, infections, or malignancies).

GLUCOSE (Gluc), BLOOD

Most carbohydrates in the diet are digested to form glucose or fructose and are taken by the portal vein to the liver, where fructose is converted to glucose. The utilization of glucose by the body cells is intimately related to the blood level of insulin, the hormone secreted from the islets of Langerhans in the pancreas.

One usually sees the following order of frequency and range for fasting blood glucose level:

1. Normal—between 80 and 100 mg/dl
2. Mild elevation—between 120 and 130 mg/dl
3. Moderate elevation—between 300 and 500 mg/dl
4. Marked elevation—greater than 500 mg/dl (associated with ketoacidosis, which is reflected by decreased CO_2 combining power)
5. Marked elevation with hyperosmolar state, without ketoacidosis
6. Below the normal accepted ranges

The normal range for fasting blood glucose values varies among laboratories and with the type of procedure used. One should consult the particular laboratory as to the normal range and the method used.

‣ Normal blood glucose

Serum or plasma: 70-110 mg/dl
  Whole blood: 60-100 mg/dl

The most commonly encountered category is a fasting blood glucose level that is within normal limits. It should be remembered that although a normal value rules out any significant diabetic problem, it does not rule out diabetes as such. Patients who have latent diabetes or prediabetes will have normal fasting blood glucose levels even though they are, by definition, diabetic. A patient has latent diabetes or prediabetes if both parents are known to be diabetic, if an identical twin is a known diabetic, or if the patient has diabetic vascular changes without an elevated blood glucose level.

Hyperglycemia

Hyperglycemia is usually equated with diabetes. In most cases any elevation in blood glucose level does indicate diabetes, whether the elevation is transitory or permanent. However, in always equating hyperglycemia with diabetes, one runs the risk of forgetting other diseases that may be associated with hyperglycemia. For example, hyperglycemia is present in Cushing's disease and in patients being treated with steroids. It is uncertain whether the hyperglycemia in the latter situation represents latent diabetes manifested as a clinical diabetes because of the excessive levels of steroids, or whether this kind of elevated blood glucose concentration represents a pathophysiologic entity that is altogether different from the well-known, inherited form of diabetes—diabetes mellitus. The uncertainty is compounded by the fact that one of the tests employed in the diagnosis of latent diabetes is the steroid stimulation test.

It is probably best simply to define diabetes mellitus as the hereditary disease associated with fasting hyperglycemia and found in the majority of hyperglycemic patients. However, it bears repeating that hyperglycemia may not necessarily mean diabetes. A reasonably diligent search for other possible causes of hyperglycemia may produce the correct diagnosis. A glucose tolerance test is indicated when blood glucose levels are borderline or there is clinical evidence of hereditary diabetes.

Mild hyperglycemia (120-130 mg/dl)

Entities (other than diabetes) associated with mild hyperglycemia are:
1. Conditions causing elevation of blood catecholamine and steroid levels. The most frequent cause is acute stress (acute infection, myocardial infarction, and the like), which may herald the onset of hereditary diabetes.
2. Pheochromocytoma, a tumor producing epinephrine (adrenaline) and norepinephrine (noradrenalin)
3. Cushing's syndrome and Cushing's disease, both of which cause hyperglycemia because of elevated glucocorticoid levels. In Cushing's syndrome, which may be caused by a pituitary adenoma, growth hormones may be involved, which definitely elevate the blood glucose level.
4. Hyperthyroidism, which is suggested when mild hyperglycemia is associated with hypocholesterolemia. The increase in blood glucose concentration is probably mediated through an increase in catecholamine levels.

5. Adenoma of the pancreas, producing only glucagon that antagonizes insulin, causing hyperglycemia
6. Diuretics, mainly the thiazide diuretics and the "loop" diuretics, most likely by inducing hypokalemia, which is known to suppress the release of insulin
7. Acute or chronic pancreatic insufficiency, the mechanism of which may be the destruction of islet cells

Moderate hyperglycemia (300-500 mg/dl)

A moderate elevation in blood glucose concentration usually leaves no doubt as to the diagnosis of diabetes mellitus. Depending on the age of the patient and other findings, a moderate hyperglycemia usually becomes a management problem.

Marked hyperglycemia (>500 mg/dl)

When a marked elevation in blood glucose level is encountered, attention should immediately be directed to the CO_2 content. This is extremely important, because if the CO_2 content is low, the patient has uncontrolled diabetes associated with ketoacidosis, a potentially dangerous situation.

A second possibility, which is relatively rare, is a marked hyperglycemia without ketoacidosis (reflected by a normal CO_2 content). This entity, also serious, is called nonketotic and nonacidotic hyperglycemia; it is not necessarily associated with diabetes. The patient is usually very ill, with significantly abnormal intermediary carbohydrate metabolism, caused by the uncoupling of oxidative phosphorylation. This condition is usually found in elderly patients with advanced vascular disease and anoxemia. There is associated dehydration with hypernatremia.

Hypoglycemia

The finding of a fasting hypoglycemia is quite unusual. However, once it is encountered the following conditions should be considered:
1. Pancreatic islet cell tumor, which independently secretes insulin without the associated check and balance of a normal metabolism
2. Large tumors of nonpancreatic origin, particularly large retroperitoneal sarcomas or large hepatomas
3. Pituitary hypofunction
4. Adrenocortical hypofunction (Addison's disease). If this is the cause, the patient will also have slight hyperkalemia and hyponatremia and a slightly elevated BUN level.
5. Acquired extensive liver disease

Other relatively rare conditions associated with hypoglycemia include glycogen storage disease; postnatal hypoglycemia, in infants of diabetic mothers; and alcoholic hypoglycemia, which is usually associated with substantial alcohol ingestion after a period of fasting.

Rarer still is hypoglycemia caused by certain amino acids (leucine hypoglycemia). One should also be aware of patients who are taking oral hypoglycemics or insulin and who may have a fasting hypoglycemia in the morning.

Reactive hypoglycemia

In functional reactive hypoglycemia, a rising blood glucose level stimulates excessive insulin secretion. In this syndrome the insulin continues to act after most of the carbohydrate has been stored or metabolized, and hypoglycemia results. A 5-hour glucose tolerance test usually shows a lowering of the blood glucose level between 3 and 5 hours. Preferably, samples should be drawn every half hour. For the 5-hour glucose tolerance test to be diagnostic, the blood glucose level must drop below 40 mg/dl and the patient must have symptoms of hypoglycemia.

PHOSPHORUS (PO$_4$)

The phosphorus level, which is usually discussed in terms of the phosphate level, is always correlated with the calcium level; the optimal ratio is 1:1, which exists when vitamin D intake is adequate. Calcium and phosphorus determinations are always ordered together because of their close relationships. As mentioned in the discussion of calcium, parathyroid hormone causes increased rates of absorption of calcium and phosphorus, and causes phosphate to be lost in the urine and calcium to be saved as a result of its effect on renal tubular reabsorption. Phosphate is a threshold substance, and as such its loss in the urine is dependent upon both its level in the serum and the level of calcium, since if either element is in excess the other will be excreted.

Of the total phosphorus, 85% is combined with calcium in the skeleton. It is found abundantly in all tissues and is involved in almost all metabolic processes.

Thus it is evident that, in the absence of significant glomerular disease (normal BUN and creatinine values), phosphate abnormalities should direct attention toward some kind of abnormality associated with the endocrine system or bone metabolism.

▶ **Normal serum phosphorus (inorganic phosphate)**

    Adults: 1.8-2.6 mEq/L
               3.0-4.5 mg/dl
  Children: 2.3-4.1 mEq/L
              4.0-7.0 mg/dl

Hyperphosphatemia

Probably the most common cause of an elevated phosphate level is chronic glomerular disease, which is indicated by elevated BUN and creatinine values. However, the importance of measuring blood phosphate and calcium levels lies in its value in diagnosing hypoparathyroidism, the hallmark of which is hyperphosphatemia in association with hypocalcemia and normal renal function.

The phosphate level may be normal or increased in both milk-alkali syndrome and sarcoidosis; in both disorders normal renal function is associated with primary abnormal calcium metabolism. In the former there will be a history of peptic ulcer disease; the latter may be suggested by hyperglobulinemia and the clinical picture.

Other endocrine conditions associated with elevated phosphate levels include hyperthyroidism and increased growth hormone secretion. Other causes may be pseudohypoparathyroidism, fractures that are in the healing stage, malignant hyperpyrexia (following anesthesia), feeding newborns with unadapted cow's milk, which has a much higher phosphate content than human milk, and hypervitaminosis D.

Hypophosphatemia

Hypophosphatemia may be the result of one of the following:

1. Hyperparathyroidism, the hallmark of which is hypophosphatemia in association with hypercalcemia. Although possibly not the most common cause of decreased phosphate concentration, this combination in the absence of significant renal disease is clinically characteristic of hyperparathyroidism.
2. Childhood rickets or adult osteomalacia, particularly if the alkaline phosphatase level is elevated. In either of these conditions, the serum calcium level may be low or normal.
3. Certain types of renal tubular acidosis, which is relatively rare and may represent a single defect of phosphate reabsorption from the distal tubules (that is, phosphate diabetes) or multiple defects (Fanconi's syndrome and the aminoacidurias). These diseases may be associated with other abnormalities of amino acid metabolism, distal tubular acidosis, and acid-base abnormalities.
4. Rapid correction of hyperglycemia and diabetic ketoacidosis
5. Chronic use of antacids containing aluminum hydroxide, which binds phosphate
6. In the absence of the above conditions, hypophosphatemia may be an indication of such conditions as malabsorption syndromes and hyperinsulinism.

TOTAL PROTEIN AND ALBUMIN/GLOBULIN RATIO
(tot prot and A/G ratio)

Plasma proteins serve as a source for rapid replacement of tissue proteins during tissue depletion, as buffers in acid-base balance, and as transporters of constituents of the blood, such as lipids, vitamins, hormones, iron, copper, and certain enzymes. The antibodies of the body are contained in the gamma globulins, and a number of the plasma proteins participate in blood coagulation. Of the total protein, between 52% and 68% is albumin. This fraction is responsible for about 80% of the colloid oncotic pressure in the serum. The capillary walls are impermeable to the proteins in plasma. The proteins, therefore, exert an osmotic force across the capillary wall (oncotic pressure) that tends to pull water into the blood.

Although the total protein and A/G ratio is still a commonly employed test, it is gradually being replaced by serum protein electrophoresis, which more clearly delineates the different albumin and globulin fractions.

Electrophoresis is the migration of charged particles in an electrolyte solution in response to an electrical current passed through the solution. The proteins move at different rates because each is different in electrical charge, size, and shape. Thus the proteins tend to separate into distinct layers.

Immunoelectrophoresis, a combination of electrophoresis and immunodiffusion, permits analysis of the various immunoglobulin fractions.

♦ Normal total protein and albumin/globulin ratio

Total: 6.0-7.8 gm/dl
Albumin: 3.2-4.5 gm/dl
Globulin: 2.3-3.5 gm/dl

Hypoalbuminemia

A depressed albumin level with a slightly elevated globulin level represents a reversal of the normal A/G ratio and suggests chronic liver disease. Thus an albumin level of 2.5 gm/dl or less, with a globulin level of 3 gm/dl and a total protein level in the range of 5.5 gm/dl, is extremely suggestive of chronic liver disease.

Other conditions associated with hypoalbuminemia are significant malnutrition (especially protein), nephrotic syndrome, and malabsorption syndromes, particularly protein-losing enteropathies.

Normal total protein, low-normal albumin, and elevated globulin

When a normal total protein level is associated with a low-normal albumin level and an elevated globulin level, the normal A/G ratio is reversed. This type of laboratory picture is suggestive of diseases that involve hypergammaglobulinemia, including the myeloproliferative diseases such as multiple myeloma, Hodgkin's disease, and leukemias, and the chronic granulomatous infectious diseases such as tuberculosis, brucellosis, collagen disease, chronic active hepatitis, and sarcoidosis.

Under the above circumstances one is obliged to use serum protein electrophoresis to determine if one is dealing with a broad band of gamma globulin or with a sharp peak in the gamma, alpha I, alpha II, or beta range. The latter situation would be indicative of variants of multiple myeloma and macroglobulinemias.

UREA NITROGEN, BLOOD (BUN)

The formation of urea, which takes place in the liver by means of the deamination of amino acids, is the primary method of nitrogen excretion. Urea, then, is the end product of protein metabolism. After synthesis, urea travels through the blood and is excreted in the urine.

♦ Normal blood urea nitrogen

8-18 mg/dl

Elevated BUN level

Renal failure, either acute or chronic, is the most common cause of high BUN levels. In prerenal failure, a diminished renal blood supply, such as occurs in congestive heart failure, leads to reduced glomerular filtration and therefore to an elevated BUN level. In renal failure, damage to the nephrons, particularly such as occurs in glomerular nephritis or pyelonephritis, leads to decreased glomerular filtration and excretion. As a result, the BUN value begins to rise when the glomerular filtration rate falls below 50 ml/min (the normal in an average-size man is approximately 125 ml/min).

Postrenal failure resulting from urinary tract obstructions can also cause uremia. Prostatic enlargement is probably the most common cause of urinary tract obstruction.

Borderline elevated levels of BUN can be caused by unusually high protein intake or by excessive body protein catabolism such as occurs with sepsis or fever and gastrointestinal bleeding.

URIC ACID

Uric acid is the end product of purine metabolism; it is cleared from the plasma by glomerular filtration and perhaps by tubular secretion. One very rarely encounters a uric acid level significantly below the normal ranges. Therefore, we will not consider hypouricemia except to state that in very rare conditions, such as Wilson's disease or Fanconi's syndrome, the uric acid level may be low. It may also be low in malabsorption states.

♦ Normal serum uric acid

   Male: 2.1-7.8 mg/dl
 Female: 2.0-6.4 mg/dl

In most instances a normal uric acid value is given no further attention. However, a normal level does not rule out gout, although it makes such a diagnosis unlikely.

Hyperuricemia

Hyperuricemia is usually equated with gout, in which there is a clinical picture of either tophi or acute arthritis with significant hyperuricemia.

However, mild hyperuricemia is most commonly idiopathic, in which case the patient is asymptomatic. It would be an unfortunate mistake to label every hyperuricemia "gout" and treat the hyperuricemia rather than the patient. Usually the blood uric acid level reflects the balance between uric acid production and excretion.

The association of idiopathic hyperuricemia with hyperlipidemia and coronary artery disease is of clinical importance, although the reason for the association is unclear.

Another common cause of hyperuricemia is chronic renal failure. Whether a patient has chronic renal failure can be ascertained relatively quickly by correlating the uric acid elevation with the creatinine and BUN levels, both of which will be elevated.

A differential diagnosis is necessary between hyperuricemia caused by chronic renal failure and that caused by gouty nephropathy with secondary chronic renal failure. In the latter condition, which is relatively rare, it would be impossible to determine through laboratory tests which came first, the gouty nephropathy or the renal failure. In this situation the clinical picture is extremely helpful.

Other causes of hyperuricemia are congestive heart failure with decreased creatinine clearance, starvation (particularly absolute starvation of obese persons for weight reduction purposes), and certain glycogen storage diseases (von Gierke's disease or Lesch-Nyhan syndrome).

Most of the conditions associated with the excessive production of uric acid belong to the lymphoproliferative or myeloproliferative diseases, such as acute or chronic leukemia, both leukocytic and granulocytic, multiple myeloma, or any other malignancy associated with rapid destruction of nucleic acid and purine products. Chemotherapy or radiotherapy in these disorders may further elevate the uric acid level.

Several drugs are associated with hyperuricemia. The most common of these are the diuretics, particularly the thiazide diuretics, which impair uric acid clearance by the kidneys.

In addition, hyperuricemia may be found in Tangier disease (alpha lipoprotein deficiency), hypoparathyroidism, primary hyperoxaluria, lead poisoning resulting from ingestion of moonshine whiskey (saturnine gout), and excessive ethyl alcohol intake.

TWO   Hematology

A routine hematology screening includes a complete blood count (CBC), which consists of the following determinations: white blood cell count (WBC), red blood cell count (RBC), hematocrit (Hct), hemoglobin (Hgb), and differential white cell count (Diff). The differential count states the number of neutrophils, lymphocytes, monocytes, eosinophils, basophils, and any abnormal cells as percentages of the total WBC count.

The hematologic examination also includes determination of the erythrocyte indices, which are mean cell volume (MCV), mean cell hemoglobin (MCH), and mean cell hemoglobin concentration (MCHC). In addition, a careful inspection of a peripheral blood smear is important, as is a determination of the sedimentation rate (Sed rate or ESR).

With accurate determinations of these values, approximately 70% to 80% of the hematologic diagnosis can be made and a significant amount of information can be gathered for the purpose either of evaluating the stages of a particular disease or of diagnosing some disease entities not directly related to the hematopoietic system.

Each hematologic measurement will be discussed separately. However, it should be emphasized that since the elements of the blood are closely interrelated, absolute values can be meaningless if the whole hematologic examination is not taken into consideration. For example, a WBC count without a differential count may be normal, even in the presence of severe sepsis. In such a case, a differential count would reveal a sharp increase in the percentage of segmented bands.

WHITE BLOOD CELL COUNT (WBC)

The white blood cell count expresses the number of white blood cells (leukocytes) in 1 microliter of whole blood. The correct WBC count can be obtained by multiplying the figure obtained from the automated Coulter counter by 1000. For example, a WBC count reported to be 7.25 should be interpreted as 7250 WBCs per microliter of whole blood.

Absolute determination of the number of leukocytes (total white blood cells) gives only partial information. Unless an accurate differential white cell count is done, significant information or pathological states can be missed, as in the case just cited.

White blood cells are either granular or nongranular. The granular leukocytes are the basophils, neutrophils, and eosinophils. The nongranular leukocytes are the lymphocytes and monocytes. (See Fig. 2-1.)

Granulocytes

Neutrophils, eosinophils, and basophils are formed from stem cells in the bone marrow. Since their nuclei have two to five or more lobes, granulocytes

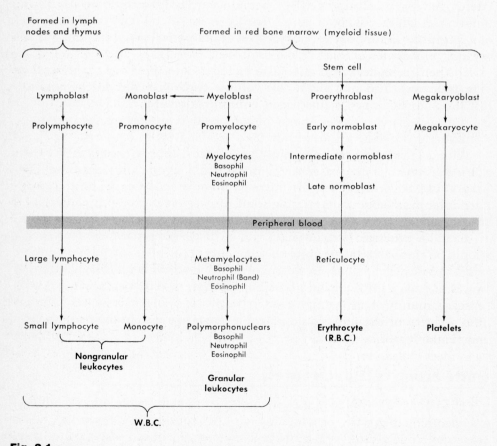

Fig. 2-1
The development of the various formed elements of the blood. In the adult, red blood cells, the granular white blood cells, monocytes, and platelets are formed in the bone marrow. The lymphocytes are formed mainly in the lymph nodes and the thymus.

are called polymorphonuclear. Neutrophils are so named because they stain with neutral dyes. Eosinophils stain with acid dyes, and basophils stain with basic dyes.

In a healthy person, the number of granulocytes is regulated at a constant level. However, when infection occurs, the number in the blood rises dramatically. When bacteria invade the body, the bone marrow is stimulated to produce and release large numbers of neutrophils, which are phagocytic. The basophils contain heparin, but their role is uncertain. Eosinophils phagocytize antigen-antibody complexes. Therefore, in patients with allergic diseases the circulating eosinophil level is often elevated.

Nongranular leukocytes

Monocytes arise in the bone marrow and migrate into inflammatory exudates, but not as rapidly as the neutrophils. Monocytosis is seen in chronic inflammatory disorders.

Lymphocytes are formed in the thymus, in lymph nodes, and in bone marrow. Lymphocytes derived from the thymus (T-cell lymphocytes) are longer-lived than those derived from the lymph nodes or the bone marrow (B-cell lymphocytes). The small lymphocytes are capable of producing a specific antibody in response to an antigenic challenge.

Normal WBC count

The normal WBC count is usually between 4500 and 11,000 cells/cu mm. The WBC count may vary in a particular individual at different times of the day. A minor variation outside the normal range is not significant as long as the differential count and the peripheral blood smear are both normal. However, an early stage of some disorder, whether infectious or myeloproliferative, is not necessarily ruled out.

Mild to moderate leukocytosis (11,000-17,000 cells/cu mm)

Mild to moderate elevation of the WBC count usually indicates infectious disease, mainly of bacterial etiology. Usually, the leukocytosis increases with the severity of the infection. However, there are exceptions to this rule—particularly in elderly patients, in whom severe sepsis can coexist with only a modest leukocytosis. As mentioned previously, the differential WBC count is of additional help.

Leukemoid reaction

Occasionally, such massive leukocytosis accompanies a systemic disease that the blood picture of leukemia is simulated. When a blood picture looks like leukemia but is not, the term "leukemoid reaction" is used. Severe sepsis, miliary tuberculosis, and other nonmalignant infectious conditions are among the more common causes.

In the differentiation between myelogenous leukemia and leukemoid reaction, determination of the leukocyte alkaline phosphatase level is helpful. The level of this enzyme is high in leukemoid reaction but low in myelogenous leukemia. Also, the presence of Philadelphia antigen is specific for the majority of cases of chronic myelogenous leukemia.

Leukopenia

A low absolute WBC count (leukopenia) can be mild (3000-5000 cells/cu mm), moderate (1500-3000/cu mm), or extremely severe (<1500 cells/cu mm), and may be associated with diminution of the WBC count as a whole, decreases in the number of neutrophils, or low levels of all the blood particles (pancytopenia).

Leukopenia associated with neutropenia

The most common causes of a mild to moderate decrease in the number of neutrophils are:
1. Familial benign neutropenia, usually accompanied by moderate monocytosis (up to 50%)
2. Acute viral infections
3. Starvation neutropenia (anorexia nervosa)
4. Primary and secondary splenic neutropenia associated with Felty's syndrome, portal hypertension, lymphoma, and some specific bacterial and protozoal infections
5. Drug-induced neutropenia, with the following drugs implicated: phenothiazines (Thorazine group), antithyroid drugs, sulfonamides, phenylbutazone, chloramphenicol, phenindione, and aminophylline, or their derivatives
6. Excessive ingestion of alcohol

Leukopenia associated with eosinopenia

The most common causes of a mild to moderate decrease in the number of eosinophils are acute and chronic stress, either emotional or somatic, and endocrine factors, such as excess adrenocorticotropic hormone (ACTH), cortisone, or epinephrine, intermenstrual period, certain diurnal variations, and acromegaly.

Granulocytopenia

From a practical point of view, one determination of neutropenia in the absence of any other sign of disease should indicate that the condition is benign, possibly diurnal, or maybe stress related. However, granulocytopenia associated with any other disease states should be evaluated to determine whether any of the following are causes:

1. Acute hypersensitivity reactions
2. Steroids (ACTH, thyroxine, epinephrine, estrogen)
3. Diurnal changes
4. Hyperthyroidism
5. Pituitary basophilism
6. Radiation therapy
7. Acute or chronic infection
8. Ovulation
9. Pregnancy
10. Aging
11. Megaloblastic anemia

The differential count

The differential count is performed on a peripheral blood smear for the purpose of identifying the different types of leukocytes. Red blood cell and platelet morphology can also be evaluated in this way.

Among the leukocytes, the neutrophils are usually the most abundant cells seen on the peripheral smear, comprising 56% of the total white blood cell count. Normally, 2.7% will be eosinophils. 0.3% will be basophils, and 34% will be lymphocytes.

When an extremely severe leukocytosis is reported, one should very carefully inspect the peripheral smear. An accurate differential count may be enough to make a diagnosis of myelogenous leukemia or lymphocytic leukemia.

A thorough examination of the peripheral blood smear should routinely include the following:

1. A diligent search should be made for abnormal lymphocytes and monocytes that may indicate some specific disease such as infectious mononucleosis. This disease is diagnosed when Downey cells are found in the peripheral smear.
2. An extreme shift to the left implies a significant number of early neutrophils and band forms rather than lobulations. This shift will indicate some kind of acute stress on the bone marrow or severe bacterial disease that is causing the release of an early granulocytic series and will, at the same time, give the interpreter some indication of the stage and severity of the disease.
3. Abnormal granulations in the leukocytes may provide an index of the toxicity generated by a specific disease (toxic granulation).
4. In examining the leukocytes, one may gain significant information by counting the lobulations of hypersegmented neutrophils. Hyperlobulation (from three to six lobules) or hypersegmentation of neutrophils is suggestive of vitamin B_{12} deficiency or folic acid deficiency.

Neutrophilic leukocytosis

The most commonly encountered causes of a mild to moderate leukocytosis of neutrophilic origin are bacterial infections, inflammatory disorders, tumors, physical and emotional stimuli, stresses, and drugs.

The bacterial infections are usually moderately severe bacterial pneumonias or systemic infections, which are sometimes coccal.

The inflammatory but noninfectious disorders causing neutrophilic leukocytosis are rheumatic fever, collagen disease, rheumatoid arthritis, vasculitis, pancreatitis, thyroiditis, and tumors and carcinomas, particularly gastric, bronchogenic, uterine, pancreatic, squamous cell, and lymphatic, and those of Hodgkin's disease. Additional conditions are burns, crush injuries, infarctions, and poisoning with carbon monoxide or lead.

Stresses that produce neutrophilic leukocytosis include extreme cold or heat, exercise, electroshock therapy, and the emotional stimuli of fear, panic, and anxiety.

Drugs that can cause neutrophilia include catecholamines, corticosteroids, lithium, methysergide, niacin, and niacinamide.

The catabolic disorders causing neutrophilia are diabetic acidosis, acute gout, thyroiditis, uremia, Cushing's syndrome, and a few hereditary conditions, such as familial neutrophilia.

Eosinophilic leukocytosis

In eosinophilic leukocytosis most of the cells causing the elevated WBC count are eosinophils—anywhere from 5% to 90%. The most frequently encountered pattern in eosinophilic leukocytosis, however, is an eosinophil count of approximately 10% to 20%. The associated diseases are the following:

1. The most common causes of an increase in the number of eosinophils are allergic disorders of nearly any kind, such as hay fever, asthma, angioneurotic edema, and serum sickness.
2. Parasitic diseases are considered second in commonality to allergic conditions. *Trichinella* is the predominant cause of such diseases in the United States. Malaria and amebiasis are also possibilities, particularly in view of widespread travel. *Ascaris* is the most common parasite in Middle Eastern countries. Other parasites associated with eosinophilia are ameba, hookworm, *Schistosoma*, and *Toxoplasma*. In the diagnosis of eosinophilic leukocytosis, particularly when parasites are a consideration, the epidemiology of the suspected associated disease and the area in which the patient has traveled become of prime importance.
3. Other, rarer conditions associated with mild to moderate eosinophilia are malignant disorders such as mycosis fungoides, brain tumors, Hodgkin's disease, and other lymphomas. Gastrointestinal causes in-

clude colitis and protein losing enteropathy. In hypoadrenocorticism, eosinophilia may be found; it may suggest the diagnosis of Addison's disease if other features of the disease are present.

4. An extremely high eosinophil count—in the range of 80% to 90%—usually indicates eosinophilic granulomatosis or eosinophilic leukemia.

Basophilic leukocytosis

An elevated WBC count associated with basophilia is uncommon; it most frequently suggests some kind of myeloproliferative disease such as myelofibrosis, agnogenic myeloid metaplasia, or polycythemia vera. A rapid fall in the basophil count may herald an anaphylactic reaction.

Lymphocytosis

Lymphocytosis may be mild to severe; it occurs in two varieties: relative, in which the total number of circulating lymphocytes is unchanged but the WBC count is low because of neutropenia, and absolute, in which the number of circulating lymphocytes increases. Relative lymphocytosis accompanies most conditions mentioned in the section on leukopenia associated with neutropenia.

The most common cause of severe lymphocytosis (80% to 90% mature lymphocytes) is chronic lymphocytic leukemia. This is associated with a marked elevation of the leukocyte count.

Marked lymphocytosis with moderate leukocytosis is found in infectious diseases, particularly pertussis, infectious mononucleosis, and acute infectious lymphocytosis.

Mild to moderate relative lymphocytosis is seen mainly in viral infections that involve exanthema, such as measles, rubella, chicken pox, and roseola infantum.

In bacterial infections, mild to moderate lymphocytosis associated with mild to moderate leukocytosis usually indicates a chronic infectious state. In addition, the overall presenting picture may suggest other disorders: brucellosis, typhoid or paratyphoid fever, or chronic granulomatous diseases such as tuberculosis.

In noninfectious disorders and nonmyeloproliferative diseases, thyrotoxicosis and adrenal insufficiency (Addison's disease) are associated with mild to moderate lymphocytosis.

Relative lymphocytosis is a normal occurrence in infants and children between 4 months and 4 years of age.

RED BLOOD CELL COUNT (RBC)

Red blood cells (erythrocytes) are formed in the red bone marrow. Their production (erythropoiesis) is inhibited by a rise in the circulating red cell level and stimulated by anemia and hypoxia. The hormone erythropoietin mediates the responses to these normal and abnormal situations. (Tissue hypoxia is the ultimate stimulus for erythropoietin production.)

The red blood cells contain a complex compound called hemoglobin, which is made up of heme, a pigmented substance containing iron, and globin, a colorless protein. Hemoglobin binds with oxygen (a reversible reaction) and can also combine with carbon dioxide. Thus the red blood cell functions primarily to transport oxygen to the tissues and to carry carbon dioxide to the lungs.

The red blood cell count represents the number of RBCs in 1 microliter of whole blood. The correct RBC count can be obtained by multiplying the figure obtained from the automated Coulter counter by 1 million. For example, an RBC count reported to be 5.11 should be interpreted as 5,110,000 RBCs in 1 microliter of blood.

In the past, the determination of the red blood cell count was tedious and occasionally erroneous. Thus the hematocrit and hemoglobin determinations were adopted for routine use. However, because of the development of automated methods, particularly the Coulter counter, routine hematologic determinations are now quick and accurate. The RBC count is, however, still not used as much as the hemoglobin and hematocrit determinations, which are also part of the Coulter panel.

Normal RBC count

The normal RBC count is 4.6 to 6.2 $\times$ 10^6 cells per microliter for men, 4.2 to 5.4 $\times$ 10^6 for women, 5.0 to 5.1 $\times$ 10^6 for infants, and 4.6 to 4.8 $\times$ 10^6 for children.

The main value of the RBC count in a routine screening examination lies in the gross evaluation of the indices, which are also obtained through automated means, either from the writeout from a Coulter counter or through an automatic analyzer.

Examining the peripheral smear
The erythrocyte indices

The relationship between the number, size, and hemoglobin content of the RBCs is important in accurately describing anemias. An index of each of these variables may be obtained from an inspection of a stained peripheral blood smear.

Terminology

hematocrit (Hct) The volume of packed red blood cells found in 100 ml of blood. For example, a value of 46% means that there are 46 ml of red blood cells in 100 ml of blood. The normal Hct in the male is 40% to 54%; in the female it is 38% to 47%.

hemoglobin (Hgb) The oxygen-carrying pigment of the red blood cells. Its level is reported in grams per 100 ml. For example, a value of 15.5 means that there are 15.5 gm of hemoglobin in each 100 ml of blood. The normal hemoglobin level in the male is 13.5 to 18.0 gm/100 ml; in the female the normal value is 12.0 to 16.0 gm/100 ml. In infants the normal hemoglobin level is 12.2 to 20.0 gm/100 ml, and in children the normal level is 11.2 to 13.4 gm/100 ml.

mean cell volume (MCV) The average volume of an individual cell. This value is usually given in the writeout from the automated system. However, it can also be calculated by dividing the volume of packed cells (hematocrit) by the number of RBCs. The result is expressed as cubic microns per red cell. The normal MCV is 82 to 98 cu μ.

mean cell hemoglobin concentration (MCHC) The amount of hemoglobin per 100 ml of RBCs. This value can be calculated by dividing the hemoglobin level, in grams, by the hematocrit and multiplying the resulting figure by 100, to produce a percentage. The normal MCHC is 32% to 36%.

mean cell hemoglobin (MCH) The average hemoglobin content of each individual red blood cell. The MCH value is calculated by dividing the hemoglobin value by the red blood cell count. The result is expressed as picograms (micromicrograms) of hemoglobin per red blood cell. The normal MCH is 27 to 31 pg.

Platelets

Platelets, which are important in blood coagulation, are visible on stained blood smears. Their absolute absence from a peripheral smear is extremely significant, indicating aplastic bone marrow. Decreased numbers of platelets (thrombocytopenia) may be caused by various conditions.

Sometimes, careful observation of a peripheral smear can provide a better indication of the platelet status than can an absolute platelet count. Such observation is easy, quick, and accurate. The shape and character of the platelets are also important. If an abnormality is noted, thrombocytopathy (abnormal-looking thrombocytes) is said to exist. Thrombocytosis is the term used when there is an unusually large number of platelets in the blood. This condition is seen most often in the blood smear in polycythemia and essential thrombocytosis, and in the blood smears of persons who have had splenectomies.

Polycythemia

Polycythemia is any condition in which the number of circulating erythrocytes rises above normal. When the red cell mass increases in response to an identifiable physiologic or pathologic stimulus, the condition is called secondary polycythemia. If no etiology can be documented, the change is considered primary, and is described as polycythemia vera (true polycythemia).

Polycythemia vera, according to some authorities, is equivalent to leukemia and in some cases does progress into one of the myeloproliferative diseases.

Secondary polycythemia has been found in persons with erythropoietin-secreting tumors, hypernephroma, renal cysts, and hepatic carcinoma. It has also been associated with chronic obstructive pulmonary disease and cyanotic congenital heart disease with hypoxemia. Secondary polycythemia is accompanied by an elevated erythropoietin level.

Erythropoietin, a hormone thought to be formed by the action of a renal factor on a plasma globulin, stimulates the proliferation and release of RBCs from the bone marrow into the peripheral circulation. One of the most sensitive ways of differentiating between primary and secondary polycythemia is the determination of the erythropoietin level. This level is diminished in polycythemia vera because the excess number of RBCs produced in this disease suppresses the production of the hormone. The level is elevated in secondary polycythemia.

In the differential diagnosis of polycythemia vera versus other polycythemias, the most important diagnostic test is measurement of the total red cell volume by the chromium tagging technique. In this test the red cell volume is increased in polycythemia vera but not in other polycythemic states.

Normal absolute RBC count and the peripheral smear

Findings on the blood film may suggest a disorder, even when the absolute RBC count is within normal limits.

1. Significant spherocytosis, polychromatophilia, and erythrocyte agglutination suggest compensated, acquired hemolytic anemia.
2. Spherocytosis with polychromatophilia is very suggestive of hereditary spherocytosis.
3. Target cells are found mainly in hemoglobin C disease and liver disease.
4. Marked hypochromia associated with target cells is suggestive of thalassemia major or thalassemia minor.
5. Erythrocytes with basophilic stipplings are characteristic of lead poisoning.
6. Macrocytosis in association with hypersegmented neutrophils suggests vitamin B_{12} and/or folic acid deficiency.
7. Rouleaux formation suggests multiple myeloma or macroglobulinemia.
8. Parasites in RBCs are the distinguishing characteristic of malaria.
9. Schistocytes and "burr" cells in association with a decreased platelet count suggest consumption coagulopathy.
10. Mechanical hemolysis is suggested by schistocytes and "burr" cells.
11. A relative increase in the number of neutrophils with increased numbers of band forms and toxic granulations suggests severe infection.
12. Atypical lymphocytes indicate the possibility of infectious mononucleosis.

13. Decreased numbers of neutrophils and increased numbers of lymphocytes suggest agranulocytosis.
14. Eosinophilia usually suggests an allergic reaction.
15. Blast (primitive) forms indicate the possibility of acute leukemia.

Anemia

Anemia, a deficiency of the total hemoglobin red cell mass, can result from many disorders. Anemias usually are classified into three broad categories:

1. Hypochromic microcytic anemia
2. Normochromic normocytic anemia
3. Macrocytic anemia, which may be normochromic, hypochromic, or hyperchromic

Terminology

normochromic Normal color (normal hemoglobin content)
hypochromic Less than normal color (decreased hemoglobin content)
hyperchromic More than normal color (increased hemoglobin content)
normocytic Normal cell size
microcytic Smaller than normal cell size
macrocytic Larger than normal cell size

Hypochromic microcytic anemia

Iron deficiency. The most frequent cause of hypochromic microcytic anemia is iron deficiency. The patient may or may not have an overt anemia. However, borderline-low hematocrit and hemoglobin values, even though the RBC count is normal, should suggest the possibility of hypochromic microcytic anemia. Although the number of cells may be within normal limits, there is a definite diminution in the size of the RBCs as well as in the hemoglobin concentration.

For a more definitive diagnosis of iron deficiency the serum iron level is checked. In an iron-deficient state the serum iron level will be low and the iron-binding capacity will be elevated. Since serum ferritin levels seem to correlate well with total body iron stores, determination of the serum ferritin level may obviate the need either for bone marrow studies for determination of total body iron stores or for liver biopsy for iron stain evaluations. A low serum ferritin level associated with a low serum iron level and a low binding capacity may indicate a decrease in total body iron levels.

Diseases associated with hypochromia and microcytosis, accompanied by low serum iron level and increased body iron stores (reflected by elevated ferritin level), include chronic infections, malignancies, and chronic kidney disease.

⬧ **Normal serum iron**

50-150 μg/dl

⬧ **Normal iron-binding capacity**

250-450 μg/dl

⬧ **Normal serum ferritin**

Female: 5-280 μg/dl
   Male: 10-270 μg/dl

The hemoglobinopathies. This term is used to describe the clinical syndromes that result from the production of abnormal types of hemoglobin for genetic reasons. The most important of these syndromes are thalassemia major and thalassemia minor (Mediterranean anemia), sickle cell anemia, and hemoglobin C disease. The blood picture in the hemoglobinopathies simulates that of iron-deficiency anemia on the peripheral smear. However, the bone marrow stores, serum iron level, and iron-binding capacity will differentiate between the two.

Normochromic normocytic anemia

The most common cause of normocytic normochromic anemia is an acute loss of red blood cell mass such as occurs in hemorrhage or hemolysis.

Another major group of normochromic normocytic anemias is the aplastic or hypoplastic anemias. In some very rare situations a combination of macrocytic and microcytic anemia may produce normal indices. Such a situation will occur in vitamin B_{12} deficiency anemia associated with carcinoma of the stomach and chronic blood loss. However, the overall clinical picture and other clues on the blood smear (multisegmented leukocytes and mild hemolysis) will suggest the correct pathologic condition.

Macrocytic anemia

In macrocytic anemia there is a decreased absolute number of RBCs per cubic microliter. However, the individual cells are larger in diameter and volume and contain more hemoglobin than normal. Consequently, the MCV and MCHC will be elevated.

The two most common diseases associated with macrocytosis with significant anemia are folic acid deficiency and vitamin B_{12} deficiency, which is also known as Addisonian or pernicious anemia. These two conditions are also associated with megaloblastic changes in the bone marrow.

Some macrocytosis is also observed in the anemia of myxedema, as well as in the anemias following acute blood loss, through either bleeding or hemolysis. The latter two conditions are not accompanied by megaloblastic changes in the bone marrow, since the macrocytosis reflects increased numbers of reticulocytes, which are slightly larger than normal RBCs.

Macrocytic normochromic anemia is also seen in some cases of chronic liver disease, hypothyroidism, and aplastic anemia.

In the differential diagnosis among folic acid deficiency, macrocytic or megaloblastic anemia, and Addisonian or pernicious anemia, the determination of the levels of B_{12} and folic acid in the blood and the Schilling test are the most widely used procedures. The Schilling test is described on p. 203.

Sedimentation rate (sed rate or ESR)

The erythrocyte sedimentation rate is the speed at which RBCs settle in uncoagulated blood. This rate is affected by factors too numerous to mention in this book. Determination of the sedimentation rate is, therefore, a nonspecific test, having neither organ nor disease specificity. Its chief value lies in the fact that a normal finding does diminish the probability of a significant disease process, giving some reassurance to the investigator. An abnormal result indicates that a more extensive search is necessary.

In addition to its general screening value, the sed rate is useful in following the progress of certain diseases such as rheumatic fever. A gradually diminishing sed rate indicates a good prognosis, while a gradually increasing rate indicates a poor prognosis.

⬥ Normal sedimentation rate (Westergren)

Men under 50 yr: <15 mm/hr
Men over 50 yr: <20 mm/hr
Women under 50 yr: <20 mm/hr
Women over 50 yr: <30 mm/hr

BLOOD TYPING AND CROSS-MATCHING

Before a blood transfusion is given, the blood group of the recipient and of the donor must be determined to ensure the similarity of the antigenic and immune properties of the blood of the two individuals. If the necessary precautions are not taken, red blood cell agglutination (clumping) and hemolysis (release of hemoglobin) may result. This situation, called a transfusion reaction, can lead to the death of the recipient.

In an emergency in which there is not time to actually determine the type of antigens on the red blood cell membranes (blood type) of the donor and of the recipient, the bloods can be cross-matched. This procedure, which indicates whether agglutination will occur, first requires mixing the cells of the donor with the defibrinated serum of the recipient. The reverse is then performed: the cells of the recipient are mixed with the serum of the donor. The antigen is contained on the red blood cells, and the antibody is contained in the serum.

Blood groups (types)

An antigen is any substance that causes the formation of antibodies. The surfaces of the red blood cells contain antigens, which determine the blood type of the individual. Normally, people do not form antibodies against the antigens of their own red cells, but if a person receives a transfusion with blood containing different antigens, antibodies will be formed against all of the foreign antigens. Among the antigens, two groups, the ABO and Rh groups, are highly antigenic and can cause transfusion reactions if they are transfused into persons with incompatible blood types.

ABO blood groups

Individuals may have A antigens, B antigens, both, or neither on their red cells. If the red cells have neither, the blood type is usually type O.

If an individual *does not* have type A red blood cells, antibodies known as "anti-A" agglutins will be present in the serum. If this person receives a transfusion with type A blood, these agglutinins will agglutinate the type A red blood cells of the donor. The same is true if an individual *does not* have type B red blood cells. The serum will contain antibodies known as "anti-B" agglutinins, which will agglutinate type B red blood cells. If the individual has both A and B (AB group) antigens on the red cells, no agglutinins (antibodies) are present and the individual can receive any type of blood ("universal recipient"). If the individual is type O, with neither A nor B antigens on the red cells, the serum will contain both anti-A and anti-B agglutinins. Both A and B blood types will be agglutinated if given to a type O individual. However, since the red cells of a type O individual cannot be agglutinated by the serum of any other blood group, these persons are called "universal donors."

Rh groups

Most individuals possess an antigen on their red cells called the Rh factor; these persons are said to be Rh positive. Persons who do not possess the factor are said to be Rh negative. Antibodies (agglutinins) to the Rh factor do not occur spontaneously as in the ABO group. If an Rh-negative individual is given Rh-positive blood, anti-Rh agglutinins develop slowly against the Rh-positive blood. This causes no ill effects unless the person subsequently receives Rh-positive blood again. Then the anti-Rh agglutinins that formed in the serum as a result of the first transfusion will agglutinate the cells of the second Rh-positive transfusion. Of course, Rh-negative blood does no harm to an Rh-positive person.

If an Rh-negative mother is carrying an Rh-positive fetus, the antigen from the blood cells of the fetus causes antibody production in the serum of the mother. The firstborn child usually shows no ill effects, but during subsequent pregnancies number of the antibodies in the mother's serum will increase to a level that is sufficient to cause agglutination and hemolysis of the red cells of the fetus, unless the mother has been exposed to RhoGam.

THREE Urinalysis

A urine examination, properly performed, may provide valuable information.

The urine that is to be analyzed should be a clean-catch (midstream) specimen collected in a clean, dry container and examined as quickly as possible, preferably within 2 hours. It should be a morning specimen, and the patient should not have had fluids for 12 hours preceding its collection. Urine that has been standing too long becomes alkaline, bacteria multiply, and leukocytes and casts disintegrate.

The standard urinalysis includes determination of pH and specific gravity, tests for the presence or absence of glucose and ketones, protein semiquantitation, and microscopic examination of the centrifuged urinary sediment.

pH (ACIDITY OR ALKALINITY)

Normal fresh urine is usually acid, with a pH of 4.6 to 8. If the specimen has not been standing too long, the pH will reflect the patient's acid-base balance.

Alkaline urine is seen in metabolic alkalosis. The exception to this statement is long-standing hypokalemic chloremic alkalosis, in which a potassium deficiency causes the renal tubular cells to secrete hydrogen ions in lieu of potassium. A paradoxical aciduria is the result. This situation (metabolic alkalosis with aciduria) may suggest generalized intracellular acidosis.

SPECIFIC GRAVITY (SG)

♦ Normal specific gravity

1.016-1.022 (normal fluid intake)
1.001-1.035 (range)

The specific gravity of a morning urine specimen voided by a fasting patient reflects the maximum concentrating ability of the kidney. In the absence of formed elements, protein, or glycosuria, the specific gravity in a clear urine specimen should be 1.025 to 1.030. Anything below this value reflects distal renal tubular disease and inability of the kidney to concentrate urine to the maximum. Endocrine disease associated with insufficient antidiuretic hormone (ADH) secretions is also a possibility.

A fixed specific gravity indicates chronic glomerulopyelonephritis.

A long-standing hypokalemic and hypercalcemic nephropathy, in which the patient has symptoms of frequency, nocturia, and polyuria, can be easily diagnosed by a proper examination of the urine for specific gravity and osmolality. The specimen should be collected after overnight fasting. If simultaneous serum and urine osmolality determinations are performed, the serum osmolality will be high while the urine osmolality will be relatively low.

GLUCOSE

When a urine specimen voided in the morning is free of glucose, diabetes mellitus is not ruled out because, normally, a blood glucose level of 130 to 140 mg/dl is necessary before traces of glucose appear in the urine.

Glucosuria means one of two things: diabetes mellitus or a low renal threshold for glucose resorption (if the blood glucose level is normal).

PROTEIN

The absence of protein in the urine, particularly in concentrated urine, rules out significant renal glomerular disease. The presence of protein in the urine indicates the possibility of any one of a large number of diseases, the differential diagnosis of which will be discussed in Chapter 7, p. 170.

When there is a trace of protein in the urine, a follow-up test for protein is indicated. However, if there is more than a trace, the 24-hour urinary excretion of protein should be ascertained. For a more specific diagnosis, a qualitative analysis of the kind of protein, be it albumin, one of the globulins, or Bence Jones proteins, should be performed.

MICROSCOPIC EXAMINATION OF SEDIMENT

Normally, a microscopic examination of the sediment in the urine will show fewer than one or two red blood cells, one or two white blood cells, and only an occasional cast. Anything more is considered pathologic. Urine microscopy is especially important in making the diagnosis of acute pyelonephritis, the classical findings in which are numerous WBCs, WBC casts, and bacteria.

Casts

Casts are formed in the kidney tubules as a result of the agglutination of protein cells or cellular debris. The presence of casts in the urine implies tubular or glomerular disorders. Because casts are cylindrical structures, their occurrence in the urine is sometimes called cylindruria. Since protein is necessary for cast formation, proteinuria often accompanies cylindruria.

WBC casts indicate pyelonephritis, and sometimes are also found in the exudative stage of acute glomerulonephritis. RBC casts may appear colorless if only a few RBCs are present. However, they are often yellow. Their presence indicates glomerulonephritis.

Epithelial casts may be difficult to distinguish from leukocyte or mixed-cell casts. When epithelial cells are seen together with red blood cell casts and lipids in casts, glomerulonephritis is suggested.

A coarsely granular cast is the result of the first step in the disintegration of a WBC cast or an epithelial cell cast. If disintegration continues, the coarse granules break down into small granules, forming a finely granular cast. The next step is the formation of what is known as a waxy cast, which is translucent and shaped by the tubule where it was formed.

Hyaline casts are clear, colorless cylinders made up of protein. They pass almost unchanged down the tubules. They may be either coarsely or finely granular, depending upon the degenerative changes that took place in the tubules. The appearance of hyaline casts alone is usually a sudden, mild, and temporary phenomenon; it must be correlated with other clinical findings.

Urine that is loaded with hyaline casts and protein is suggestive of the nephrotic syndrome.

Red blood cells

The appearance of red blood cells in the urine is an indication of bleeding that is occurring after the urine has passed through the glomeruli and tubules, such as would occur with hemorrhagic cystitis or calculi in the renal pelvis. Another possibility is disease of the renal collecting and tubular systems, such as tuberculosis or tumors.

Telescoping

The phenomenon in which urine sediment shows different stages of glomerular nephritis (acute and subacute) and also has the findings of the nephrotic syndrome is called "telescoping" of the urine. Such a sediment is seen in lupus nephritis.

Crystals

The types of crystals found in normal urine vary with the pH of the specimen. Calcium oxalate, uric acid, and urate crystals may be seen in acid urine. Phosphate and carbonate crystals and amorphous phosphates are often seen in alkaline urine.

Calcium oxalate crystals, if numerous, may suggest hypercalcemia.

APPEARANCE

The color of the urine is not usually reported in a routine urinalysis. It should be specifically requested if a rare diagnosis is suspected.

Normal urine is golden yellow. A darker color suggests hematuria, hemoglobinuria, bilirubinuria, urobilinuria, or porphyria. Tests specifically directed toward the cause of these entities should be ordered.

Urine that changes to a bright burgundy red when exposed to the light is highly suggestive of porphyria.

Tea-colored urine that stains the underwear indicates the possibility of obstructive jaundice, which would result in the presence of urobilinogen in the urine.

The fruity aroma of the urine of persons who have diabetes and the red discoloration of the urine of persons who are taking pyridium are two well-known diagnostic clues commonly encountered in the emergency room.

Common variances in the results of the routine screening panels and their clinical implications

This appendix contains some of the most common variances found in the routine screening examinations and the clinical implications or potential disease states that may exist. Generally speaking, a variance in the result has more significance when it is compared with the results of all three examinations.

This appendix has been provided so that you can more easily determine what further action is indicated when there is a variance from a normal value. The last column in each table refers you to the page on which additional tests for the evaluation or confirmation of a suspected disease entity are discussed.

BLOOD CHEMISTRY

Test	Abbreviation	Normal value	Variance	Clinical implication	Subsequent laboratory studies, comments, and/or conclusive symptoms
Alkaline phosphatase (total serum)	Alk phos	Adults: 1.5-4.5 U/dl (Bodansky) 4-13 U/ml (King-Armstrong) 0.8-2.3 U/ml (Bessey-Lowry) 15-35 U/ml (Shinowara-Jones-Reinhart) Children: 5.0-14.0 U/dl (Bodansky) 3.4-9.0 U/ml (Bessey-Lowry) 15-30 U/dl (King-Armstrong)	↑ (marked) with liver disease (bilirubinemia)	Early obstructive jaundice	pp. 209-212
			↑ (marked) without liver disease	Paget's disease of bone	Bone x-ray
			↑ (marked)	Carcinoma with bone metastasis	Bone scan
			↑ (moderate) with liver disease	Cholangiolitic hepatitis	p. 212
			↑ (mild) with liver disease	Liver cirrhosis with active hepatitis	pp. 212-217
			↑ (mild) without liver disease and with hypercalcemia	Hyperparathyroidism	p. 236
			↑ (mild to moderate) with N or ↓ Ca	Osteomalacia	History, physical, and x-rays
Bilirubin (serum)		Up to 0.3 mg/dl (direct or conjugated) 0.1-1.0 mg/dl (indirect or unconjugated) Total: 0.1-1.2 mg/dl Newborn total: 1-12 mg/dl	↑ indirect or unconjugated, with reticulocytes, absent urine bilirubin	Low-grade hemolytic disease	pp. 271-277
			↑ indirect or unconjugated with normal liver function	Gilbert's disease	p. 213
			↑ direct or conjugated with abnormal albumin, globulin, and enzymes	Parenchymal liver disease, obstructive liver disease	pp. 209-212
			↑ (marked) indirect or unconjugated	Massive hemolysis	pp. 271-277
			↑ (marked) direct or conjugated	Obstructive jaundice: obstructive phase of hepatitis, cholangitis, lower biliary tract obstruction (carcinoma or calculus)	pp. 209-212

N = normal
↑ = elevated
↓ = depressed

Continued.

BLOOD CHEMISTRY—cont'd

Test	Abbreviation	Normal value	Variance	Clinical implication	Subsequent laboratory studies, comments, and/or conclusive symptoms
Calcium (serum)	Ca	Ionized: 4.2-5.2 mg/dl 2.1-2.6 mEq/L or 50%-58% of total	N with marked ↓ albumin	Hypercalcemia	See hypercalcemia p. 236
			N with ↑ BUN	Primary hyperparathyroidism, secondary hyperparathyroidism	
		Total: 9.0-10.6 mg/dl 4.5-5.3 mEq/L Infants: 11-13 mg/dl	↑ with ↓ phosphorus and N BUN	Hyperparathyroidism	p. 236
			↑ with ↑ gamma globulin	Sarcoidosis, multiple myeloma, malignancies with possible metastasis to bone	Biopsy
			↑ with metabolic alkalosis	Milk-alkali syndrome	History of peptic ulcer disease p. 226
			↑	Severe thyrotoxicosis	
			↑	Malignant tumors with or without bone metastasis	X-ray; alkaline phosphatase
			↑	Bone fractures	History, physical, and x-ray
			↑ with ↑ alk phos	Paget's disease of bone	X-ray
			↑ with ↓ albumin fraction of serum protein	Pseudohypocalcemia	X-ray
			↓ with ↑ phosphorus, N BUN, N creat	Hypoparathyroidism	p. 237
			→	Osteomalacia (adults), rickets (children)	History, physical, and x-rays
			→	Malabsorption syndrome	p. 204
			→	Acute pancreatitis	p. 220
			→	Pregnancy	History and physical
			→	Diuretics	History
			→	Respiratory alkalosis	Blood gases, p. 147
Carbon dioxide content (plasma, serum, venous)	CO_2 content	24-30 mM/L	↑ without chronic obstructive lung disease and frequently with ↓ K and ↓ Cl	Hypokalemic-chloremic alkalosis (serum alkalosis and intracellular acidosis)	24-hr Cl

Test	Abbr	Normal value	Change	Condition	Reference
Chloride	Cl	95-103 mEq/L	→	Uremic acidosis	Blood gases, p. 147
			→	Diabetic ketoacidosis	Glucose tolerance test
			→	Lactic acidosis	Serum lactic acid levels
			→ with ↓ K and ↑ Cl	Renal tubular acidosis	Anion gap, p. 170
			→	Respiratory alkalosis (hyperventilation syndrome)	p. 149 (blood pH)
			↑ with ↓ CO_2 content, and ↓ K	Renal tubular acidosis, iatrogenic (tube feeding and inappropriate IV fluids)	Anion gap, p. 170
			↓ with ↑ CO_2 content, and N K	Potassium-saving diuretics	History
			↓ with ↑ K and ↑ CO_2 content	Hypokalemic-chloremic alkalosis	24-hr Cl
Cholesterol (total serum)	Chol	150-250 mg/dl (varies with diet and age)	↑ (marked) with ↑ alk phos and ↑ bilirubin	Liver disease with biliary obstruction	pp. 212-217
			↑ (marked) with ↑ BUN and ↑ creat	Nephrotic stage of glomerulonephritis	p. 182
			↑ (marked)	Familial hypercholesterolemia	pp. 94-96
			↓ (marked)	Diet and malnutrition	History and physical
			↓ (marked)	Extensive liver disease	pp. 212-217
			↓ (marked)	Hyperthyroidism	p. 236
Creatinine	Creat	0.6-1.2 mg/dl	↑	Kidney disease with >50% destruction of nephrons	p. 170
Blood glucose	Gluc	70-110 mg/dl	↑	Diabetes mellitus	History and glucose tolerance test
		60-100 mg/dl	↑ mild with ↑ blood catecholamines	Acute stress, pheochromocytoma	History, p. 248
			↑ (mild) with ↑ glucocorticoids	Cushing's syndrome (hyperadrenalism), Cushing's disease (secondary hyperadrenalism)	p. 246

N = normal
↑ = elevated
↓ = depressed

Continued.

BLOOD CHEMISTRY—cont'd

Test	Abbreviation	Normal value	Variance	Clinical implication	Subsequent laboratory studies, comments, and/or conclusive symptoms
Blood glucose—cont'd			↑(mild) with ↓cholesterolemia	Hyperthyroidism	p. 236
			↑(mild)	Diuretics	History
			↑(mild)	Acute and chronic pancreatic insufficiency	Malabsorption, p. 204
			↑(moderate)	Diabetes mellitus	History and glucose tolerance test
			↑(marked) with ↓CO_2 content	Uncontrolled diabetes and ketoacidosis	Electrolytes
			↑(marked) with N CO_2 content and hypernatremia	Nonketotic, nonacidotic hyperglycemia	Electrolytes
			↓	Pancreatic islet cell tumor	p. 219
			↓	Large nonpancreatic tumor	IVP and laminograms
			↓	Pituitary hypofunction	p. 251
			↓ with hyperkalemia, hyponatremia, and ↑BUN	Addison's disease (adrenocortical hypofunction)	p. 248
			↓	Extensive liver disease	pp. 212-217
			↓	Reactive hypoglycemia	5-hour glucose tolerance test, p. 257
Lactic dehydrogenase (serum)	LDH	80-120 Wacker units 150-450 Wroblewski units 71-207 IU/L	↑(marked)	Myocardial infarction	pp. 69-71; 90-94
			↑(marked)	Hemolytic disorders (pernicious anemia)	p. 271
			↑(mild)	Chronic viral hepatitis	p. 217
			↑(mild)	Pneumonia, pulmonary emboli	Chest x-ray, pp. 140-141
			↑(mild)	Generalized viral infections	p. 217
			↑(mild)	Low-grade hemolytic disorders	p. 271
			↑(mild)	Cerebral vascular accident	p. 283 (spinal tap)
			↑(mild)	Renal tissue destruction	p. 170
Phosphorus (serum)	PO_4	Adults: 1.8-2.6 mEq/L 3.0-4.5 mg/dl	↑ with ↑BUN, ↑creat	Chronic glomerular disease	p. 170
			↑ with ↓Ca, N BUN, N creat	Hypoparathyroidism	p. 237

Test	Status	Disease/Condition	Diagnostic Aid
Children: 2.3-4.1 mEq/L 4.0-7.0 mg/dl	N or ↑ with N BUN, N creat	Milk-alkali syndrome	History of peptic ulcer disease
	N with ↑ Ca and ↑ gamma globulin	Sarcoidosis	Biopsy
	↓ with ↑ Ca, N BUN, N creat	Hyperparathyroidism	p. 236
	↓ with N or ↓ Ca and ↑ alk phos	Rickets (children), osteomalacia (adults)	History, physical, and x-rays
	↓	Renal tubular acidosis	Anion gap, p. 170
	↓	Malabsorption syndrome	p. 204
Potassium (plasma) K	3.8-5.0 mEq/L		
	↑	Renal failure	p. 170
	↑ with hypovolemia and ↑ BUN	Addison's disease	p. 248
	N with ↓ total body K and ↑ CO_2 content	Chronic diuretic use, alkalosis	History, p. 147
	↓ with ↑ CO_2 content	Cushing's syndrome	p. 246
	↓	Primary and secondary hyperaldosteronism with chronic congestive heart failure	History and physical, p. 246
	↓	Liver disease with ascites	History and physical, pp. 212-217
	↓	Excessive licorice ingestion (hypertension)	History
	↓	Antiinflammatory drugs	History
	↓	Malignant hypertension, hypertensive disease, unilateral renal vascular hypertension	↑ reninemia, pp. 185-187
	↓	Poor diet	History
	↓	Chronic stress	History
	↓	Chronic diarrhea	History
	↓	Malabsorption syndrome	p. 204
	↓	Diaphoresis	History
	↓	Chronic fever	History and physical
	↓ with ↑ Cl and ↓ CO_2 content	Renal tubular acidosis	Anion gap, p. 170

Continued.

N = normal
↑ = elevated
↓ = depressed

BLOOD CHEMISTRY—cont'd

Test	Abbreviation	Normal value	Variance	Clinical implication	Subsequent laboratory studies, comments, and/or conclusive symptoms
Total protein and albumin/globulin ratio (serum)	Tot prot and A/G ratio	Total: 6.0-7.8 gm/dl Albumin: 3.2-4.5 gm/dl Globulin: 2.3-3.5 gm/dl	↓ with ↓ albumin (<2.5 gm) and ↑ globulin (3 gm) (reversed A/G ratio)	Chronic liver disease	pp. 212-217
			N with ↓ albumin and ↑ globulin (reversed A/G ratio)	Myeloproliferative diseases, chronic granulomatous infectious diseases	Serum protein electrophoresis
Sodium (serum)	Na	136-142 mEq/L	↑	Iatrogenic	History
			↑ with hyperglycemia	Hypothalamic lesion, head trauma, and hyperosmolar states	History and physical
			↓ with dehydration (slight ↑ BUN)	Addison's disease (primary adrenocortical deficiency)	p. 248
			↓ with N or ↑ BUN	Chronic sodium-losing nephropathy	24-hr urine Na
			↓ with ↓ Cl	Vomiting, diarrhea, or tube drainage	History
			↓	Diaphoresis, burns	History and physical
			↓	Diuretics (mercurial and chlorothiazide)	History
			↓ with ↑ BUN, ↑ creat	Chronic renal insufficiency with acidosis	p. 170
			↓	Starvation with acidosis, diabetic acidosis	pH
			↓	Paracentesis, thoracentesis	History
			↓ ↓	Dilution hyponatremia: diuretics with Na restriction, secondary hyperaldosteronism, hepatic failure with ascites, excessive water administration, acute or chronic renal insufficiency	History and physical (see index for specific tests)

Test	Abbr.	Normal value	Change	Associated conditions	Reference/diagnostic test
			↓ with inappropriate ADH syndrome (↑ S. G. and ↓ Na)	(oliguria), hypothermia, lobar pneumonia	
				Bronchogenic carcinoma, pulmonary infections, and porphyria	Chest x-ray
Serum glutamic-oxaloacetic transaminase	SGOT	8-33 U/ml	↑ (marked)	Acute severe fulminating hepatitis, severe liver necrosis, and acute myocardial infarction	pp. 69; 212-217
			↑ (moderate)	Myocarditis, cardiomyopathies	
			↑ (mild)	Cirrhosis, cholangiolitic jaundice, metastatic liver disease, skeletal muscle disease, trauma, generalized infections, dissecting aneurysm, pulmonary infarction, shock, pericarditis	Chapter 4 History and physical (see index for specific tests)
Blood urea nitrogen	BUN	8-18 mg/dl	↑	Acute or chronic renal failure, congestive heart failure with decreased renal blood supply, and obstructive uropathy	p. 170
Uric acid (serum)		Male: 2.1-7.8 mg/dl Female: 2.0-6.4 mg/dl	↑ with acute arthritis	Gout	X-ray and 24-hour urine excretion of uric acid
			↑ (mild)	Idiopathic	
			↑ with ↑ BUN, ↑ creat	Chronic renal failure	p. 170 History and physical
			↑	Starvation	Liver biopsy or bone marrow biopsy
			↑	Glycogen storage disease	
			↑	Diuretics	History

N = normal
↑ = elevated
↓ = depressed

HEMATOLOGY

Test	Abbreviation	Normal value	Variance	Clinical implication	Subsequent laboratory studies, comments, and/or conclusive symptoms
White blood cell count	WBC	4500-11,000/microliter	↑ (mild to moderate)	Infectious disease, mainly bacterial and moderate	History, physical, and differential
			↑ (mild to moderate)	Severe sepsis in elderly patients	History, physical, and differential
			↑ (marked)	Severe sepsis	History, physical, and differential
Red blood cell count	RBC	Male: 4.6-6.2 × 10⁶/microliter Female: 4.2-5.4 × 10⁶/microliter	↑ (primary)	Polycythemia vera (equivalent to leukemia)	↓ erythropoietin level
			↑ (secondary)	Chronic obstructive lung disease, cyanotic congenital heart diseases with hypoxemia	p. 161 and ↑ erythropoietin level
THE DIFFERENTIAL WBC COUNT					
Neutrophils		Mean %: 56% Range of absolute counts: 1800-7000/microliter	↑ (mild to moderate)	Bacterial infections, inflammatory disorders, tumors, physical and emotional stimuli, stresses (heat, extreme cold, exercise, electroshock therapy, emotional stimuli), and drugs (catecholamines, corticosteroids)	History and physical, and cultures
			↓ (mild to moderate) with monocytosis (up to 50%)	Familial benign neutropenia	History
			↓ (mild to moderate)	Acute viral infections, anorexia nervosa (starvation), primary and secondary splenic neutropenia, drug induced, and excessive ingestion of alcohol	History and physical
Eosinophils		Mean %: 2.7%	↑	Allergic disorders, parasitic diseases	History and physical, pp. 327-329; 346

Range of absolute counts: 0-450/microliter	↑ (90%) ↓	Eosinophilic leukemia Acute and chronic stress (emotional or somatic), endocrine causes (excess ACTH, cortisone, epinephrine, intermenstrual period, diurnal variations, and acromegaly)	p. 259 History, p. 246
Basophils — Mean %: 3%	↑	Myeloproliferative disease	p. 259 (bone marrow, serum protein electrophoresis) Serology
Range of absolute counts: 0-200/microliter	↓ with granulocytopenia	Anaphylactic reaction Acute hypersensitive reactions, steroids, diurnal changes, hyperthyroidism, pituitary basophilism, radiation therapy, acute and chronic infection, ovulation, pregnancy, and aging	History and physical (see index for specific tests)
Lymphocytes — Mean %: 34% Range of absolute counts: 1000-4800/microliter	↑ (80%-90%) with ↑ (marked) leukocytes	Chronic lymphocytic leukemia	p. 259
	↑ (marked) with ↑ (moderate) leukocytes	Infectious diseases: pertussis, infectious mononucleosis, and acute infectious lymphocytosis	p. 259 (bone marrow, peripheral smear)
	↑ (mild to moderate relative)	Viral infections with eczemas	History and physical
	In bacterial infections: ↑ (mild to moderate) with ↓ (mild to moderate) leukocytes	Chronic infectious state	History and physical
	↑ (mild to moderate) in noninfectious and nonmyeloproliferative disease	Thyrotoxicosis, adrenal insufficiency (Addison's disease)	p. 248

Continued.

N = normal
↑ = elevated
↓ = depressed

HEMATOLOGY—cont'd

Test	Abbreviation	Normal value	Variance	Clinical implication	Subsequent laboratory studies, comments, and/or conclusive symptoms
THE PERIPHERAL SMEAR					
Platelets		290,000/mm (140,000-440,000) Brecher-Cronkite method)	Absolute absence	Aplastic bone marrow, thrombocytopenia (various etiologies)	p. 259
			↑	Polycythemia, essential thrombocytosis, persons who have had splenectomies	↓ hemopoietin, history
Hemoglobin	Hbg	Male: 13.5-18.0 gm/dl Female: 12.0-16.0 gm/dl	↓	Anemia	p. 259
			↓ (borderline) with ↓ (borderline) Hct and N RBC count	Hypochromic microcytic anemia: iron deficiency, thalassemia major and minor, sickle cell anemia, and hemoglobin C disease	p. 259 (bone marrow), ↓ serum iron level, Hgb electrophoresis, p. 275
			↓	Normochromic normocytic anemia	History, reticulocyte count
			↓ with ↑ MCV and ↑ MCHC	Macrocytic anemia: folic acid deficiency, vitamin B_{12} deficiency (pernicious anemia)	p. 259

ADDITIONAL FINDINGS ON THE PERIPHERAL SMEAR

Spherocytosis, polychromatophilia, and erythrocyte agglutination	Compensated, acquired hemolytic anemia	p. 259
Spherocytosis with polychromatophilia	Hereditary spherocytosis	Fragility test
Basophilic stipplings	Lead poisoning	Peripheral smear for lead
Macrocytosis and hypersegmental neutrophils	Vitamin B_{12} and/or folic acid deficiency	Serum folate, RBC folate
Rouleaux formation	Multiple myeloma or macroglobulinemia	p. 259 (bone marrow, serum protein electrophoresis)
Parasites in RBCs	Malaria	p. 327
Schistocytes and "burr" cells with ↓ platelet count	Consumption coagulopathy	Fibrinogen degradation product
Schistocytes and "burr" cells	Mechanical hemolysis (prosthetic valves)	History
↑ neutrophils, ↑ band forms and toxic granulations	Severe infection	History and physical
Atypical lymphocytes	Infectious mononucleosis	p. 327
↓ neutrophils and increased lymphocytes	Agranulocytosis	p. 259
Eosinophilia	Allergy reaction	History
Blast (primitive) forms	Acute leukemia	p. 259

N = normal
↑ = elevated
↓ = depressed

URINALYSIS

Test	Abbreviation	Normal value	Variance	Clinical implication	Subsequent laboratory studies, comments, and/or conclusive symptoms
pH (acidity or alkalinity)		4.6-8.0	↑ (alkaline) with ↑ CO_2 content ↓ (aciduria) with metabolic alkalosis, ↓ K, ↓ Cl	Metabolic alkalosis Generalized intracellular acidosis	p. 147
Specific gravity	SG	1.016-1.022 (normal fluid intake) 1.001-1.035 (range)	↓ with ↓ K, ↓ Ca, ↑ Cl Fixed SG (isosthenuria) ↓ with ↑ Ca, ↓ K	Distal renal tubular disease Chronic renal disease Hypokalemic and hypercalcemic nephropathy	p. 183 p. 170 p. 173, osmolality
Glucose (quali-tative)	Gluc	Negative	Glycosuria with ↑ blood glu-cose Glycosuria with ↓ blood glu-cose	Diabetes mellitus Low renal threshold for glucose re-sorption	Gluc tolerance test Gluc tolerance test
Protein (quali-tative)		Negative	Proteinuira (trace) Proteinuria (more than a trace)	Follow-up indicated 24-hour urine quantitative analysis indicated	p. 170

MICROSCOPIC EXAMINATION

Casts	Negative	WBC casts	Pyelonephritis	p. 312
		RBC casts	Glomerulonephritis	p. 181
		Hyaline casts with proteinuria	Nephrotic syndrome	pp. 182-183
Red blood cells RBCs	Negative	Hematuria	Hemorrhagic cystitis or calculi in the renal pelvis, tuberculosis or tumors of the renal collecting and tubular system	pp. 177-180
Crystals	Negative	Present with amorphous substances and ↑ uric acid	Possible gouty nephropathy	pp. 28-30
		Calcium oxalate crystals with ↑ serum calcium	Suggests hypercalcemia	pp. 4-5
Color	Golden yellow	Darker color	Hematuria, bilirubinuria, hemoglobinuria, urobilinuria, and porphyria	See index
		Color changes when exposed to light	Porphyria	Measurement of porphyrins pp. 209-212
		Tea-colored and staining (urobilinogen in urine)	Possible obstructive jaundice	

N = normal
↑ = elevated
↓ = depressed

Evaluative and diagnostic laboratory tests for specific diseases

Unit 1 dealt with the routine screening of patients through laboratory tests. In Unit Two additional tests are discussed. This unit is intended to provide guidelines for ordering and understanding the tests that will lead to a more definitive diagnosis when an abnormality is detected in a screening examination.

The anatomy and physiology of the organ or system that is involved in a disease process are discussed before specific laboratory tests are described, so that the rationale behind the tests, the nomenclature, and the limitations of the tests may be better understood. The laboratory tests are then described in detail, followed by discussions of specific clinical entities. The most important diseases are defined, and the diagnostic laboratory steps are listed in sequence of performance.

FOUR Diagnostic tests for cardiac disorders

The heart is a muscular pump that contains four chambers and four valves. The heart is innervated by the autonomic nervous system, it receives its blood supply from the coronary arteries, and it possesses a marvelous conduction system.

The course of the blood through the four chambers of the heart, the valves, and the great vessels is shown in Fig. 4-1. The blood enters the two atria simultaneously, unimpeded by valves. The right atrium receives venous blood through the inferior and superior venae cavae. The left atrium receives arterial blood through the four pulmonary veins. During diastole both the atria and the ventricles fill. During atrial systole an extra complement of blood is pushed into the ventricles. When ventricular systole begins, the two valves (mitral and tricuspid) guarding the atria close (S_1), and blood is pumped to the lungs from the right ventricle (via the pulmonary artery) and to the systemic circulation from the left ventricle (via the aorta). When diastole begins, the valves (pulmonary and aortic) guarding the two ventricles close (S_2).

The two coronary arteries (right and left) spring from the root of the aorta. During diastole the coronary arteries fill, supplying the myocardium with oxygenated blood.

The conduction system of the heart is shown in Fig. 4-2. The sinus node, which paces the heart, lies in the superior portion of the right atrium. The atrioventricular (AV) node lies in the lower posterior part of the right atrium. Its function is to receive the impulse from the sinus node and delay it slightly so that the atria will have time to pump their contents into the ventricles before they contract, thus complementing cardiac output.

Since there is a fibrous ring separating the atria from the ventricles, the bundle of His is the sole muscular connection between these two parts of the

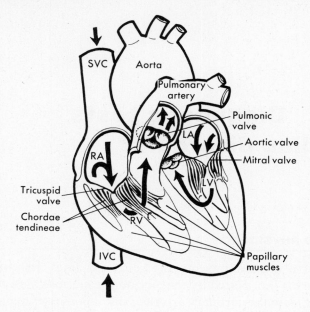

Fig. 4-1

Heart chambers, valves, papillary muscles, and course of blood flow. (From Tilkian, A., and Conover, M.: Understanding heart sounds and murmurs, Philadelphia, 1980, W.B. Saunders Co.)

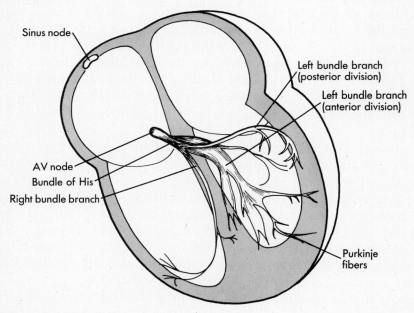

Fig. 4-2

The conduction system.

heart. The impulse enters the AV node and is conducted down the bundle of His, the bundle branches, and the Purkinje fibers to the ventricular myocardium. The right bundle branch serves the right side of the heart, and the left bundle branch, which is divided into an anterior division and a posterior division, serves the left side.

The conduction system of the heart enables the impulse to travel six times faster than would be possible without it.

GENERAL DIAGNOSTIC TESTS

The electrocardiogram (ECG)

This brief section on electrocardiography will not teach the performance or the interpretation of electrocardiograms. It is hoped that it will increase appreciation of the value and the limits of this diagnostic test and will provide motivation for further study of the subject. Subsequent sections of this book will assume that the reader has a working knowledge of the vocabulary used in electrocardiography. Although the electrocardiogram is used in almost all types of heart disease, this section will emphasize those areas in which the test has been found most useful.

Coronary artery disease

The electrocardiogram is indispensable in the proper diagnosis and treatment of coronary artery disease. Valuable information can be obtained about both the asymptomatic person, who has a normal resting electrocardiogram (as shown by means of stress electrocardiography—see the section on exercise electrocardiography), and the patient with acute myocardial infarction.

Electrocardiographic changes in coronary artery disease include the following.

"Nonspecific ST-T abnormalities." This is one of the most common electrocardiographic interpretations made. This vague interpretation can frustrate the beginner or one who expects a diagnostic label to result from every ECG. This is not always possible. Nonspecific ST-T abnormalities are what the term says they are. They are changes of the S-T segment and the T waves that are outside the range of what is considered normal, and this renders the electrocardiogram abnormal. These changes can be seen in a variety of disorders, cardiac or noncardiac, and do not necessarily signify heart disease. Still, these deviations may be the earliest manifestations of coronary artery disease.

S-T depressions. S-T depressions may indicate myocardial ischemia and are more specific changes, being flat or down-sloping 1 mm or more. Although not diagnostic of coronary artery disease, S-T depressions are quite characteristic of it. Digitalis and electrolyte abnormalities can accentuate or even mimic these changes.

S-T elevations. Marked S-T elevations in well-localized leads in a 45-year-old man clutching his chest in an emergency room characterize the onset of acute myocardial infarction. But an unqualified diagnosis of acute myocardial infarction would be incorrect. Such a tracing may reflect early changes in acute myocardial infarction ("hyperacute") or may revert to normal in a matter of minutes, at which time the tracing would be characteristic of variant (Prinzmetal's) angina, reflecting massive but totally reversible myocardial ischemia secondary to reversible coronary artery spasm. Thus an unqualified diagnosis of myocardial infarction, either acute or chronic, cannot be based upon an abnormality of ST-T waves, regardless of the severity of the changes. Abnormal Q waves (see the section on QRS changes) must be present before such a diagnosis is made. S-T elevations that remain unchanged over many weeks following an acute myocardial infarction may point to a ventricular aneurysm.

T inversions. Prominent or giant T inversions may reflect diffuse myocardial ischemia or possibly subendocardial infarction but are by no means specific. Central nervous system lesions, usually caused by massive damage or subarachnoid hemorrhage, can produce marked T wave inversions that can easily be confused with those of severe coronary artery disease.

QRS changes. Changes of the QRS complex are commonly seen in coronary artery disease. Abnormal Q waves are the hallmark of myocardial infarction. By also observing the associated changes in the ST-T segment, one can make a reasonable estimate of the age of the infarction—that is, determine whether it is recent or old. It is generally accepted that the more leads in which the Q waves are seen, the larger the infarction. Also, most Q waves persist indefinitely, but it is not uncommon for an electrocardiogram with diagnostic Q waves to lose the Q waves or even revert to normal months or years following an infarction.

Pathologic Q waves do not necessarily signify coronary artery disease or myocardial infarction. They can also be seen in infiltrative myocardial disorders, such as amyloidosis.

P waves. The diagnostic usefulness of the P waves in coronary artery disease is limited. In patients who have atrial infarctions or who have heart failure accompanied by elevated pressures in the left atrium, P waves may become abnormal.

U waves. U waves are seen in normal people, become more prominent in electrolyte disorders (hypokalemia), and may be inverted in myocardial ischemia.

P-R segment. The P-R segment is commonly normal in coronary artery disease. A prolonged P-R segment (first-degree heart block) is frequently seen in patients with myocardial infarction, especially of the inferior wall, and may also be the result of digitalis excess.

Q-T interval. The Q-T interval in coronary artery disease with myocardial ischemia may be prolonged. This fact is helpful in differentiating the ST-T abnormalities caused by ischemia (which is accompanied by Q-T prolongation) from those caused by digitalis (which is commonly accompanied by Q-T shortening). The QT interval may also be prolonged as a result of the administration of cardiac drugs (quinidine, and others) or as a result of brain damage. Marked Q-T prolongation can lead to ventricular tachycardia or fibrillation.

Valvular heart disease

Valvular heart disease is commonly reflected in the electrocardiogram by either increased voltage or ST-T abnormalities, indicating enlargement or hypertrophy of the affected cardiac chambers. Common examples include the following: *Aortic stenosis* or *aortic insufficiency* can cause left ventricular hypertrophy and enlargement. This condition is reflected in the electrocardiogram by increased voltage and ST-T abnormalities. *Mitral stenosis* produces increased pressure in the left atrium, causing this chamber to hypertrophy and dilate, and the result is reflected as a broad notched P wave in leads II and III (P mitrale), indicating left atrial enlargement. Similar examples can be extended to all other valvular lesions. *Hypertension* acts in a manner that is similar to that of aortic stenosis, since it also causes a pressure overload of the left ventricle, producing left ventricular hypertrophy. It should be noted that left ventricular hypertrophy identified by electrocardiogram does not necessarily mean a fixed increase of the muscle mass of the left ventricle, since treating the hypertension may improve the electrocardiogram, and in some cases may cause it to revert to normal.

Congenital heart disease

Congenital heart disease in infants, as well as in adults, is commonly accompanied by an abnormal electrocardiogram. The electrocardiogram is characteristic but can lead to an exact diagnosis in only a few conditions, such as endocardial cushion defect, atrial septal defect of the ostium primum type, and transposition of the great vessels with ventricular inversion. More frequently, the abnormality helps in localizing the disease to the right or the left side of the heart. Of course, in infants and children the set of criteria used for normals is different from that used in adults.

Arrhythmias

Although an astute examiner can sometimes make a specific diagnosis of a rhythm disorder by examining the radial pulse, the jugular venous pulsations, and the quality of the heart sound, the simplest and most accurate method of arrhythmia diagnosis is electrocardiography. In some cases, further investigations, by intracardiac electrophysiologic studies, may be necessary before a definite diagnosis can be established. Any deviation from the arbitrarily set sinus rhythm of 60 to 100 beats/min is considered to be an arrhythmia; however, some arrhythmias are considered to be usual elements of a normal heart, such as sinus arrhythmia or sinus tachycardia.

Extrasystoles. *Atrial premature beats* can be seen in an otherwise normal heart. If they are frequent, they may indicate atrial disease and may precipitate atrial fibrillation.

Junctional premature beats, when seen in normal individuals, have no clinical significance. Frequent junctional premature beats may be associated with digitalis toxicity, myocardial infarction, or the mechanical stimulation of the bundle of His by a prosthetic tricuspid valve. Occasionally, junctional extrasystoles are concealed and may cause unexpected conduction prolongation or nonconduction, mimicking first-degree AV block or second-degree AV block, types I and II.

Ventricular premature beats may be considered benign if they are seen in a healthy young individual without other evidence of cardiac disease. They may herald ventricular tachycardia or fibrillation, especially if they are seen in a setting of myocardial ischemia, severe heart disease, or acute myocardial infarction, in all of which the ventricular fibrillatory threshold is lowered. Premature ventricular contractions in the presence of organic heart disease are thought to be malignant if they are multiform, appear in pairs, or are early and appear on the T wave of the preceding complex. When three or more ventricular extrasystoles are present, the condition is commonly designated ventricular tachycardia. In the presence of organic heart disease, usually coronary artery disease, any of these arrhythmias increases the risk of sudden death.

Atrial fibrillation. Atrial fibrillation is the most common sustained atrial arrhythmia. Its presence frequently indicates organic heart disease, usually mitral valve disease or coronary artery disease. Although the diagnosis can be suspected because of an irregular pulse, an electrocardiogram is essential for an accurate diagnosis. Frequent premature beats can mimic the pulse of atrial fibrillation, while a regular pulse may be seen in atrial fibrillation with a high degree of AV block. This latter condition may indicate digitalis excess. See p. 75 for discussion of atrial fibrillation in WPW syndrome.

Atrial flutter. Atrial flutter is another common atrial arrhythmia that usually indicates the presence of organic heart disease. It is frequently seen in acute pericarditis.

Paroxysmal supraventricular tachycardia (PSVT). This type of tachycardia is sometimes referred to as "reciprocating"; it may be initiated by a premature atrial, junctional, or even ventricular beat. This form of tachycardia is sustained by a reentry mechanism within the AV node or by an AV reentry mechanism using two anatomically separate pathways—the AV node and an accessory bundle (WPW syndrome). AV nodal reentry may be seen in otherwise-healthy young people who are free of significant heart disease. However, when an accessory pathway forms part of the reentry circuit, recurring, persistent tachycardia may develop; this condition may be very debilitating and may precipitate atrial fibrillation or flutter. If the effective refractory period of the accessory pathway is short, the resulting rapid ventricular response to the atrial fibrillation may deteriorate into ventricular fibrillation.

Junctional rhythms. If the junctional rate exceeds 60 beats/min but is less than 100 beats/min, the condition is referred to as an accelerated rhythm, which is one of the common causes of AV dissociation, especially in the clinical setting of acute myocardial infarction, acute myocarditis, or digitalis excess. If this ectopic rhythm exceeds 100 beats/min, the condition is called junctional tachycardia. This condition, the result of enhanced automaticity, must be differentiated from PSVT, which results from a reentry mechanism.

Ventricular tachycardia. Ventricular tachycardia is rarely seen in an otherwise normal heart. Since it usually indicates severe heart disease, it requires prompt and accurate diagnosis and treatment. Occasionally, ventricular tachycardia cannot be distinguished from supraventricular tachycardia with aberrant ventricular conduction on the surface electrocardiogram. In such a situation, if permitted by the clinical setting, an intracardiac electrocardiogram provides a definitive diagnosis.

Ventricular fibrillation. Ventricular fibrillation is the end stage of severe organic heart disease, but it can also be induced by drugs (such as digitalis), electrolyte abnormalities (marked hypokalemia and marked hypomagnesemia), or electrocution. Ventricular fibrillation is the most common immediate cause of sudden death. This extreme rhythm disorder permits no effective cardiac output. Irreversible brain damage and subsequent death result if effective resuscitative measures are not instituted in 3 to 5 minutes. As a rule, one should not wait to make an electrocardiographic diagnosis of ventricular fibrillation before instituting such measures.

Sinoatrial (SA) block and sinus arrest. These are relatively rare arrhythmias. A marked increase in vagal tone can cause sinus arrest and prolonged asystole. Extreme fright, a hypersensitive carotid sinus, and an exaggerated diving reflex are some of the causes of this increase. Atropine administration is effective therapy, but in recurrent cases pacing may be a necessity. Airway obstruction and hypoxia—as in sleep apnea syndrome (see p. 336)—are another cause of SA block and sinus arrest. Inflammatory or ischemic involvement of the SA node can cause SA block, but in such a setting an escape junctional or ventricular rhythm frequently emerges.

Atrioventricular (AV) block. Atrioventricular block exists when conduction from atria to ventricles is interrupted because of a pathologic condition. Atrioventricular block is commonly classified as first, second, or third degree. Care should be taken not to confuse physiologic refractoriness with true AV block and thus run the risk of overdiagnosing and overtreating the patient. Before nonconduction is diagnosed, one should make sure that the opportunity to conduct is present, by noting the R-P intervals and considering the possibility of concealed junctional or fascicular extrasystoles.

First-degree AV block. First-degree AV block is generally defined as a prolongation of AV conduction time (P-R greater than 0.20 second). It may be secondary to increased parasympathetic tone, or may reflect digitalis excess, myocarditis, or infiltration of the myocardium by tumor or amyloid. By itself, first-degree AV block causes no hemodynamic compromise and warrants no treatment.

Second-degree AV block. Second-degree AV block is present when one or more, but not all, atrial impulses fail to reach the ventricles because of impaired conduction. Second-degree AV block can be of two types. In type I (Wenckebach) there is progressive prolongation of the P-R interval preceding a nonconducted P wave; in type II the P-R interval is constant.

Type I second-degree AV block can be benign, resulting from a marked increase in parasympathetic tone. When seen in trained athletes or only during sleep, it can be a normal finding. Digitalis excess and diaphragmatic myocardial infarction are common pathologic causes.

Type II second-degree AV block is indicative of organic heart disease; frequently it indicates involvement of the His-Purkinje system. Common causes are anteroseptal myocardial infarction and degenerative or infiltrative disease of the myocardium. Pacemakers are commonly necessary.

Third-degree (complete) AV block. Complete AV block is present when the opportunity for conduction exists but conduction does not take place. Thus, before this diagnosis can be made numerous factors must be taken into consideration, including the refractoriness of the AV junction, autonomic influences, drugs, the atrial rate, the ventricular rate, and the level of the escape pacemaker.

Complete AV block is usually caused by degenerative disease of the conduction system. Coronary artery disease is the second most common cause. This arrhythmia can also be seen in traumatic or inflammatory disease or drug toxicity. Newly acquired complete AV block in adults usually causes significant hemodynamic impairment and can cause syncope (Stokes-Adams syndrome) or death. As a rule, permanent demand ventricular pacing is used in all adult patients. In congenital complete heart block with stable, narrow QRS complexes and an adequate ventricular rate, a pacemaker may not be necessary if close follow-up care is available.

Newer pacemakers, which permit synchronous pacing of the atria and the ventricles (atrioventricular sequential pacers), are physiologically superior to standard demand ventricular pacers, and in the future will probably be used more frequently in this setting.

Bundle-branch block

Bundle-branch block has traditionally been classified as right bundle-branch block (RBBB) or left bundle-branch block (LBBB), but in recent years anterior and posterior branches of the left bundle have been recognized. In the presence of left bundle-branch block, a diagnosis of myocardial infarction or ventricular hypertrophy may be difficult or impossible to make. Right bundle-branch block does not mask a diagnosis of myocardial infarction and may be the clue to silent coronary artery disease. It is commonly seen postoperatively, especially after repair of ventricular septal defect, or in the presence of atrial septal defect. Bifascicular block (right bundle-branch block and left anterior hemiblock or left posterior hemiblock) in the presence of acute myocardial infarction usually indicates massive myocardial damage with a poor prognosis. Although pacemakers have been used electively (or prophylactically) in these patients, their use has not substantially improved survival. In chronic bifascicular block, pacemakers are effective in preventing recurrences of syncope caused by intermittent second-degree or complete heart block.

Wolff-Parkinson-White (WPW) syndrome

Congenital defects may exist in the form of extra muscular tracts (accessory pathways) between the atria and the ventricles. Such tracts provide an anatomic link for AV reentry tachycardia, which may be precipitated by either atrial or ventricular premature beats. If conduction during atrial fibrillation occurs exclusively over an accessory pathway with a short refractory period, the ventricular rates can be very high (160-300 beats/min) and the rhythm may degenerate into ventricular fibrillation. The classical ECG features of the originally described syndrome are a short P-R interval and a broad QRS. Other features are a delta wave (the initial slurring of the QRS), secondary T wave changes, and abnormal Q waves. It is important to note, however, that the ECG may be completely normal, or show only minimal preexcitation, in the presence of an accessory pathway, and yet the patient may be subject to the same life-threatening arrhythmias as in the overt syndrome.

Effects of drugs and electrolytes on the electrocardiogram (see Table 4-1)

Digitalis, which is commonly used in patients with heart disease, can mimic many of the diagnostic changes of the electrocardiogram. It is important to be familiar with the usual electrocardiographic abnormalities produced by this drug. In usual therapeutic doses digitalis causes sagging of the S-T segment with flattening of the T waves, shortening of the Q-T interval, and slight prolongation of the P-R interval (Table 4-1). In the presence of atrial fibrillation, digitalis also slows the ventricular rate. In digitalis excess the following arrhythmias are commonly noted: marked P-R prolongation, second- and third-degree AV block, junctional extrasystoles, sinus bradycardia, accelerated junctional rhythm, and atrial tachycardia with AV block. Digitalis toxicity should be strongly suspected in the presence of bigeminal ventricular extrasystoles, multifocal ventricular extrasystoles, pairs of ventricular extrasystoles, or runs of ventricular tachycardia. In the presence of atrial fibrillation, digitalis excess may produce a regular pulse because of high-degree AV block and/or an accelerated junctional focus. Arrhythmias suggesting digitalis toxicity appear earlier if there is concurrent potassium and/or magnesium depletion.

Quinidine in therapeutic doses can cause prolongation of the Q-T interval, with widening and notching of the P waves. There could be some depression of the S-T segment and flattening or inversion of the T waves. When therapeutic levels in the blood are exceeded, the toxic effects noted are varying degrees of AV block, widening of the QRS complexes over 50% of normal, and ventricular arrhythmias, including ventricular tachycardia or fibrillation—thus the term "quinidine syncope."

Occasionally, ventricular tachycardia or fibrillation is precipitated in the absence of drug toxicity. Usually, marked Q-T prolongation or U waves precede the onset of the characteristic arrhythmias ("torsades de pointes").

Ventricular tachycardia or fibrillation secondary to marked Q-T prolongation can also be caused by procainamide (Pronystyl) and disopyramide (Norpace).

Propranolol (Inderal), metoprolol (Lopressor), nadolol (Corgard), and atenolol (Tenormin) belong to the group of drugs known as *beta blockers*. These drugs slow the sinus rate, producing sinus bradycardia with slight P-R prolongation. The Q-T interval is shortened, and the T wave may remain normal or be slightly higher (Table 4-1). In atrial fibrillation, beta blockers slow the ventricular response.

Phenytoin (Dilantin) is used in the treatment of digitalis toxicity. This drug shortens the P-R and Q-T intervals without having a significant effect on the QRS complex (Table 4-1). This characteristic of phenytoin makes it the drug of choice in the treatment of digitalis toxicity in the presence of prolongation of the P-R interval or first- or second-degree AV block.

Disopyramide (Norpace), like quinidine, in high doses may cause prolongation of the P wave, QRS complex, and P-R interval.

Lidocaine has little effect on the electrocardiogram. Studies have shown increased conduction delay in ischemic tissue without any effect on normal tissue.

Verapamil (Isoptin, Calan) is a calcium channel blocking agent with important antiarrhythmic properties. Verapamil produces a dose-related block at the AV node; it is therefore used in the treatment of paroxysmal supraventricular tachycardia. Verapamil also slows the ventricular rate in atrial fib-

Table 4-1

Effects of drugs and electrolytes on the electrocardiogram

Drug or electrolyte	P-R	QRS	Q-T$_c$	Sinus rate	Waveform changes
Amiodarone	0	0	+	−	
Aprindine	+	+	+	−	
Atropine	−	0	0	+	T changes
Bretylium tosylate	Sl+	0	0	−	
Daunomycin	0	0	0	0	− QRS voltage; ST-T changes
Digitalis	+	0	−	−	S-T sags; T flattens
Diltiazem	+	0	0	−	
Disopyramide	0	Sl+	+	Sl+	
Doxorubicin HCl	0	0	0	0	− QRS voltage
Encainide	+	+	Sl+	0	
Ethmozin	Sl+	Sl+	Sl−	Sl−	
Hypercalcemia	Sl+	Sl+	−	0	T widens and rounds
Hyperkalemia	+	+	0	0	P widens; S-T depresses; T wave tall and peaked
Hypocalcemia	0	0	+	0	
Hypokalemia	0	Sl+	0	0	U prominent; S-T sags; T notches, then inverts
Imipramine HCl	Sl+	Sl+	Sl+	Sl+	T changes
Lithium	0	0	0	0	T flattens
Minoxidil	0	0	0	0	T changes; +QRS voltage
Phenothiazines	0	0	+	0	T changes
Phenytoin	Sl−	Sl−	Sl−-	0	
Procainamide	Sl+/−	+	+	0	ST-T changes
Propranolol (and other beta blockers)	Sl+	0	Sl−	−	T changes
Quinidine	Sl+/−	+	+	0	S-T depresses: T flattens or inverts; U wave
Tocainide	0	0	0	Sl−	
Verapamil	+	0	0	−	

0 = no significant change; + = increase; − = decrease; Sl+ = slight increase; Sl− = slight decrease.

rillation and can cause various degrees of AV block. It does not alter the rest of the ECG. *Diltiazem (Cardiem)* is another calcium channel blocking agent; its action on the AV node is similar to that of verapamil.

Lithium in therapeutic doses can cause flattening and inversion of the T waves. Sinus node dysfunction with SA block can result from lithium treatment, usually when a lithium compound is given in toxic doses.

Hyperkalemia is reflected in the electrocardiogram in the following manner: The first electrocardiographic manifestation of hyperkalemia occurs when blood concentrations of potassium enter the range of 5.5 to 6.5 mEq/L. At this level the T waves become characteristically tall and peaked. With further elevations in the plasma potassium concentration, there is a decreased amplitude of the R waves, with increased S waves, S-T depressions, and prolongation of the QRS duration and the P-R interval. When the plasma potassium concentration exceeds 7.5 mEq/L, intra-atrial conduction disturbances develop and are reflected in broad, low-amplitude P waves and P-R interval prolongation. At still higher potassium levels, the P wave disappears altogether, and the QRS becomes markedly widened and moves into a smooth diphasic (sine) wave. The final stage, if the hyperkalemia is untreated, consists of ventricular tachycardia, flutter, fibrillation, and standstill.

Hypokalemia initially causes an apparent prolongation of the Q-T interval. This results from the appearance of a U wave that merges with the T wave and may cause notching of the T wave. T wave inversion follows, and then sagging of the S-T segment. Ventricular arrhythmias—premature beats, tachycardia, and fibrillation may occur. The administration of potassium reverses these changes rapidly.

Hypercalcemia characteristically shortens the S-T segment of the Q-T interval and may also widen and cause a rounding of the T waves.

Hypocalcemia causes a prolongation of the Q-T interval.

Hypermagnesemia can cause P-R prolongation and intraventricular conduction delay, with QRS widening. These changes may occur at magnesium levels of 10 mEq/L. Complete heart block, cardiac arrest, and asystole may occur if the plasma magnesium concentration exceeds 15 mEq/L.

Hypomagnesemia can cause P-R prolongation, broadening and lowering of T waves, and Q-T prolongation. These changes may resemble the changes of hypokalemia and may be secondary to intracellular potassium depletion. Ventricular premature beats, ventricular tachycardia, and ventricular fibrillation can also occur.

Computer interpretation of the electrocardiogram

Computer assistance in the interpretation of electrocardiograms is available. Several programs now in use provide immediate interpretation and facilitate preparation of final written reports. Computer programs are excellent in differentiating normal from abnormal tracings and in listing the abnormalities present in a tracing. The limitations of these programs include difficulty in recognizing artifacts and generally poor performance in the diagnosis of complex arrhythmias. Improvements in these areas are expected. Computer ECG interpretations are generally checked by physicians.

Important points to remember

A normal electrocardiogram does not rule out severe organic heart disease. Severe obstructive disease of all major coronary arteries without myocardial infarction or active ischemia of the heart is one situation that could exist in spite of a perfectly normal electrocardiogram.

A definitely abnormal electrocardiogram does not necessarily signify heart disease. Many abnormalities, even pronounced, can result from CNS lesions or autonomic influences, or can be produced by drugs, electrolytes, or other causes.

Electrocardiographic interpretations should be made in the context of the clinical situation. Serious errors will be made if the clinical data are not used in interpreting an electrocardiogram.

The limitations of the standard resting electrocardiogram should be recognized. It is at most a 1-minute record of the heart's electrical activity, and it is recorded at rest, without stressing the heart. Whenever necessary, further tests should be used, such as the Holter monitor for arrhythmia diagnosis or stress electrocardiography for diagnosis of coronary artery disease. These will be discussed in the following sections.

Ambulatory electrocardiography (Holter monitoring)

Ambulatory electrocardiography is an extension of the resting electrocardiogram. A portable recorder is worn by the patient, and the electrocardiogram is recorded continuously on magnetic tape during unrestricted activity. The tapes are scanned rapidly by electrocardioscanners, and abnormalities or selected areas of interest are printed out in real time. Computers and microprocessors are utilized in the rapid processing of tapes. This permits detailed and quantitative analysis of the data.

Clinical value

The clinical uses of ambulatory electrocardiography are many. It enables a much larger sample of the heart's electrical activity to be recorded; instead of the 30 to 50 complexes noted on the usual resting electrocardiogram, this procedure samples 50,000 to 100,000 beats on a 10- to 24-hour record. Resting, unrestricted activity, and sleep recordings are made. Many abnormalities that have in the past gone undetected because they occurred during the patient's sleep are now being recognized.

Indications

1. *Diagnosis of arrhythmias.* In patients complaining of dizziness or palpitations or actually having episodes of syncope, the ambulatory electrocardiogram is an invaluable diagnostic tool. If the rhythm disorder *and* the symptoms are shown to be coincident, then an exact diagnosis of an elusive disorder can be made.
2. *Monitoring of high-risk patients.* Holter monitoring is especially useful when a patient is discharged from the hospital soon after a myocardial infarction.
3. *Evaluation of the effectiveness of drug treatment of arrhythmias*
4. *Diagnosis of ischemic heart disease.* Not uncommonly, ischemic S-T depressions can be noted on an ambulatory electrocardiogram during periods of stress, be it caused by exertion, emotions, heavy meals, or cigarette smoking. Sometimes, ischemic changes are recorded during a patient's sleep; these are commonly associated with periods of rapid-eye-movement sleep (during which dreams occur), sinus tachycardia, and possibly a rise in the blood pressure.

Prinzmetal's angina causes S-T elevation during angina and is associated with proximal high-grade coronary artery obstructive lesions and/or coronary spasm. An exercise electrocardiogram (see following discussion) may be negative, showing no ischemic S-T changes or pain. In such a case an ambulatory electrocardiogram can be very useful in detecting the S-T abnormalities that may occur during rest—or sleep.

Contraindications and limitations

There are no absolute or relative contraindications for ambulatory electrocardiography; however, the limitations are several.

Initial systems were able to monitor only one lead, causing difficulties in recognizing artifacts and detecting ST-T changes. Also, the timing devices were crude and inaccurate. Newer models have a much improved design, and two-lead systems are standard now. One major limitation is inherrent in the technique. Arrhythmias are detected and recorded, but this information is generally not available to the physician for 24 hours, after the recording has been completed and the tape scanned. Several innovative techniques have recently been developed to permit earlier—or immediate (real time)—transmission of the ECG signal to a monitoring station, using telephone lines. Once they have been standardized and tested, these new techniques will further enhance the value of ambulatory monitoring.

The major risk of ambulatory electrocardiographic monitoring remains the potential for misdiagnosis (failure to recognize artifacts) or overdiagnosis (detection of benign arrhythmias), with the subsequent initiation of unnecessary and potentially hazardous therapy.

Exercise electrocardiography

The exercise electrocardiogram was initially a twelve-lead electrocardio-gram performed after the patient had stepped up and down a set of stairs of a standard height a certain number of times (Master's test). Today the test con-sists of gradually increasing the level of exercise on a motorized treadmill or a bicycle ergometer, while the electrocardiogram is being monitored. All twelve leads can be monitored. Newer models incorporate automatic rate meters and S-T segment analyzing computers. Various investigators have proposed protocols for gradually increasing the work load; the most widely used is that proposed by Robert Bruce. Valuable information obtained includes (1) the minutes of exercise—(given a standard load, the maximum oxygen consumption can be estimated), (2) the heart rate and blood pressure achieved at the peak of exercise (heart rate × blood pressure "double product" provides a good approximation of myocardial or heart work), (3) the degree of S-T depression that relates to myocardial ischemia, and (4) arrhythmias provoked during exercise or, more often, during the early part of the recovery period.

Clinical value

The values of exercise electrocardiography are many. In coronary artery disease, a resting electrocardiogram may be normal, or show nonspecific changes. In this situation the exercise electrocardiogram is commonly abnor-mal and frequently quite diagnostic, by indicating flat or down-sloping isch-emic S-T depression.

Another value of exercise testing is in diagnosis of arrhythmias. Although ambulatory monitoring remains the method of choice in detecting suspected arrhythmias, exercise electrocardiography can also be used for this purpose, especially if the arrhythmias are suspected to occur during exercise. These arrhythmias could be provoked during exercise electrocardiography in a con-trolled setting, with facilities available for immediate treatment.

This test is also useful in the evaluation of a patient's functional capacity or "physical fitness." In addition, it is useful in evaluating methods of ther-apy, including drugs or surgery, such as coronary artery bypass surgery, as well as in obtaining an objective evaluation of a patient's disability in situa-tions in which a history is confusing or difficult to obtain. The exercise ECG is also useful in prescribing exercise for the rehabilitation of patients follow-ing myocardial infarction or cardiac surgery.

In patients with combined heart and lung disease, or when the presenting problem is effort dyspnea or fatigue with no clear cause, a *combined cardio-pulmonary exercise test* is valuable. In addition to monitoring the heart rate, blood pressure, and heart electrical activity, one can collect expired gases, monitor oxygen consumption and oxygen saturation, and collect samples for blood gas determinations at key points during exercise in an attempt to physiologically define the causes of a patient's symptoms.

Indications

The indications for exercise (or stress) electrocardiography are many. Like resting electrocardiography, it can be considered an extension of the physical examination. Specific indications were discussed in the section on the value of the test.

Contraindications

This test, unlike resting electrocardiography and ambulatory electrocardiography, does have some contraindications. Among these are any acute cardiac illness, specifically acute myocardial infarction or myocarditis, or severe arrhythmias. Other contraindications are uncompensated congestive heart failure and drug toxicity.

In acute coronary insufficiency or unstable angina the test is best avoided; if the diagnosis is clear, the test is probably superfluous; if the diagnosis is in doubt, cardiac catheterization and angiography may be the diagnostic test of choice (p. 116). After stabilization and therapy one may proceed to an exercise ECG to assess the effect of therapy.

Limitations

The major limitation of stress electrocardiography is the high level of false-positive and false-negative results in the diagnosis of ischemic heart disease. False-negative results, even when a maximal heart rate is achieved, may be seen in as many as 25% of patients with coronary artery disease. Massive coronary occlusion with myocardial infarction can occur in patients whose maximal exercise electrocardiograms were normal only days or weeks prior to the insult. False-positive results—for example, ischemic S-T depression in the absence of coronary artery disease—can also occur. Possible causes of this particular situation include digitalis administration, electrolyte abnormalities, cardiomyopathies, left ventricular hypertrophy, and left bundle-branch block.

Myocardial perfusion imaging using thallium 201 following exercise helps decrease the frequency of false-positive and false-negative results (see p. 112). Also, computer analysis of an exercise ECG may further improve the diagnostic accuracy of the test.

Pitfalls

Digitalis and electrolyte abnormalities, specifically hypokalemia, can produce or accentuate ischemic ST changes. Thus, ST depression that is not flat or down-sloping 1 mm or more can be misdiagnosed as ischemia.

Nitroglycerin enables a patient with coronary artery disease to perform a higher level of exercise, and it possibly results in the production of fewer arrhythmias. Thus a patient's drug history immediately prior to testing should be noted.

If careful attention is not given to details of the testing—for example, if the patient uses the handrail for support—conclusions can be erroneous.

Another pitfall is that patients do learn how to perform the test and very commonly perform better on a second test, without any intervention. Usually this learning does not progress from a second to a third test and so on.

Risks

One in 10,000 tests leads to the death of the patient, usually as a result of ventricular fibrillation from which the patient was not successfully resuscitated. Complications necessitating hospitalization are in the range of 0.2% and include myocardial infarction, prolonged bouts of chest pain, severe arrhythmias, and hypotensive and hypertensive episodes. These risks can be minimized by screening patients by means of a history and physical examination and a resting electrocardiogram prior to testing, and through the availability of, and the familiarity of personnel with, resuscitative equipment.

Informed consent is not routinely obtained for this test, but is advisable in high-risk patients.

Vectorcardiography (VCG)

The vectorcardiogram was introduced by Frank Wilson in 1938. While the ECG displays electrical forces of the heart at a given time and point, the VCG displays all of these forces at any instant. A vectorcardiogram involves a plot of voltage against voltage in three-dimensional space; it is a useful addition to the scalar ECG, reinforcing and making the understanding of scalar electrocardiography more complete.

Clinical value

The VCG has diagnostic advantages over the ECG in the following situations:

1. In determining the cause of slowing of electrical waveforms. Specifically, VCG is helpful in the diagnosis of the initial slowing that occurs in WPW syndrome and in the differentiation of bundle-branch block from other causes of widened QRS complexes.
2. In establishing the differential diagnosis between inferior wall myocardial infarction and left anterior hemiblock when there are S waves with embryonic r waves in leads II, III, and aV_F
3. In differentiating RBBB from right ventricular hypertrophy

4. In detecting left ventricular hypertrophy in the presence of **LBBB**. Analysis of the vector angle and magnitude can be helpful.
5. As an adjunct to scalar electrocardiography, increasing the diagnostic yield by approximately 10%

Routine radiographic examination of the heart

A chest x-ray examination in two projections, posterior-anterior (PA) and lateral, provides valuable information about the size and contour of the heart. Anatomic changes of individual chambers are seen in the right and left

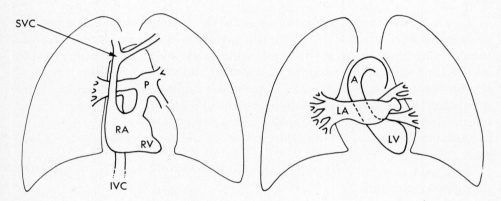

Fig. 4-3
X-ray film of the chest in the posterior-anterior projection. *SVC,* Superior vena cava. *IVC,* Inferior vena cava. *RA,* Right atrium. *RV,* Right ventricle. *P,* Pulmonary artery. *LA,* Left atrium. *LV,* Left ventricle. *A,* Aorta.

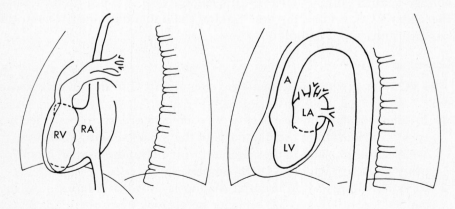

Fig. 4-4
X-ray film of the chest in the left lateral projection.

anterior oblique projections. These projections are shown in Figs. 4-3 to 4-6. Before the advent of echocardiography, radiographic examination was the simplest, most accurate way of assessing cardiac size, a fact that made percussion of the chest for heart size in the physical examination almost a lost art.

The cardiothoracic ratio

The simplest and most frequently used measurement of the heart is the cardiothoracic ratio. This ratio is obtained by first adding the longest dis-

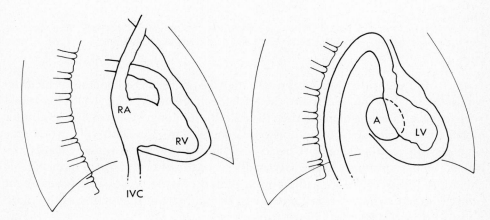

Fig. 4-5
X-ray film of the chest in the right anterior oblique projection.

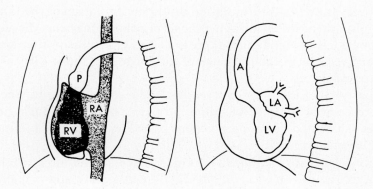

Fig. 4-6
X-ray film of the chest in the left anterior oblique projection.

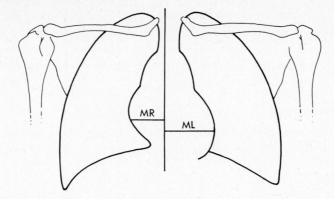

Fig. 4-7
The cardiothoracic ratio, which is derived by adding the midright *(MR)* and midleft *(ML)* measurements. The sum is then divided by the longest transverse diameter of the chest.

tance from the midline of the chest to the right side of the heart and the longest distance from the midline to the left side of the heart (Fig. 4-7). This transverse diameter of the heart is then divided by the longest transverse diameter of the chest to arrive at a cardiothoracic ratio. This is a relatively crude way of assessing cardiac size, but because the cardiothoracic ratio is easily obtained, it is commonly used. Generally, a cardiothoracic ratio over 50% is considered indicative of cardiac enlargement. Some reasonable assessment of individual chamber enlargement can be made from inspection of the plain chest film in the PA and lateral projections.

Inspection of the lung fields

One looks for overcirculation or undercirculation, pulmonary vein patterns, and edema.

An observation of overcirculation or undercirculation of the lung fields is most helpful in the differential diagnosis of congenital heart diseases. In the presence of a left-to-right shunt there are signs of increased circulation in the pulmonary vessels; in the presence of a right-to-left shunt there is evidence of undercirculation.

The patterns of the pulmonary veins, their size and prominence, as well as the presence or absence of pulmonary lymphatic markings, help in the diagnosis of elevated pulmonary venous pressure, which is a common sign of congestive heart failure.

Pulmonary edema can be of two kinds, alveolar and interstitial. Alveolar edema is characteristic of acute left-sided heart failure and is manifested by bilateral confluent densities that start centrally and spread peripherally. This is commonly referred to as the *butterfly-wing pattern.* In interstitial edema, fluid accumulates in the interstitial tissues of the lungs and produces a generalized haziness and clouding of the vascular shadows. When such fluid collects in the interlobular septa of the lung, septal lines are formed that are referred to as *Kerley's lines*.

Inspection of the pleural spaces

Approximately 250 ml of pleural effusion is necessary for an accurate radiologic diagnosis. Pleural effusion is usually manifested as blunting of the costophrenic angle. Larger effusions, 1 liter or more, can also accumulate; such an effusion may be an accompaniment of congestive heart failure, or it may be independent of heart disease and indicate the presence of lung disease. Occasionally, pleural effusions are hidden under the lung (subpulmonic effusion) and therefore do not obliterate the costophrenic angle. Such effusions can be detected by obtaining film with the patient in the lateral position (lateral decubitus film). Pleural fluid examination is discussed on p. 158.

Inspection of the rib cage

Inspection of the rib cage may provide a clue to the existence of coarctation of the aorta, in which condition collateral circulation from enlarged intercostal arteries would produce characteristic deformity or notching of the rib margins.

Cardiac series

The ability to make an accurate diagnosis of the enlargement of a specific chamber is enhanced by obtaining a cardiac series, in which a bolus of barium is swallowed by the patient, opacifying the posterior-lying esophagus. In addition to the PA and lateral films, two oblique films are obtained. In a cardiac series an enlarged left atrium or even an enlarged aorta could be noted because it would displace the barium-filled esophagus (Fig. 4-8). This, along with additional projections, would aid in the diagnosis of left or right ventricular enlargement.

Cardiac fluoroscopy

Cardiac fluoroscopy is most useful in detecting calcifications of various parts of the heart. Introduction of image intensifiers has decreased the overall radiation hazard of this test and has improved the quality of the images. Cardiac fluoroscopy is also useful in detecting calcification in the coronary artery system. Although the diagnostic method of choice for detection and semiquantitation of coronary artery disease is selective coronary angiography (see p. 116), cardiac fluoroscopy is a useful *screening* tool for this purpose. Approximately 75% of patients with coronary artery disease have calcification of the coronary artery system, but 20% of patients (especially older

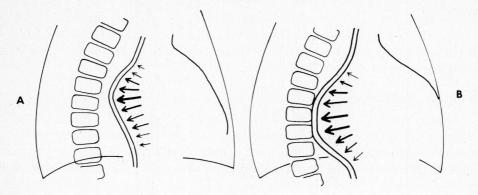

Fig. 4-8
X-ray film of the chest obtained after a patient has swallowed barium (a "cardiac series"). Note the moderate, **A,** and marked, **B,** degrees of left atrial enlargement, which are reflected in the displacement of the atrium by the barium-filled esophagus. This is a right anterior oblique projection.

patients) with no obstructive coronary disease also have calcification of the coronary arteries. Calcification of the various valves of the heart, specifically the aortic and mitral valves, is unequivocal evidence of disease of these valves. Although heavy calcification suggests more advanced disease of the valves (usually narrowing), an exact correlation cannot be made. Other cardiac diseases in which calcification is helpful in the diagnosis are tumors of the heart, constrictive pericarditis (evidenced by calcification of the pericardium), and old myocardial infarction or trauma (evidenced by calcification of the myocardium).

CO₂ injection

Carbon dioxide (CO_2) may be injected into a peripheral vein for the diagnosis of pericardial effusion. After a brief period, x-ray films are taken with the patient in the left lateral position. The carbon dioxide acts as a contrast material within the right atrial chamber, defining the thickness of the right atrial and pericardial walls. (This technique has now been replaced by echocardiography, which is simpler and has greater diagnostic accuracy.)

Indications

The chest x-ray examination and the cardiac series are used almost as extensions of the physical examination; they are performed on patients with all kinds of cardiac disease, as well as on patients without cardiac disease, for screening purposes. Cardiac fluoroscopy is indicated when calcification of various parts of the heart is suspected.

Contraindications

There is no absolute contraindication, since the risk is limited to a minimal exposure to ionizing radiation—a risk that increases, however, with repeated exposures. This risk becomes more important in young children and in pregnant women, in whom studies should be performed only when absolutely necessary; the gonads or the fetus should routinely be shielded.

Limitations

The heart can appear perfectly normal on chest x-ray film, even in the presence of severe organic disease of the heart. The information revealed is mainly of a static nature, with the dynamic aspects of the working heart not detected.

Variations of heart size in systole as compared with diastole also diminish the accuracy of x-ray detection of cardiac enlargement.

Pitfalls

In radiographic examination of the heart, diagnostic errors can result either from the recording technique or from the interpretation of the information.

Technical errors. Films exposed during expiration may produce a false impression of an enlarged heart and pulmonary vascular congestion. This impression also may be produced in films of an obese patient, who will have a high diaphragm and excessive pericardial fat. In addition, overpenetration of x-rays may cause the disappearance of pulmonary vascular markings. Rotation of a patient may produce a false appearance of enlargement or may result in the magnification of various vessels.

Errors of interpretation. In the presence of a pectus excavatum deformity of the chest, the heart may be displaced posteriorly, producing a false impression of cardiomegaly. In pectus carinatum deformity of the chest, the anterior-posterior diameter is increased and possible enlargement of the right ventricle may go undetected. Patients with a straight dorsal spine may appear to have cardiomegaly, especially in a lateral projection. In patients with severe kyphoscoliosis, accurate assessment of cardiac size and pulmonary vasculature may be impossible. A portable chest x-ray examination cannot be used to assess cardiac size, although it can be helpful in assessing the degree of pulmonary congestion.

Further pitfalls in the interpretation of x-ray films of the chest are many, but discussion of them would be beyond the scope of this book.

Computerized tomographic imaging of the heart

Computerized tomographic imaging (CAT scan) of the heart, by means of x-rays (transmission tomography) or positron-emitting radio tracers (emission tomography) is still in the developmental stage. Its role in clinical cardiac diagnosis remains to be defined.

Digital fluoroscopy

Digital fluoroscopy is a newly developing diagnostic tool, utilizing computer processing of radiographic images. This technique permits visualization of pulmonary arteries, cardiac chambers, and major systemic arteries, following *intravenous* injection of contrast material. When fully developed, this technique will decrease the need for selective arteriographic studies.

Determination of blood levels of cardiac enzymes

Enzymes are proteins that act as catylists in chemical reactions. The blood levels of various enzymes are noted in the diagnosis of many pathologic states, one of which is acute myocardial infarction. Normally, these enzymes are present in the blood in small amounts. But following injury or infarction to an organ the levels of various enzymes increase in the blood, in proportion to the organ's enzyme content and the extent of injury. Different organs have different enzyme contents.

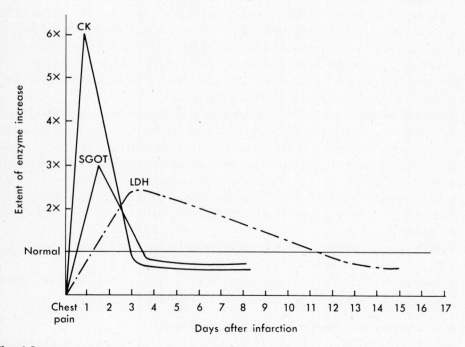

Fig. 4-9
Typical changes in serum enzyme levels following myocardial infarction.

Clinical value of enzyme level determinations

Careful scrutiny of the pattern and time course of changes in enzyme levels in the blood can help to verify a diagnosis of acute myocardial infarction that is based on history and physical examination and an electrocardiogram. The pattern and time course of increases and decreases in enzyme levels following myocardial infarction are depicted in Fig. 4-9.

Enzyme level determinations also permit the diagnosis of an extension of an infarction or of a reinfarction. In addition, within certain limitations, the degree of elevation of enzyme levels correlates with the degree of myocardial injury.

Attempts are under way to use enzyme techniques in *quantitating* myocardial infarction and assessing the value of various treatment interventions. Various enzymes have been used in the past in the diagnosis of myocardial infarction, but the discovery of the isoenzymes of creatine kinase (CK) and lactic dehydrogenase (LDH) has made the use of other enzymes obsolete. Work is in progress to further improve the laboratory diagnosis of acute myocardial infarction; this work involves the measurement of urinary and plasma levels of myoglobin and the use of highly sensitive assays for CK-MB and CK-B fractions.

In the diagnosis of acute myocardial infarction, the clinical setting and time of presentation determine the significance of increases or decreases in the levels of the various enzymes. At one extreme, when the ECG shows unequivocal diagnostic features, enzyme level determinations may be superfluous. At the other extreme, when electrocardiographic changes are nondiagnostic, the levels of both CK and LDH isoenzymes may be monitored every 12 hours to make a specific diagnosis. In most hospitals, a cardiac enzyme *panel* includes determinations for CK and LDH (and their isoenzymes) and SGOT (mostly for historical reasons). This panel of tests is done on admission and daily for 3 days.

Creatine kinase (CK)

Measurement of serum levels of CK and its isoenzymes is useful in the diagnosis of acute myocardial infarction, because the total CK activity in myocardial tissue is high and because one of the CK isoenzymes (MB) is found in significant amounts only in the heart muscle.

CK activity is greatest in skeletal muscle, and second greatest in myocardium. The CK activity in brain, bladder, stomach, and colon is about half that in myocardium.

CK isoenzymes. There are three known CK isoenzymes: MM, MB, and BB. Methods for measuring their levels are readily available.

Heart muscle is the only tissue in which a significant fraction of the CK activity results from isoenzyme MB. The CK in skeletal muscle is over 98%

MM but may contain some MB. Brain, bladder, stomach, and colon contain primarily isoenzyme BB (see Table 4-2).

Clinical implications of elevated CK isoenzyme levels. Following the onset of acute myocardial infarction, elevated CK-MB and total CK values are detected in the blood in 3 to 5 hours. At 6 to 12 hours more than 98% of patients with acute myocardial infarction will show an abnormal rise. In most of these patients, the high level will persist for about 24 hours. After 30 hours many persons who have had myocardial infarctions have no MB elevation. CK-MB levels at various hours after the onset of symptoms are shown in Fig. 4-10.

Eighty percent of myocardial CK consists of the MM fraction, which persists in the blood longer than the MB fraction. Therefore, it is possible to have an elevated CK level, all MM fraction, secondary to myocardial infarction, especially if the sampling is done more than 24 hours after acute infarction. The CK-MM level, although sensitive to myocardial injury, is not specific for it, since the level can be elevated after trauma to any muscle.

Serial CK-MB determinations remain the best single laboratory aid to the *early* diagnosis of acute myocardial infarction. The CK-MB level may be elevated in Duchenne's muscular dystrophy, dermatomyositis, and polymyositis. The clinical distinction between acute myocardial infarction and one of these conditions should be relatively easy. Elevated CK-MB levels are oc-

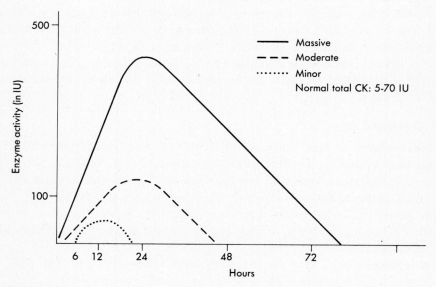

Fig. 4-10
Typical curve of CK-MB levels after acute myocardial infarction.

casionally seen in pericarditis, myocarditis, and sustained tachyarrhythmias. It is not clear whether these elevations result from prolonged ischemia or from actual cell necrosis.

Lactic dehydrogenase (LDH)

Elevation of serum total LDH levels and a characteristic isoenzyme pattern are almost always found in patients who have had acute myocardial infarctions. The serum total LDH level is also high after injuries involving liver, skeletal muscle, kidney, lung, or erythrocytes.

LDH isoenzymes. Five LDH isoenzymes are known; they are usually given the designations LDH_1 through LDH_5 (see Table 4-3).

LDH_1 has the greatest activity in heart muscle, renal cortex, and erythrocytes.

LDH_2 has the greatest activity in normal serum, with LDH_1 second ($LDH_2 > LDH_1$). Following acute myocardial infarction this ratio in the

Table 4-2

Tissue location of CK isoenzymes

CK isoenzyme	Tissue
BB	Brain, smooth muscle, thyroid, lung, prostate
MB	Cardiac muscle, tongue, diaphragm; trace amounts in skeletal muscle
MM	Skeletal muscle, cardiac muscle

Table 4-3

Tissue location of LDH isoenzymes

Principal LDH isoenzymes	Tissue
LDH_1, LDH_2	Heart Kidney Brain Red blood cells
LDH_3	Thyroid Adrenal gland Lymph nodes Pancreas Thymus Spleen Leukocytes
LDH_4, LDH_5	Liver Skeletal muscle

serum is reversed ($LDH_1 > LDH_2$); this situation is sometimes referred to as a "flipped ratio."

LDH_5 is the major isoenzyme in liver and muscle.

Clinical implications of elevated LDH isoenzyme levels. Following the onset of symptoms of acute myocardial infarction, increases in the LDH level above the normal range are usually seen in 12 hours, with peak activity occurring about the third day. After 6 to 8 days values usually return to normal, but they may remain elevated for 14 days.

During the first 12 hours after an acute myocardial infarction, the LDH isoenzyme ratio usually remains normal ($LDH_2 > LDH_1$). Twelve to 24 hours after the infarction a characteristic pattern of myocardial infarction appears ($LDH_1 > LDH_2$), and may persist for about 12 days, even when total LDH values have returned to normal. Refer to Table 4-4 for a summary of LDH isoenzyme patterns in disease states.

Glutamic-oxaloacetic transaminase (GOT)

Increases in serum GOT levels are seen 8 to 12 hours after the onset of acute myocardial infarction. The elevation usually peaks at 18 to 36 hours, and the level is close to normal by 3 to 7 days. Damage to liver, skeletal muscle, lungs, or kidneys may elevate GOT levels, limiting the specificity of the test. No heart-specific isoenzymes exist.

Determination of levels of blood lipids

Elevated blood lipid levels have received much attention in relation to coronary artery disease. The association between serum cholesterol level and coronary artery disease is unequivocal. Less strong is the association between triglyceride levels and coronary artery disease. The blood lipids (cholesterol, triglycerides, and phospholipids) circulate in the plasma, in which they are bound to protein; thus the term "lipoproteins." Electrophoresis is the method used to separate the lipoproteins; from this procedure the following classification has evolved:

1. *Chylomicrons*—primarily exogenous triglycerides
2. *Very-low-density lipoproteins (VLDL)*—primarily endogenous triglycerides
3. *Intermediate-density lipoproteins (IDL)*—transitional forms, with 30% cholesterol and 40% triglycerides
4. *Low-density lipoproteins (LDL)*—50% cholesterol
5. *High-density lipoproteins (HDL)*—may serve to remove cholesterol from tissues

LDL has a strong and direct association with coronary artery disease, while HDL has been *inversely* associated with the risk of coronary artery disease. High levels of HDL thus have a protective role. Determination of the *total cholesterol* level is therefore not sufficient for the assessment of coronary risk. It is important to determine whether elevated cholesterol levels are caused by an increase in the concentration of LDL (high risk of coronary artery disease) or the concentration of HDL (low risk of coronary artery disease). Generally accepted normal values for these lipids are listed in Table 4-5.

Hyperlipidemia

The association between hyperlipidemia (specifically, high levels of LDL) and coronary artery disease is well established; this association is most striking in the younger population. Although there is no conclusive proof at this

Table 4-4

LDH isoenzyme patterns in various disease states

LDH isoenzyme pattern	Disease state
LDH_1 and LDH_2 elevated generally; $LDH_1/LDH_2 > 1$	Myocardial infarct Pernicious anemia Acute renal damage Hemolysis
LDH_5 elevated	Liver damage
$LDH_1 > LDH_2$; LDH_5 elevated	Myocardial infarct with liver congestion
LDH_2 and LDH_3 elevated	Lymphoproliferative disorders Pulmonary infarct
Elevation of levels of all isoenzymes	Heart failure Crush syndrome Neoplastic disease

Table 4-5

Normal values for plasma lipoproteins (mg/dl)

Age	Total cholesterol	Triglycerides	LDL cholesterol	HDL cholesterol
<24	125-200	50-146	73-138	32-57
25-39	140-250	60-250	90-180	32-60
40-49	161-260	70-250	100-185	33-60
50-64	170-265	75-200	105-190	34-70
>64	175-280	70-200	105-200	33-75

Adapted from Levy, E.I. and Feinleib, M.: Risk factors for coronary artery disease and their management. In Braunwald, E., editor: Heart disease, Philadelphia, 1980, W.B. Saunders Co., pp. 1254-1255.

time that lowering abnormally elevated lipid levels will stop or retard the progression of coronary artery disease, it is prudent to detect these elevations and to use dietary and, if indicated, drug measures to bring these levels within the normal range or at least to lower them. It is generally agreed that the lower the blood lipid levels, the smaller the chance of acquiring coronary artery disease.

Pitfalls

There are two common pitfalls in the measurement of blood lipid levels: the patient has to be fasting if useful information is to be obtained, and there can be marked fluctuations from day to day in the same patient. Therefore, a patient should have several measurements before a definite diagnosis of hyperlipidemia is made and dietary and/or drug therapy is instituted.

Blood glucose level and glucose tolerance test (GTT)

An abnormal glucose tolerance test result is commonly associated with hyperlipidemia and obesity, and is an additional risk factor for coronary artery disease. Fasting blood glucose measurements will verify the presence of diabetes in an overtly diabetic patient. The value of the glucose tolerance test in detecting diabetes in an asymptomatic patient lies in recognizing the risk factor for coronary artery disease. Generally, no treatment is necessary except weight reduction in the obese.

Pitfalls

A patient should not have a below-average carbohydrate intake before the test, and the test should not be done too soon (days to weeks) after a myocardial infarction, since glucose levels are elevated following infarction.

Measurement of blood drug levels

Monitoring of blood levels of various cardiac drugs is essential to their successful and safe use. Of the commonly used drugs, assays for blood levels are presently available for digoxin, quinidine, procainamide, phenytoin, lidocaine, and propranolol. The therapeutic and potentially toxic blood levels for these and other cardiac drugs are shown in Table 4-6. This table is to be used as a *general guide.* The cardiac condition, clinical context, and electrolyte status of a patient have to be considered in interpreting blood levels of these drugs. For example, serum digoxin levels of 1.5 ng/ml may be associated with clinical toxicity and arrhythmias in a setting of severe myocardial disease or in a setting of hypokalemia, hypomagnesemia, and hypercalcemia. But serum levels of digoxin higher than 4 or 5 ng/ml may be necessary in rare instances to slow down the ventricular rate in atrial fibrillation.

Table 4-6

Therapeutic and potentially toxic blood levels of cardiac drugs

Drug	Therapeutic blood level (per ml)	Potentially toxic blood level (per ml)
Amiodarone (Cordarone)	1-10 μg*	Not known
Digitoxin	20-35 ng	Over 40 ng
Digoxin (Lanoxin)	1-2 ng	Over 3 ng
Diltiazem (Cardiem)	100-200 ng*	Not known
Disopyramide (Norpace)	2-4 μg	Over 6 μg
Lidocaine	1.4-5 μg	Over 6 μg
Mexiletine	0.5-2 μg	Over 3 μg
N-Acetylprocainamide (NAPA)	2-22 μg	Not known
Nifedipine (Procardia)	50-100 ng*	Not known
Phenytoin (Dilantin)	10-18 μg	Over 18 μg
Procainamide (Pronestyl)	4-8 μg	Over 8 μg
Propranolol (Inderal)	20-85 ng	Over 150 ng
Quinidine	2.5-5 μg	Over 5 μg
Theophylline	10-20 μg	Over 20 μg
Tocainide	6-12 μg	Over 14 μg
Verapamil (Isoptin, Calan)	100-200 ng	Not known

*Preliminary data.

Miscellaneous blood tests

The complete blood count (CBC) is useful in detection of anemias, which may (1) present as angina in a patient with coronary artery disease, (2) aggravate congestive heart failure, (3) constitute a diagnostic clue in subacute bacterial endocarditis, or (4) constitute evidence of hemolysis in patients with prosthetic valves.

The white blood cell count (WBC) is elevated in patients with myocardial infarction, bacterial endocarditis, or the postmyocardial infarction (Dressler) syndrome.

The sedimentation rate is elevated in acute myocardial infarction, bacterial endocarditis, Dressler's syndrome, and in many other diseases that cause inflammation. It is considered to be characteristically low in congestive heart failure.

Abnormalities of electrolytes are common in patients with heart disease. These abnormalities can result from congestive heart failure, or they can occur as side effects of drug therapy for this condition. Chronic congestive heart failure causes total-body, as well as myocardial, potassium and magnesium depletion. Diuretics used as treatment for congestive heart failure may further increase these losses. Accurate diagnosis of an electrolyte abnormality requires determination of the tissue (intracellular) levels of these cations. Serum levels, which are routinely measured, *may* reflect intracellular deficits.

In both congestive heart failure and myocardial infarction scrupulous attention to electrolyte balance (sodium, potassium, and magnesium, as well as calcium and phosphorus) will decrease the number and severity of problems with arrhythmias and drug (especially digitalis) toxicity.

In severe congestive heart failure, creatinine clearance may fall and the blood urea nitrogen and serum creatinine levels may rise.

Antistreptolysin-O (ASO) titer is elevated after streptococcal infections and can be the clue to diagnosis of acute rheumatic fever.

The *VDRL test*, discussed on p. 286, can be the clue to syphilitic heart disease, usually presenting as aortic insufficiency or disease of the ostia of the coronary arteries.

A test of *prothrombin time* is used in initiating and maintaining anticoagulation therapy with oral anticoagulants (drugs such as Coumadin). Usually the prothrombin time is kept within 2 to 2.5 times the normal, and that is generally comparable to 20% to 30% of the normal prothrombin activity. The partial thromboplastin time (PTT) and the clotting time are used in following the cases of patients receiving heparin; 2 to 2.5 times the normal is the therapeutic range.

Anticoagulation therapy with heparin, and subsequently with Coumadin-type drugs, is used in pulmonary embolism, deep venous thrombosis, cerebral embolism, and acute peripheral arterial embolism and is felt to be beneficial in patients with acute myocardial infarction with congestive heart failure, during the period of bed rest. Many drugs interfere with the metabolism and action of the Coumadin-type anticoagulants. Frequent measurements of the prothrombin time and careful checks of the interaction of drugs are important in minimizing the risk of hemorrhage in patients receiving anticoagulant drugs.

Blood cultures are crucial in the diagnosis of infective endocarditis. It is important to obtain an adequate number of cultures. Generally, six is considered adequate. The specimens should be obtained by sterile technique, with inoculation preferably being done at the bedside. The specimens should be cultured on aerobic, anaerobic, and microaerophilic media.

The common pitfalls in the diagnosis of endocarditis from blood cultures are (1) contamination, causing a false-positive diagnosis, and (2) the presence of antibiotics in the patient's serum or treatment with antibiotics prior to the blood culture, which may lead to false-negative results.

Arterial blood gas determinations are discussed on p. 197. Patients with myocardial infarction or congestive heart failure commonly have abnormalities of the arterial blood gases. Patients who have hypoxemia or desaturation secondary to altered ventilation/perfusion ratios usually benefit from oxygen administration in an attempt to keep their oxygen saturation 90% or higher. Patients who have myocardial infarctions, especially with pulmonary congestion or edema, commonly hyperventilate, with subsequent lowering of the PCO_2 and mild respiratory alkalosis. In the presence of severe pulmonary edema, hypoventilation with elevation of the PCO_2 and mild respiratory acidosis may occur.

Some drugs used in the treatment of myocardial infarction, especially morphine, produce a predictable drop in the rate and depth of respiration and may, in excessive doses, precipitate hypoventilation with respiratory acidosis. Therefore, in patients who are receiving larger than usual doses of morphine or morphine along with other respiratory suppressants, arterial blood gas determinations are indicated to detect and/or avoid respiratory depression.

Nitroglycerine and nitroprusside may decrease arterial oxygen saturation. The mechanism is poorly understood, but it probably involves an increase in the degree of mismatch between ventilation and perfusion. In a marginally compensated patient, such a decrease in oxygen saturation may be clinically important.

The carbon monoxide level is elevated in moderate to heavy smokers, as well as in persons living in areas of heavy industrial pollution; such an elevation may precipitate or exacerbate angina pectoris in a person who has coronary artery disease. Measurement of carbon monoxide levels in the blood thus can be helpful in identifying factors that are contributing to a patient's angina pectoris.

Urine examination

Measurement of the volume of urine through 24 hours is helpful in the diagnosis of cardiac disorders, since in heart failure the night volume may be from 30% to 50% more than the day volume. Such nighttime elevation is referred to as nocturia.

The presence of red cells in the urine may be evidence of infective endocarditis or embolic disease of the kidneys.

Mild proteinuria, 1 to 2 gm of protein per day in the urine, can be seen in congestive heart failure. Patients with marked elevation of venous pressure, constrictive pericarditis, or tricuspid insufficiency may present with massive proteinuria, and even with the nephrotic syndrome.

Recently, the detection of myoglobin in the urine (myoglobinuria) has been found useful as a sensitive test in the diagnosis of myocardial infarction, but clinical experience with this test remains limited.

NONINVASIVE SPECIALIZED DIAGNOSTIC METHODS IN CARDIOLOGY

The following is a discussion of the more important specialized tests used in cardiovascular diagnosis. These tests are grouped together because they are noninvasive; that is, they do not break the patient's skin or interfere with or alter the events that are being observed. They also pose no risk or significant discomfort to the patient and can be repeated at frequent intervals with absolute safety. Great advances have been made in such testing procedures over the past decade. Further advances in technology and more sophisticated use of microprocessors and computers in data analysis will certainly be forthcoming during the next decade.

M-mode echocardiography

M-mode echocardiography (ultrasound cardiography) was first introduced to clinical cardiology in the early 1970s. In the brief span of 10 years it has become an indispensable tool, being the most frequently used test after the electrocardiogram. M-mode echocardiography utilizes echoes (reflected ultrasound) from pulsed high-frequency sound waves to locate and study the movements and dimensions of various cardiac structures. The technique permits direct recordings of the motion of the mitral, aortic, tricuspid, and pulmonic valve leaflets, the intraventricular septum, and the right and left ventricular walls. In addition, the technique provides accurate measurements of the size of the cardiac chambers and the changes in their dimensions during the cardiac cycle, and it allows recognition of abnormal filling defects, as in atrial tumors. Because the ultrasound beam tracks the motion of various cardiac structures over a period of time, it provides a time-motion study of the heart (hence the term M [motion]-mode echocardiography). (See Figs. 4-11 and 4-12.)

Real-time, two-dimensional, cross-sectional echocardiography (2-D echo)

Two-dimensional echocardiography represents a further development of ultrasound technique. While in M-mode echocardiography the angle of the ultrasound beam is kept stationary, in 2-D echocardiography this angle is rapidly moved within a sector (usually 45-86 degrees), producing a "sector scan." Images produced by this technique are presented in a more familiar format, comparable to that in angiography. The ability of 2-D echo to appreciate spatial anatomic relationships makes this test more versatile than the M-mode technique. (Also, many of the limitations inherent in M-mode echocardiography can be eliminated by using both techniques simultaneously.) The sound beam can be moved with a mechanical device (mechanical sector scanner) or by electronic systems (phased array scanner). Both types of 2-D echo scanners provide good-quality two-dimensional images of cardiac structures (chambers, walls, valves, and so on) in real time. The images, along with the electrocardiogram, are recorded on videotape to permit later viewing. All 2-D echo machines also have the capability for simultaneous M-

Text continued on p. 104.

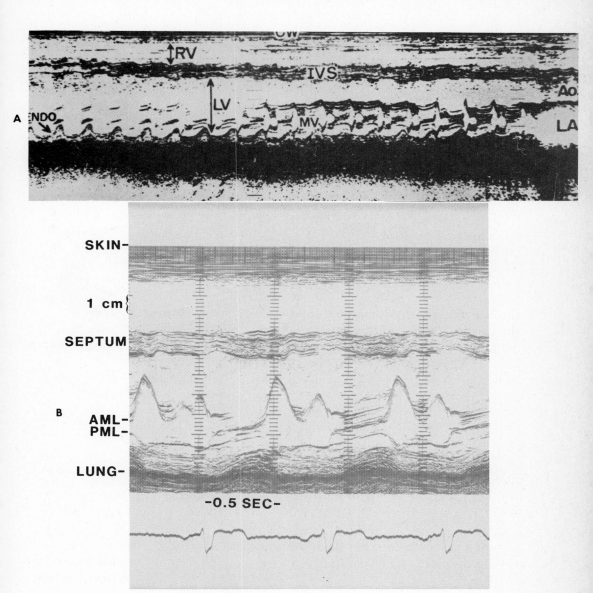

Fig. 4-11
A, M-mode scan from the left ventricle (LV) to the aorta (Ao) and left atrium (LA) in a normal person.
RV, Right ventricle. *IVS,* Interventricular septum. *ENDO,* Left ventricular free posterior wall endocardium. *CW,* Chest wall. *MV,* Mitral valve. **B,** M-mode echocardiogram of a normal mitral valve. *AML,*
Anterior mitral leaflet. *PML,* Posterior mitral leaflet. (From Linhart, J.W., and Joyner, C.R., editors:
Diagnostic echocardiography, St. Louis, 1982, The C.V. Mosby Co.)

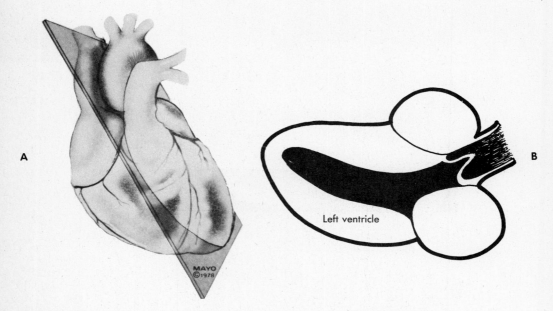

Fig. 4-12
A, The long-axis plane of the left ventricle extends along an imaginary line from the right shoulder to the left flank. The scan begins at the base of the heart and continues toward the apex of the left ventricle (long axis of the heart). **B,** Diagrammatic representation of the long-axis plane of the left ventricle. **C,** Resultant two-dimensional ultrasonic image in the long-axis plane (parasternal, long-axis plane, left ventricle). *AV,* Aortic valve. *RV,* Right ventricle. *VS,* Ventricular septum. *LV,* Left ventricle. *LA,* Left atrium. *PW,* Posterior wall. *A,* Anterior. *P,* Posterior. *I,* Inferior. *S,* Superior. (**A** and **C** from Seward, J.B., and Tajik, A.J.: Med. Clin. North Am. **64:**177, March 1980.)

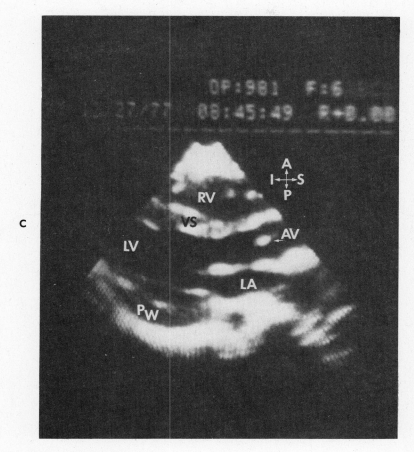

Fig. 4-12, cont'd
For legend see opposite page.

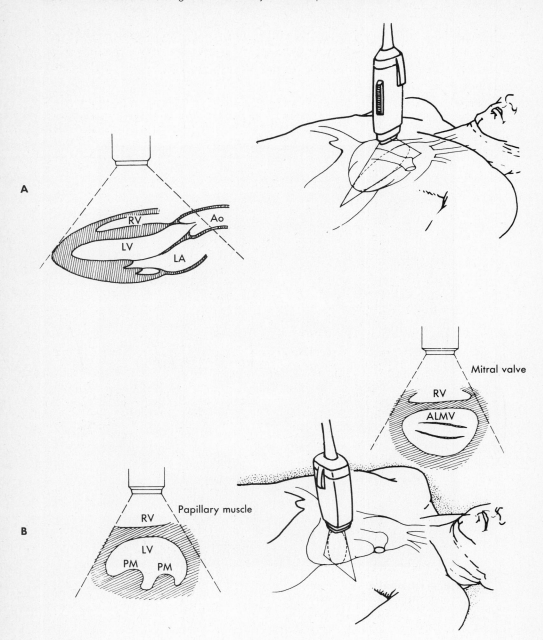

Fig. 4-13
Two-dimensional echocardiogram. **A,** Conventional precordial long-axis view. **B,** Short-axis view.
RV, Right ventricle. *LV,* Left ventricle. *LA,* Left atrium. *Ao,* Aorta. *ALMV,* Anterior leaflet mitral valve.
PM, Papillary muscle. (From Carr, K.W., and others: Measurement of left ventricular ejection fraction
by mechanical cross-sectional echocardiography, Circulation **59:**1196-1206, 1979. By permission of
the American Heart Association, Inc.)

mode recordings on strip charts. Newer recorders are compact in size, permitting bedside examinations. Computer processing of images for quantitation and for 3-dimensional reconstruction of structures is being attempted, but is not generally used yet.

A complete two-dimensional examination includes long- and short-axis views. Figs. 4-13 and 4-14 show the transducer in the parasternal position and apical two- and four-chamber views.

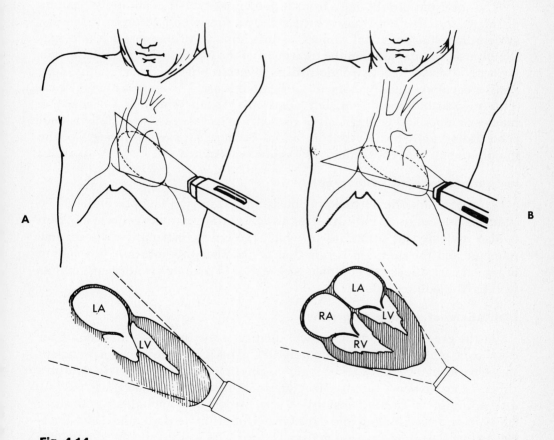

Fig. 4-14
A, Apical two-chamber, two-dimensional echocardiogram (axial). **B,** Four-chamber view (hemiaxial). Views are obtained with the transducer located at the apex and directed toward the right shoulder. *LA*, Left atrium. *LV*, Left ventricle. *RA*, Right atrium. *RV*, Right ventricle. (From Carr, K.W., and others: Measurement of left ventricular ejection fraction by mechanical cross-sectional echocardiography, Circulation **59:**1196-1206, 1979. By permission of the American Heart Association, Inc.)

Exercise echocardiography

Attempts have been made to extend the echocardiographic examination to include exercise. The concept is valid, since frequently the left ventricular wall motion and ejection fraction may appear normal at rest but be abnormal during exercise. Exercise echocardiography therefore can provide valuable information. However, the technical difficulty involved in obtaining good images during exercise (and motion) has limited the usefulness of exercise echocardiography. Nuclear cardiac studies seem to be more suited to this purpose (p. 110).

Clinical value of echocardiography

The information obtained from a good-quality 2-D echo study permits definitive treatment, including surgery, of persons who have mitral stenosis, pericardial effusion, atrial tumors, or mitral valve prolapse. Such information is also very valuable in the treatment of the following conditions: valvular heart disease, infective endocarditis, hypertrophic cardiomyopathy, congestive cardiomyopathy, congenital heart disease, coronary artery disease with myocardial infarction, left ventricular aneurysm, and intracardiac masses or clots. In the diagnosis of coronary artery disease, two-dimensional echocardiography has severe limitations because satisfactory images of the major coronary arteries cannot be regularly obtained.

Indications for echocardiography

Any of the disorders listed previously, or a suspicion that one of these disorders is present, is an indication for an echocardiogram. An echocardiogram is also indicated in situations in which the only abnormality is a cardiac murmur and the question is raised as to whether this murmur is a sign of organic heart disease. A complete study should include two-dimensional as well as M-mode recordings.

Limitations of echocardiography

At the present time the technical quality of the images is inadequate for diagnostic purposes in approximately 10% of patients. Technicians proficient in the performance of the test, as well as physicians able to expertly interpret the tests, are in short supply. The equipment is costly, ($60,000 to $110,000), and a complete two-dimensional study, which also includes an M-mode study, is time consuming and expensive. Quantitative data analysis—determination of ejection fraction and valve areas—is still in the developmental stage. The resolution of present echocardiographic systems approaches 2.5 to 3 mm. Better focusing techniques and high-frequency transducers may improve this situation.

Pitfalls in echocardiography

There is no contraindication to echocardiography, since there is no inherent risk in the procedure. There are, however, pitfalls in the performance of the technique, and obtaining consistently high-quality echocardiograms and interpreting these records properly can be difficult. A possible risk to the patient exists in the potential for misdiagnosis or wrong therapeutic decisions as a result of poor-quality echocardiograms. It can be unequivocally stated that poorly done or inadequately interpreted echocardiography is worse than no echocardiography.

Phonocardiography and external pulse recording
Phonocardiography

Phonocardiography is the graphic recording of sounds that originate in the heart and the great vessels. Such a recording may be obtained by placing microphones on the surface of the body or by introducing special apparatus into the heart (intracardiac phonocardiography). This discussion will be limited to the former.

Phonocardiography is an extension of auscultation of the heart as performed with a stethoscope, in that it generally records only the sounds that can be heard by the clinician. The phonocardiogram is, however, superior to the stethoscope in recording low-frequency sounds (gallop sounds), while the stethoscope is better in appreciating high-frequency sounds (murmurs). The

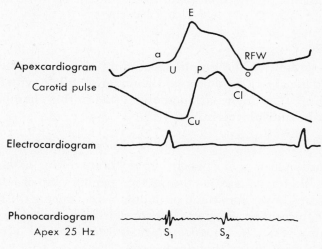

Fig. 4-15
Normal phonocardiogram and external pulse recordings displayed with an ECG.

phonocardiogram can record the four components of the first sound, systolic murmurs, the two components of the second sound (aortic and pulmonic), the opening snap of mitral stenosis, the third and fourth heart sounds, and clicks. It can also give information about the *relative* loudness of these events. A normal phonocardiogram is displayed in Fig. 4-15.

A phonocardiogram is commonly produced simultaneously with tracings of other external pulses, which can serve as references for timing various sounds. These other procedures are carotid pulse tracing, jugular pulse tracing, and apexcardiography.

Carotid pulse tracing

Carotid pulse tracing is the graphic recording of the displacement of the carotid artery produced by each heartbeat; this tracing reflects small volume changes in a segment of this artery. The recording is obtained by applying a pressure-sensitive transducer to the neck, over the point of maximal pulsation of the carotid artery. Information thus gained includes the rate of rise of the displacement curve, its duration, and its overall contour. Although records obtained in this manner closely resemble tracings obtained by pressure transducers inside vessels, carotid pulse tracings cannot be used to measure absolute pressures. A normal carotid pulse tracing appears in Fig. 4-15.

Jugular pulse tracing

Jugular pulse tracing is performed in a manner similar to carotid pulse tracing, except that the recording is obtained over the jugular venous system. This tracing yields information about events in the right atrium and right ventricle.

Apexcardiography

Apexcardiography is the graphic recording of the displacement of the chest wall produced by the motion of the underlying left ventricle. Analysis of this record provides information about events in this chamber. A normal apexcardiogram is displayed in Fig. 4-15.

Clinical uses

A phonocardiogram is most useful for accurate *timing* of various sounds and murmurs. Examples include timing the opening snap of mitral stenosis, timing the closing of the aortic and pulmonic valves during the second sound (A2-P2), and determining whether clicks are ejection clicks (early in systole) or late systolic clicks. The phonocardiogram is also useful in recording the shapes of various murmurs that are heard.

A carotid pulse tracing provides information about the functional state or the performance of the left ventricle. This information can be obtained by measuring the various components of the curve that is produced (systolic time intervals). Also, the general evaluation of the contour of the curve can give information about aortic stenosis, aortic insufficiency, mitral insufficiency, and idiopathic hypertrophic subaortic stenosis (IHSS).

A jugular pulse tracing serves as a reference for the phonocardiogram; it yields information about right ventricular hypertrophy, elevated pressure in the right atrium, tricuspid regurgitation, and constrictive pericarditis; and it aids in the analysis of complex arrhythmias. In complete heart block it displays the cannon A wave that is observed at the bedside examination.

Apexcardiography is helpful in timing various heart sounds, especially the opening snap of mitral stenosis. It is also useful as a reference tracing for locating the fourth heart sound, or the atrial gallop, and in distinguishing the origin of the gallop (right or left side). The evaluation of the contour of the tracing yields information about left ventricular hypertrophy, possible aortic or mitral stenosis, or idiopathic hypertrophic subaortic stenosis.

These four tests—phonocardiography, carotid pulse tracing, jugular pulse tracing, and apexcardiography—are valuable because they provide permanent, objective records that are far superior to handwritten descriptive records and because they can be used in serial comparisons in the same patient. These procedures are also superb devices for teaching the physical examination and auscultation of the heart.

Indications

These graphic methods are indicated whenever a permanent, objective record is important, as well as when specific information about various auscultative findings and their timing is not otherwise available.

Equipment presently available permits the simultaneous production of an electrocardiogram, echocardiograms, multiple phonocardiograms, carotid pulse tracings, jugular pulse tracings, and apexcardiograms. The value of each individual test is usually enhanced when these tests are performed together.

Advances in echocardiography and nuclear cardiology (p. 110) have in large measure replaced pulse tracings in cardiac diagnosis. Of course, these tracings continue to be superb teaching aids.

Limitations

There are major limitations to the clinical use of these tests. They serve as extensions of the physical examination; what cannot be heard through a stethoscope usually cannot be recorded on a phonocardiogram. A specific diagnosis can rarely be made *only* by inspection of graphic records. Much skill and time are necessary to perform the tests properly, and the information obtained is of a qualitative nature.

Nuclear cardiology

Radioactive tracer techniques are being used in cardiovascular diagnosis with increasing frequency. These tests generally qualify as "noninvasive" because they are safe and can be performed repeatedly; the total radiation exposure is considered minimal. Nevertheless, they do involve the intravenous injection of a tracer material.

The general technique in all such tests consists of injecting a radioactive tracer material into a vein and recording the radioactivity emitted over a specific area of the body. By using various types of tracers as well as different recording techniques, vastly different types of information can be obtained. Among the diagnostic tests employing radioactive tracer techniques are lung perfusion scanning, angiocardioscanning, myocardial scanning during rest and after exercise, and resting and exercise wall-motion studies of the right and left ventricles.

Improvements in instrumentation and radioactive tracers, as well as increasingly more sophisticated use of computer methods in analysis and quantitation of data, have increased the clinical usefulness of these techniques.

Lung perfusion scanning

In lung scanning, technetium 99, tagged to albumin, is injected intravenously; it subsequently becomes trapped in the lung capillaries and provides information about the status of pulmonary perfusion.

In scanning for right-to-left shunts, the radioactive material, instead of being trapped in the pulmonary vasculature, is passed to the left side of the heart and trapped in systemic capillaries (for example, in the kidney or the spleen), where radioactivity will be seen. In such a situation an angiocardioscan (nuclear angiocardiogram) can further localize the shunt.

The lung scan is most helpful in the diagnosis of a pulmonary embolus when the x-ray film of the chest is normal or near normal, and when the test is interpreted in conjunction with a ventilation scan, which would detect the presence of parenchymal lung disease. This is discussed on p. 145.

In the presence of grossly abnormal x-ray films of the chest resulting from parenchymal lung disease, such as those normally seen in chronic obstructive lung disease or pneumonia, the diagnostic accuracy of a lung scan is markedly diminished. In questionable or doubtful cases it is necessary to use selective pulmonary angiography to obtain a definite diagnosis. Occasionally, a lung scan will reveal absolutely no perfusion on one side of the lung. This could be the manifestation of a large pulmonary embolus, or it may indicate a congenitally absent or atretic right or left pulmonary artery.

Nuclear angiocardiography

A bolus of radionuclide is injected intravenously, and its course through the circulatory system is followed with a scintillation camera. The size, shape, and sequence of filling of the various chambers of the heart can then be studied. This procedure is most useful in the detection of an intracardiac shunt or complex congenital heart diseases. It is also helpful in evaluating a surgically performed shunt in congenital heart disease. The radionuclide used is technetium 99m (^{99m}Tc). Its passage through the heart is monitored, using a scintillation camera and a computer. Right and left ventricular function can be assessed, the wall motion of both ventricles can be reconstructed, and the ejection fraction (index of ventricular function) can be calculated. Such a study is called a "first pass" or "first transit" study. The technetium 99m can be tagged to albumin or to red cells, thus preventing its rapid exit from the vascular pool. This will permit "equilibrium studies," in which all cardiac chambers are visualized simultaneously. The ECG is used to time systole and diastole; multiple counts are obtained over a period of time, providing an "equilibrium blood pool study" or "equilibrium study." Such studies will give information about regional as well as overall ventricular function. Also, ventricular aneurysms and clots can be identified. Computers can generate time (systolic and diastolic) activity (count) curves for the right and left ventricles, permitting calculation of the ejection fraction.

The *ejection fraction (EF)* is calculated by dividing the stroke volume (end-diastolic volume minus end-systolic volume) by the end-diastolic volume. It is assumed that counts in the ventricle are directly proportional to the volume of blood, and therefore end-diastolic counts (EDC) and end-systolic counts (ESC) are used to estimate the ejection fraction (EF):

$$EF = \frac{EDC - ESC}{EDC}$$

The ejection fraction is a sensitive index of ventricular function. Normal hearts generally have an ejection fraction greater than 55%. Combining such a study with exercise further increases the value of the test. Normally, exercise will cause an increase in ejection fraction. A drop in ejection fraction because of exercise is abnormal and clearly reflects ventricular dysfunction.

Clinical uses. Radionuclide wall-motion studies are used in the noninvasive evaluation of left ventricular function. They provide both a regional and a global assessment of ventricular function at rest and during exercise. In patients with myocardial infarction, cardiomyopathy, or valvular heart disease, serial evaluations are possible.

Limitations. Frequent ectopic beats or atrial fibrillation may cause errors in the timing of systole and diastole and therefore in the counts obtained. In equilibrium studies if the right and left ventricles are not separated adequately, the data may be inaccurate.

Equipment is expensive, and the test involves intravenous injection and some minimal exposure to radiation.

Myocardial perfusion studies

Myocardial perfusion, and therefore, indirectly, coronary obstructive disease, can be evaluated by means of radioactive tracer techniques. Currently, the most popular tracer is thallium 201 (^{201}Tl), an analogue of potassium. After intravenous injection, thallium 201 will accumulate in various regions of the myocardium in direct proportion to regional myocardial blood flow and extraction of the thallium by the myocardial cells. A viable myocardial cell, with intact cell membrane function, is necessary in order for this extraction to occur. Thus, in the presence of severe coronary artery narrowing and decreased blood flow to a given region of the heart, the accumulation of thallium in that region will be decreased. Such an abnormality is accentuated if the study is combined with exercise. Total occlusion of a vessel, with infarction of the left ventricular muscle supplied by that vessel, will result in no uptake of thallium.

Photons emitted by the thallium 201 are detected by an Anger camera, and recorded on film and in a computer. By comparing the relative densities of these photons, a physician can make assumptions about myocardial blood flow (normal, decreased, or absent) (see Fig. 4-16).

Clinical uses. Resting thallium 201 myocardial perfusion studies are most helpful for the diagnosis of myocardial infarction, either acute or chronic. An infarct will appear as an area of markedly decreased or absent perfusion (Fig. 4-16). An exercise thallium 201 perfusion study is more helpful in the diagnosis of coronary artery disease and myocardial ischemia in which a perfusion defect is identified during exercise but disappears over time (4 to 24 hours). Combining thallium 201 perfusion imaging with an exercise electrocardiogram (p. 112) increases the diagnostic yield of the exercise treadmill test.

Limitations. Myocardial perfusion studies *do not* visualize the coronary arteries; they provide *indirect* evidence of coronary artery narrowing or obstruction. Therefore if such narrowing is not very severe or if there is adequate collateral flow, a study may be normal. Quantitation of regional perfusion may increase the diagnostic value of a study.

Both the equipment used and the thallium 201 are expensive.

Technetium 99m pyrophosphate imaging

This test is used as an aid to the diagnosis of acute myocardial infarction. Infarcted tissue will have an increased uptake of the isotope. Various bony structures will also take up the isotope. Studies done within 1 to 8 days of infarction are frequently positive. The size of a myocardial infarction can also be estimated.

The clinical usefulness of this type of imaging for the diagnosis of myocardial infarction remains limited. Cardiac amyloidosis may be suspected if there is diffuse uptake of the isotope by both the right and left ventricles.

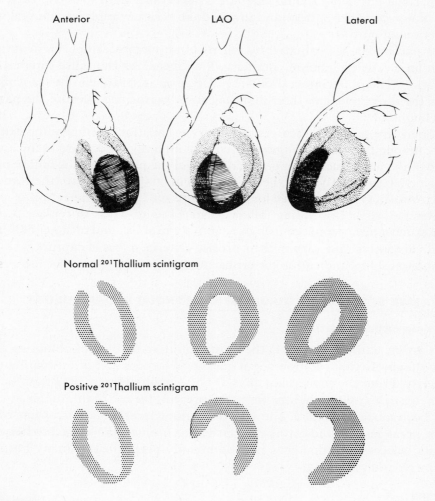

Fig. 4-16
Change in configuration of thallium 201 scintigrams with rotation of the heart. Top row: location of left ventricular myocardium (dotted area) in anterior, LAO, and left lateral projections. Linear shading denotes area of anterior wall infarction. Middle row: normal thallium 201 images. Bottom row: anterior wall defects in thallium 201 images caused by anterior myocardial infarction. (From Parkey, R.W., and others: J. Nucl. Med. **17:**771, 1976.)

Pacemaker evaluation

All pacemakers rely on batteries of one type or another to generate the pulse for pacing. Battery exhaustion is the most common cause of pacemaker failure. Thus the purpose of pacemaker evaluation is to obtain the longest possible use of a pacemaker pulse generator without exposing the patient to the risk of pacemaker failure. Rather than relying on the arbitrary limit set by the manufacturer to determine how long a pacemaker will function properly, a physician should evaluate a pacemaker both to detect early failure of a pacemaker battery and to avoid unnecessary replacement of a well-functioning unit.

A pacemaker is evaluated by means of an electrocardiograph equipped with an electrical interval counter, which measures the pulse interval and duration. The pulse interval or the pulse generator rate can be transmitted over the telephone, and thus analysis can be performed without the patient leaving home.

There are several indicators of battery exhaustion or impending exhaustion. Among these are changes in the pulse interval, a decrease in the amplitude of the pulse, a change in the duration of the pulse, and the failure of the sensing circuit. Analysis of these variables in conjunction with the standard electrocardiogram to detect loss of capture will permit detection of pacemaker failure or impending failure. Criteria as to when to replace a pacemaker have been proposed using the above variables, and although different medical centers may vary in their precise criteria, a loss of capture is considered an absolute indication for replacement.

INVASIVE SPECIALIZED DIAGNOSTIC METHODS IN CARDIOLOGY

Cardiac catheterization

Cardiac catheterization is the most definitive method of obtaining accurate diagnostic information about cardiac disorders and of evaluating their severity. From the pioneering days of Forssmann, who in 1929 positioned a catheter in his own right atrium, to the present, the use of this diagnostic test has been much expanded. The selective catheterization of all cardiac chambers, great vessels, and coronary arteries has been accomplished so frequently and successfully that it is now commonly performed in many hospitals with remarkable safety.

Method

Cardiac catheterization and angiography are performed by specially trained personnel (usually cardiologists and radiologists in cooperation) in a cardiac catheterization laboratory, where, besides the special equipment for diagnostic uses, complete resuscitative equipment is available.

In its simplest form the procedure includes introduction of a cardiac catheter into the right side of the heart through an arm vein (basilic or cephalic vein) or a leg vein (the femoral vein). The catheter is advanced through the vena cava, the right atrium, the right ventricle, and the pulmonary artery. Then for a brief period it is advanced further, to the distal pulmonary artery wedge position. On the left side of the heart the catheter is introduced through an artery, either the brachial artery or the femoral artery. It is advanced through the arterial system to the ascending aorta, through the aortic valve into the left ventricle, and if necessary to the left atrium.

The cutdown technique can be used for both of these routes. In this method, the veins are usually tied at the end of the procedure while the arteries are repaired. Cardiac catheterization also can be performed percutaneously, a method in which the vessels are not isolated and all catheters are introduced over guide wires and needles.

In the various chambers, pressures are recorded, and blood is sampled and analyzed for its oxygen content, ordinarily during rest as well as exercise. This information, coupled with measurement of the patient's rate of oxygen consumption, which is obtained by collecting gases expired by the patient, reveals (1) the patient's cardiac output (the amount of blood pumped per minute), (2) the presence and size of a right-to-left or left-to-right shunt within the cardiac chambers, and (3) the presence and severity of stenosis (narrowing of various valves). The information also makes possible the calculation of the resistance of the various vascular beds. Additional information is obtained using the indicator dilution test, angiography, and selective arteriography.

Indicator dilution test. An indicator is a substance that can be harmlessly introduced into the cardiovascular system and detected with appropriate sensing apparatus. The substance commonly used for determining cardiac output is indocyanine green, which is introduced on the venous side and sampled by means of a densitometer (an instrument that is sensitive to optical changes of the blood). Curves that are thus obtained are used to calculate cardiac output, blood flow, and the size of shunts.

A slight modification of this principle involves the use of hydrogen gas that is introduced into the patient's system by inhalation. The gas is diffused into the circulation at the level of the pulmonary capillaries. Left-to-right shunts at various levels within the heart chambers can be detected by specially designed platinum-tipped electrode catheters positioned at specific sites.

Specialized catheters with thermistor (temperature-sensing) tips can be used to detect changes in temperature in various chambers after the injection of fluid at temperatures lower than the temperature of the body. This information can be used to calculate cardiac output (thermodilution techniques).

Angiography. Angiography is a modification of the basic catheterization technique. The catheter tip is positioned in a specific area of the cardiovascular system, and a contrast substance is injected to permit opacification of the area. Concomitant x-ray filming provides a permanent graphic record. Injection of contrast material into the right atrium is useful in detection of pericardial effusion and also for visualization of the tricuspid valve. Injection into the right or left ventricle gives information about the size and contraction of the respective chambers, as well as information about the tricuspid and mitral valves. Injection into the pulmonary artery makes the pulmonary arterial system visible and is the most definitive way of diagnosing a pulmonary embolus.

Selective coronary arteriography. Selective injection into the coronary arteries is performed in selective coronary arteriography. This technique was introduced in 1962 and has since served as the cornerstone for the evaluation of coronary artery disease. It has also made possible the development of surgical revascularization procedures. For selective coronary arteriography, various catheters are positioned at the coronary ostia, where contrast material is injected, and cinematographic films are taken. In selected cases in which coronary artery spasm is suspected and obstructive coronary artery disease is absent or minimal, provocative tests with intravenous ergonovine maleate are sometimes used to induce coronary artery spasm. Such spasm is promptly reversed by sublingual, intravenous, or intracoronary administration of nitroglycerine or nifedipine.

Results of vein bypass grafting are evaluated by injection of dye into the graft that is interposed between the aorta and the coronary arteries.

Transluminal coronary angioplasty. This is a therapeutic extension of the technique of selective coronary arteriography. In certain cases specifically designed balloon catheters can be introduced through a coronary catheter and positioned across the stenotic segment of a coronary artery. By means of controlled inflation of the balloon, such stenotic segments can be dilated.

Transluminal coronary recanalization. Another therapeutic extension of catheter techniques has been the introduction of fibrinolytic agents into a coronary artery that has become thrombotic, resulting in acute myocardial infarction. Clots can be lysed and occluded vessels can be recanalized. The role of such methods of treatment of coronary artery disease and myocardial infarction is under intensive evaluation.

Intracardiac electrophysiologic studies. Intracardiac electrophysiologic studies can be added to standard cardiac catheterization with the use of specially designed catheters that have recording and stimulating electrodes at their tips. When these catheters are introduced into the right and left atria and ventricles, supraventricular and ventricular arrhythmias can be induced and analyzed. The functional properties of the SA and AV nodes and accessory pathways can be evaluated. The actions of various types of pacemakers, as well as the effects of various drugs on arrhythmias, can be assessed. Clinical intracardiac electrophysiologic studies have recently gained in popularity because of their potential for identifying patients who are prone to ventricular fibrillation, as well as for permitting a rational choice of antiarrhythmic therapy.

Indications

The indications for cardiac catheterization are many but well defined. The procedure, because of its cost and inherent hazards, should not be performed before careful consideration is given to the indications and to alternative ways of obtaining the desired information.

The most common indication is clinically diagnosed congenital or acquired heart disease requiring surgical therapy. In most patients noninvasive diagnostic methods are adequate in making an exact diagnosis and also in deciding on the advisability of surgery. But preoperative cardiac catheterization should almost always be performed anyway, to confirm the diagnosis and to evaluate cardiac function. Occasionally, cardiac catheterization will reveal an unsuspected cardiac lesion or will be helpful in determining the type of surgical procedure required.

Cardiac catheterization is indicated for patients with heart disease of unknown etiology in which an exact diagnosis would improve or change the mode of therapy.

Evaluation of operative results, another indication, applies to both congenital heart disease and acquired heart disease in adults. The following could be evaluated: the status of prosthetic valves and of shunt procedures, the results of corrective procedures for congenital heart disease, and the adequacy and patency of grafts for coronary artery disease.

Presently, the largest number of catheterizations and angiograms are being performed on patients with coronary artery disease—first to diagnose the presence of coronary heart disease and then to select patients for surgical revascularization.

The indications for selective coronary arteriography are continuously being redefined, but at present the commonly accepted indication is the presence of symptomatic coronary artery disease, with angina pectoris, that has not responded well to medical therapy. Some advocates of this catheterization technique believe that all patients with suspected coronary artery disease should undergo coronary arteriography.

An uncommon indication for cardiac catheterization is the need to evaluate cardiac status for a reason that is primarily nonmedical. Such evaluations might be done in athletes with poorly defined murmurs who need permission for unrestricted activity or in airline pilots who have vague chest pains or mild electrocardiographic abnormalities and who need complete clearance to continue flight status.

Contraindications

There is no absolute contraindication to cardiac catheterization and angiography. Severe, uncontrolled congestive heart failure, severe arrhythmias, and a history of allergy to the dye are relative contraindications. If a study is essential in a person who is allergic to the dye, the study can be carried out if appropriate premedication is given and precautions are taken (see Appendix E, p. 394).

Limitations

These techniques are invasive and therefore pose some discomfort as well as small but definite risks to a patient's life or well-being. In addition, the tests are costly to perform, both in personnel and equipment; a team of highly trained, technically capable people is needed. Another limitation or disadvantage of the test is that the contrast medium itself can cause changes in the cardiovascular system.

Pitfalls

Individual discussion of the pitfalls in cardiac catheterization is beyond the scope of this book. To avoid serious errors, if a diagnosis from a cardiac catheterization laboratory is at variance with the clinical diagnosis, the catheterization diagnosis should not automatically be accepted. The catheterization data, as well as the clinical data, should be critically reviewed.

Risks

Catheterization of the right side of the heart has essentially no mortality and a morbidity of less than 1%, which is limited to arrhythmias or minor bleeding. Catheterization of the left side of the heart, combined with cardiac angiography, is somewhat more hazardous; it carries the risk of myocardial infarction, cerebrovascular accident, arterial bleeding, and arterial thrombosis with possible loss of limb.

The risk of death varies among catheterization laboratories and among procedures. The procedure with the highest risk of death is selective coronary arteriography. In this procedure the risk of mortality varies from less than 0.1% to 1% or even higher, depending on the patient population studied and the experience of the catheterization team.

It is mandatory that there be written, informed consent in the patient's record prior to any type of cardiac catheterization.

Patient preparation and care

The patient remains fasting prior to cardiac catheterization, since the contrast media may cause nausea and vomiting. Sedation is given, although some physicians avoid any medications because of the possible effect on hemodynamics. After the procedure vital signs are monitored and bed rest is maintained for 12 to 24 hours. (In low-risk patients the study can be done on an outpatient basis, with the observation continued at home.)

An arterial puncture site should be checked for bleeding, and pulses distal to the site should be checked frequently. Vascular insufficiency secondary to embolization is manifested by sudden pain and by cold, white, blotchy skin. Immediate intervention is required.

A venous puncture site should be checked for warmth, pain, swelling, and redness, since thrombophlebitis may be a complication.

For preparation of patients known to be allergic to contrast material, see Appendix E.

Diagnostic pericardiocentesis

When pericardial effusion is present in large quantities or has accumulated rapidly in smaller quantities, life-threatening complications can result: tachycardia, hypotension, and shock with elevated venous pressure (a combination characteristic of cardiac tamponade). In such a situation, therapeutic pericardiocentesis is performed to remove fluid and relieve pressure on the heart. In some situations in which pericardial fluid is present without causing cardiac tamponade, diagnostic pericardiocentesis is performed to remove a small sample of the fluid for laboratory examination. This procedure is usually performed with the patient in a semisitting position. A pericardiocentesis needle is introduced via the subxiphoid approach into the pericardial space, under continuous electrocardiographic monitoring. The V lead of the ECG is connected to the needle, and the ECG is monitored to prevent puncture of the heart. S-T segment elevation indicates needle contact with the epicardium and necessitates withdrawal of the needle. The fluid removed is studied for chemical content (protein, sugar, LDH), malignant cells, or infection (bacterial, fungal, tubercular, or viral), or for other purposes as indicated. Catheters can be introduced in the pericardial space for continuous drainage and introduction of medications.

When echocardiography is being used in the evaluation of pericardial effusion, no air should be introduced, but if x-ray films are to be used for follow-up study, a volume of air equal to the volume of fluid removed may be introduced to better define the pericardial space. Monitoring right atrial pressures before and after pericardiocentesis yields hemodynamic information that is useful in the diagnosis of cardiac tamponade or coexistent pericardial constriction.

Clinical value

Diagnostic pericardiocentesis is useful in the detection of infective pericarditis and hemopericardium. This test is also helpful in diagnosing tumors or immunologic disorders such as systemic lupus erythematosus (SLE) or rheumatoid arthritis.

Indications

The main indications for diagnostic pericardiocentesis are infective pericarditis and suspected carcinomatous infiltration of the pericardium.

Contraindications

An absolute contraindication is an uncooperative, uncontrollable patient, since this situation would markedly increase the risk of laceration of the heart. A bleeding disorder or anticoagulant therapy should also be considered a contraindication to elective diagnostic pericardiocentesis. Puncture of a cardiac chamber under such circumstances may precipitate uncontrollable bleeding in the pericardial sac with cardiac tamponade.

Limitations

Pericardiocentesis may be ineffective if pericardial effusion is loculated or if it is mainly posterior without free-flowing anterior effusion. Surgical exploration may be necessary in such a situation.

Pitfalls

Among the many pitfalls encountered in the performance of this test is the danger of puncturing and entering the right atrial chamber by directing the needle too far toward the right shoulder. In this situation elevation of the S-T segment may not be seen, but there may be elevation of the P-R interval, a clue that the right atrial chamber has been entered. Aspirated blood that clots normally and that has the patient's usual hematocrit indicates that a cardiac chamber has been entered. Air should not be injected until the operator is absolutely certain that the needle is in the pericardial space and not in the cardiac chamber.

Risks

The risks of this procedure include arrhythmias (atrial or ventricular), puncture of a cardiac chamber (usually the right atrium or the right ventricle), coronary arterial puncture, pneumothorax (puncture of the lung), and possible introduction of infection. With careful attention to technique and with experience, the risk of complications is minimal. Informed consent is necessary before the procedure.

Cardiac biopsy

The cardiac biopsy is probably the most invasive diagnostic test in cardiac disorders, other than open surgical exploration for diagnostic purposes. Generally, two approaches are used. Transthoracic needle biopsy of the left ventricular myocardium is the older method and is generally considered to have a higher risk of complications. Percutaneous transvenous endomyocardial biopsy is a newer and safer technique. In this procedure forceps are introduced through a vein, usually the internal jugular or the femoral, and through the right atrium into the right ventricle. The biopsy specimen is obtained from the right ventricular apex or the septum. A similar technique for biopsy of the left ventricular endomyocardium has also been developed.

Indications

Endomyocardial biopsy is indicated in the diagnosis of rejection of a transplanted heart, active inflammatory carditis, or diffuse infiltrative disorders of the heart (amyloidosis or tumors of the heart). It is the most specific method of evaluating the effect of cardiotoxic drugs (such as Adriamycin). Other conditions in which a biopsy has been useful are primary myocardial disease (cardiomyopathies), hypertrophic obstructive cardiomyopathy (idiopathic hypertrophic subaortic stenosis), hypothyroidism, some of the storage diseases (glycogen storage disease), hemochromatosis, and others.

Contraindications

Bleeding disorders, anticoagulation therapy, and an uncooperative patient are among the contraindications for this procedure.

Limitations

The disease process must be diffuse to be diagnosed by the biopsy, since the sampling is very small. The transvenous endomyocardial biopsy, the more common method used, samples the right ventricle and the right ventricular septum, but does not sample the left ventricle. The risk of the procedure, although very low in initial reports, may increase as the procedure is popularized and performed in more medical centers.

Risks

Complications of endomyocardial biopsy include right-sided pneumothorax immediately after the procedure, usually a self-limiting, inconsequential problem; arrhythmias (isolated ventricular contractions, premature contractions, atrial fibrillation, flutter, or supraventricular tachycardia); and, in rare cases, evidence of right ventricular puncture that presents as intrapericardial bleeding with cardiac tamponade.

Consent is obtained, as in cardiac catheterization.

FIVE Diagnostic tests for vascular disorders

Major advances have been made during the past 5 years in the noninvasive diagnosis of peripheral vascular disease. These advances have been possible through the use of improved graphic techniques, sonography, and nuclear studies. Many patients in whom peripheral vascular disease is suspected, or who are at high risk for such disease, can now be safely screened with these studies. In addition, these tests are suitable for repeat studies to help evaluate the results of surgical treatment and to follow the progression of disease. Invasive angiographic studies can thus be reserved for patients who need surgical intervention or for situations in which noninvasive studies have yielded equivocal data.

ANATOMY AND PHYSIOLOGY

The circulation is a closed, continuous loop; the blood that is pumped by the heart must flow through each subdivision of the circuit. If blood is displaced from one segment, another segment must expand to accommodate it. Fig. 5-1 shows the principal arteries and veins.

Hemodynamics is the study of the dynamics of blood circulation. It is concerned with the physical characteristics of blood and with pressure, resistance, and flow.

Blood is composed of plasma and cells, of which more than 99% are red cells. The *hematocrit* of blood is the volume percentage of blood that consists of red cells; the hematocrit determines the viscosity of blood. Plasma is similar to interstitial fluid, except that plasma contains more protein.

Blood pressure is the force exerted by the blood against any unit area of a vessel wall. It is usually measured in millimeters of mercury. When the heart contracts and ejects blood into the aorta, the proximal part of the aorta distends because of the pressure. A pressure wave is transmitted down the aorta, picking up speed as it reaches the less compliant vessels and finally arriving in the peripheral arteries. The pressure that exists during this rise in pressure in the arterial system after cardiac systole is called systolic pressure; the minimum pressure, which occurs late in diastole, is called diastolic pressure. The difference between the two is known as pulse pressure.

The rate of flow of blood through a vessel is determined by the pressure difference between the two ends of the vessel and by vascular resistance to the flow. Blood flows from the area of high pressure to the area of low pressure.

Vessels are distensible, veins more so than arteries. Veins are called the storage areas of the circulatory system, because with a given rise in pressure, 6 to 10 times more blood fills a vein than an artery of the same size. The term *compliance* refers to the ability of a vessel to increase its volume in response to a given increase in pressure. The compliance of the venous system is about 24 times greater than that of the arteries.

Resistance to blood flow is measured indirectly; it is expressed in *peripheral resistance units*. In the arteries there is little resistance to blood flow, but in the arterioles and the capillaries the resistance is considerable. In order for blood to be pumped into these small vessels, the arterial pressure must be high. The arterioles, which have strong muscular walls, are able either to close off completely or to dilate severalfold and thus to control the amount of blood going into the capillaries, which have very thin, permeable walls to permit the exchange of fluids and nutrients between the blood and the interstitial spaces. The venules gradually turn into veins, which transport the blood back to the heart.

Blood flow is the amount of blood (in milliliters or liters) passing a given point in the circulatory system each minute. *Cardiac output* represents the amount of blood pumped by the left ventricle into the aorta each minute. *Venous return* is the amount of blood flowing from the veins into the right atrium each minute.

The amount of blood that can pass through a vessel in a given time at a given pressure difference changes dramatically with slight changes in vessel diameter and resistance. Complex neural and humoral controls exist. Blood flow slows as arterial pressure falls. If arterial pressure falls to a certain point, blood flow ceases entirely. At this point (critical closing pressure) the arterioles close completely.

The blood returns very efficiently from the lower extremities, against gravity. There are valves in the veins that permit the blood to flow only toward the heart, and every time the legs are moved, muscles contract and squeeze the veins, providing a "muscle pump" to help propel venous blood back to the heart. When this muscle pump is not operating (as when a person is standing at absolute attention), venous pressure in the lower leg increases, fluid leaks into the tissue, and blood volume diminishes.

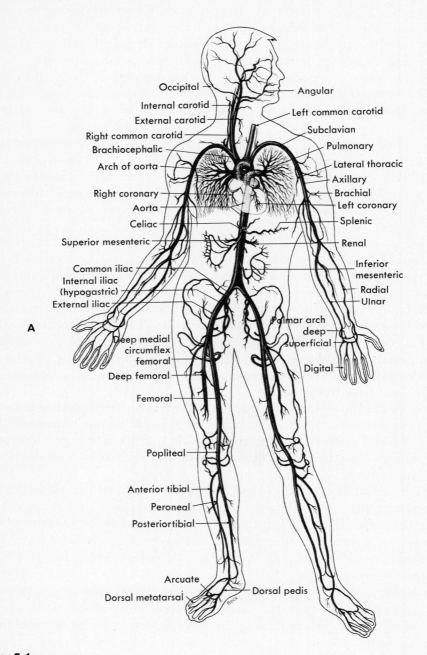

Fig. 5-1
A, The arterial system. **B,** The venous system. (From Anthony, C.P,. and Kolthoff, N.J.: Textbook of anatomy and physiology, ed. 9, St. Louis, 1975, The C.V. Mosby Co.)

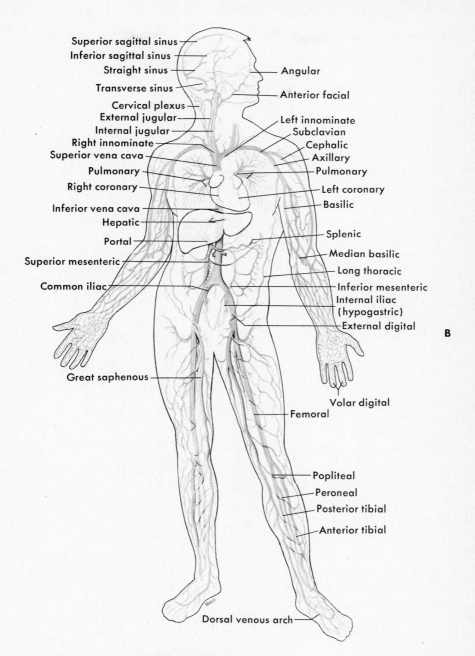

Superior sagittal sinus
Inferior sagittal sinus
Straight sinus
Transverse sinus
Cervical plexus
External jugular
Internal jugular
Right innominate
Superior vena cava
Pulmonary
Right coronary
Inferior vena cava
Hepatic
Portal
Superior mesenteric
Common iliac

Great saphenous

Angular
Anterior facial
Left innominate
Subclavian
Cephalic
Axillary
Pulmonary
Left coronary
Basilic
Splenic
Median basilic
Long thoracic
Inferior mesenteric
Internal iliac
(hypogastric)
External digital

Volar digital
Femoral

Popliteal
Peroneal
Posterior tibial
Anterior tibial

Dorsal venous arch

B

Fig. 5-1, cont'd
For legend see opposite page.

NONINVASIVE DIAGNOSTIC STUDIES

Carotid phonangiography (CPA)

Carotid phonangiography, also called carotid audiofrequency analysis, is an extension of the technique of auscultation. The concepts and techniques are similar to those of phonocardiography (p. 107). Special microphones are positioned over areas of bruits—usually the carotid arteries. The sound picked up is displayed on an oscilloscope and photographed. The sound frequency pattern is analyzed with the help of computers. In general, the longer the duration of the bruit, the greater the degree of stenosis. If the bruit extends into diastole, it usually signifies severe stenosis. The presence or absence of heart sounds and the frequency of the sounds recorded also provide diagnostic clues.

Clinical value

This test is helpful in documenting the presence and location of carotid bruits and in estimating the degree of stenosis. Also, transmitted cardiac murmurs can be differentiated from cardiac bruits.

Limitations

Meticulous attention to technique is necessary. In very severe degrees of narrowing (>90% closure—that is, subtotal or total occlusion of a vessel), no bruit may be recorded. Thus CPA is not reliable in the diagnosis of severe carotid stenosis. It remains a screening method and an adjunct to other noninvasive tests.

Oculoplethysmography (OPG) and oculopneumoplethysmography (OPPG)

In OPG, fluid-filled contact lenses or cups are applied to the eyes following a local anesthetic. Cyclic changes in the volume of this fluid are recorded; these changes reflect pulsatile flow in the ophthalmic artery—the first branch of the internal carotid artery (Fig. 5-2). Narrowing of an internal carotid artery will cause a delay in the pulse wave and changes in the blood volume. The pulse wave in the ipsilateral ear lobe—which reflects external carotid artery pulses—is used for reference. Twenty milliseconds or more of delay in the pulse wave in the ophthalmic artery (which reflects internal carotid pulse) is considered abnormal, signifying stenosis of that vessel.

In OPPG, air-filled transducers are applied to the lateral aspects of the sclerae; negative pressure of up to 300 mm Hg is then applied in an attempt to obliterate the ophthalmic artery pressure form and thereby estimate the systolic pressure in the ophthalmic artery. This method is felt to be more accurate than OPG.

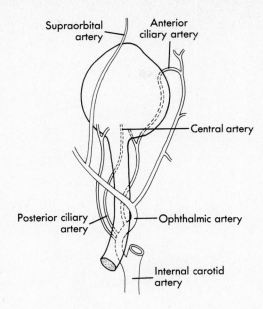

Fig. 5-2
Ophthalmic artery and its branches.

Clinical value

OPG and OPPG provide additional graphic methods of screening for internal carotid artery stenosis or occlusion. When information obtained from these tests is combined with the information obtained from CPA, the risk of a false-positive or false-negative result is as low as 5%.

Limitations

Mild to moderate narrowing of carotid arteries—or bilateral narrowing, if the narrowing is of approximately the same magnitude on each side—can be missed with OPG. OPPG, being more sensitive, may be able to detect these conditions.

Precautions

OPG and OPPG are contraindicated in patients with conjunctivitis, uncontrolled glaucoma, history of retinal detachment, recent eye surgery (within 2 months), or allergy to topical anesthetics.

Occasional side effects may include subconjunctival edema or ecchymosis, for which no special treatment is needed.

Impedance plethysmography

In impedance plethysmography a pneumatic cuff is applied to a limb for the purpose of occluding the venous return. As the blood volume in the

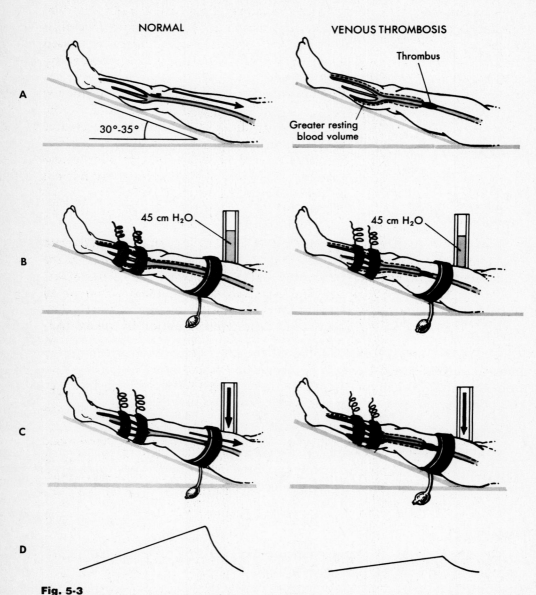

Fig. 5-3

Impedance plethysmography. **A,** The resting blood volume is greater in the leg with venous thrombosis than in the normal leg. **B,** Two electrodes are applied, to deliver a weak electrical current, and the cuff is inflated to 45 cm H_2O to occlude venous return. In the leg with venous thrombosis, there is a smaller increase in blood volume and less resistance to the current. Thus the tracing (**D**) does not rise as high as for the normal leg. **C,** When the cuff is deflated, the decrease in electrical resistance, recorded in **D,** is smaller in the leg with venous thrombosis than in the normal leg.

limb increases, so does the electrical resistance; by measuring the electrical resistance, a physician can obtain information about blood flow. Two electrodes are applied to the limb, and a very weak electrical current is passed through it. The resistance of the limb to this current is then recorded on ECG graph paper.

In patients with venous thrombosis the resting blood volume in the leg is greater than normal. Therefore, when venous return is occluded by the cuff, the increase in blood volume and the increase in electrical resistance are smaller than normal; and after the cuff is deflated, the decrease in blood volume and the decrease in electrical resistance are smaller than normal.

Fig. 5-3 illustrates this procedure and compares the results from a normal leg with those from a leg with venous thrombosis.

Clinical value

Impedance plethysmography is helpful in the diagnosis of deep-vein thrombosis and other types of obstruction to venous flow. The cause of the obstruction (thrombus, pregnancy, tumor) should be clinically determined.

Impedance plethysmography is indicated when clinical suspicion of deep-vein thrombosis exists, but needs confirmation. In approximately 20% of cases, the test is nondiagnostic and definitive evaluation by venography is necessary.

Ultrasound arteriography

Two types of ultrasound instruments can be used to demonstrate the anatomy of the arteries—the pulsed Doppler imaging instrument and the B-mode scanner.

The pulsed Doppler imaging instrument uses echoes of the moving blood column to produce images of the outline of a vessel wall. It takes 10 to 20 minutes to construct these images, which are static. The B-mode scanner provides instant images of a vessel wall in real time, with a resolution of 0.5 to 1 mm.

Clinical value

The two instruments provide different information and tend to be complementary. (In addition, technology now exists that combines the two methods [duplex systems]). This type of imaging is applied most frequently to the carotid bifurcation and the internal carotid artery, although it is also used to study arteries that lead to the lower extremities. Thus, ultrasound arteriography is very useful in the noninvasive evaluation of patients who have had strokes, transient ischemic attacks, asymptomatic bruits, or claudication. High-grade narrowing of an internal carotid artery can be reliably diagnosed; the test is essentially diagnostic for total occlusion.

The future of ultrasonic imaging of vessels is very bright. The combined utilization of real-time, B-mode imaging and pulsed Doppler techniques permits visualization of plaque and analysis of the flow disturbance it creates. Improved signal processing methods and the use of computerized pattern recognition systems should make such studies even more reliable than they are now.

Fig. 5-4 shows the evidence of internal carotid artery obstruction provided by bruit recording, contrast arteriography, and ultrasonic arteriography. Fig. 5-5 shows how a duplex scanner visualizes and analyzes blood flow at a carotid bifurcation.

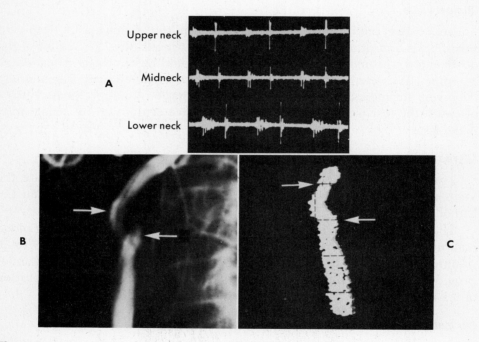

Fig. 5-4
Noninvasive studies of an occluded internal carotid artery yielded varying amounts of information, but in combination were as conclusive as contrast arteriography. **A,** Microphone recordings along the neck revealed a bruit only in the lower neck. **B,** Contrast arteriogram showed total occlusion of proximal interval carotid artery (right arrow) and a patent external carotid artery (left arrow). **C,** Ultrasonic arteriogram gave corresponding image (arrows mark same arteries). (From Strandness, D.E.: Noninvasive evaluation of carotid artery disease, J. Cardiovasc. Med., September 1980, p. 841.)

Limitations

Great precision and experience with ultrasound methods are required if the results are to be of diagnostic value. Also, calcification of the wall of an artery will interfere with ultrasound imaging, by simulating defects or "blanks" in the lumen where none may exist.

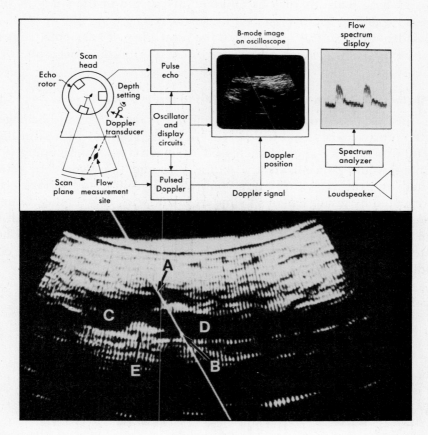

Fig. 5-5
Top, Electronic-component diagram showing an ultrasonic duplex scanner processing pulse echo information to provide a real-time B-mode image of the carotid bifurcation. In addition, pulsed Doppler signals are used to measure flow velocity at specific sites, providing both an audible output via a loudspeaker and a display of the analyzed flow spectrum. *Bottom,* In this enlarged B-mode image, the diagonal line *(A)* indicates the path of the Doppler beam along which flow at point *B* is being analyzed. In the imaged view of the bifurcation, a plaque *(E)* is seen at the mid-portion of the bulb, between the common carotid *(C)* and the internal carotid *(D)* arteries. (From Strandness, D.E.: Noninvasive evaluation of carotid artery disease, J. Cardiovasc. Med., September 1980, p. 841.)

INVASIVE DIAGNOSTIC STUDIES

Radionuclide phlebography (venography)

This test is used in the diagnosis of deep-vein thrombosis. Technetium 99m–labeled albumin is injected into a vein, and its flow is photographed with a scintillation camera, which provides images of the vein. After injection, the albumin will be trapped in the pulmonary capillaries, and thus a perfusion lung scan can also be obtained at the end of the study. A simultaneous leg and lung scan is therefore feasible.

Disadvantages of this test include the possibility of false-positive results because of valve incompetence. Tagged human albumin microspheres can be used to try to improve the yield.

^{125}I-Fibrinogen uptake test (FUT) or fibrinogen leg scanning

In this test, 100 microcuries of iodine 125–tagged human fibrinogen is injected intravenously, and the patient's legs are scanned with scintillation detectors to identify sites of increased radioactivity. A developing (fresh) thrombus would concentrate the iodine 125, and thus would be reliably detected by external scintillation counting. Thyroid gland uptake should be prevented by giving Lugol's iodine 24 hours prior to scanning. Counting is done with a portable rate meter at previously marked sites on both legs, 1 to 2 hours after the injection. The counting may be repeated in 24 hours or later. A persistent 20% increase in count rate compared with the corresponding position is considered indicative of a fresh thrombus.

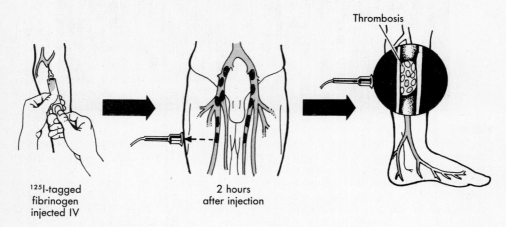

^{125}I-tagged
fibrinogen
injected IV

2 hours
after injection

Thrombosis

Fig. 5-6
Procedure for diagnosis of venous thrombosis by leg scanning.

Fig. 5-6 shows the procedure for the diagnosis of venous thrombosis by leg scanning.

Since iodine 125 is prepared from blood donors, its use carries a *small* risk of transmitting hepatitis. In addition, the test exposes a patient to radiation, although in small amounts.

Limitations of FUT include built-in delays in the performance of the test, the possibility of false-positive results in the presence of inflammation and hematoma, and the inability of the test to evaluate the high femoral and iliac veins. Also, if heparin has been used 24 to 48 hours prior to the test, the results are unreliable.

Contrast venography (phlebography)

A contrast medium is injected into a superficial vein of the foot or ankle, and sequential radiologic visualization of the veins is done by means of rapid serial radiography. The technique may also be applied to a vein in an upper extremity.

Clinical value

Contrast venography is the *definitive* way of diagnosing venous thrombosis; it is done when noninvasive studies yield equivocal results.

Limitations

Careful attention to technique is necessary to prevent extravasation, insufficient injection of contrast medium may give false-positive results, and the test can be painful. Informed consent is required.

Contrast arteriography

Contrast arteriography remains the "gold standard" in vascular diagnostic imaging. The techniques are similar to those of cardiac catheterization and angiography (p. 116); they may be applied to any vessel. Most studies are done by percutaneous techniques, but a vessel cutdown technique may be used. As in the case of coronary studies, special catheters can be used to penetrate and dilate narrowed vessels (transluminal angioplasty).

Small risks are present in *all* arteriographic studies. These include the complications relating to bleeding, thrombosis, or embolism. The potential for loss of limb or even life, although very remote, exists. Informed consent is necessary.

Digital fluoroscopy

Digital fluoroscopy, a very promising new imaging technique, permits adequate visualization of the pulmonary and systemic arteries after the *intravenous* injection of contrast material. This technique, when fully developed, will probably be the most useful imaging method for screening patients who have carotid or cerebrovascular disease, pulmonary embolic disease, or abnormalities of the renal or peripheral arteries.

The morbidity related to the procedure is very low and is limited to that associated with venous puncture and reaction to contrast media.

SIX Diagnostic tests for bronchopulmonary disease

ANATOMY AND PHYSIOLOGY

The lung is an organ of gas exchange. The exchange of gases occurs between air and blood at the level of the alveoli, where pulmonary capillary vessels are in contact with blood (Fig. 6-1). The interaction of the respiratory muscles with the chest wall and the mechanical properties of the lung provide the driving force for air flow, permitting gas exchange.

Respiratory muscles

The diaphragm, the external intercostals, and the parasternal intercartilaginous muscles are the chief muscles of respiration, with the diaphragm accounting for more than two thirds of the air entering the lung during quiet breathing. When the inspiratory muscles contract, the chest expands, pleural pressure, which is always subatmospheric, becomes more so, alveolar pressure changes from atmospheric to subatmospheric, and the lungs fill with air. Inspiration ends when alveolar pressure reaches atmospheric level. The muscles that overcame the elastic recoil of the lung during inspiration now relax; the resulting recoil of the lung causes the alveolar pressure to exceed atmospheric pressure, and air flows out of the lung. Thus expiration during quiet breathing occurs passively, with expiratory muscles coming into play only during heavy breathing, talking, singing, coughing, or defecation, or when the movement of air out of the lungs is impeded. The primary muscles of expiration are the internal intercostal muscles, the external and internal oblique abdominal muscles, and the transversus and rectus abdominis muscles, the contraction of which depresses the ribs. At the end of expiration, when the respiratory muscles are at rest, the elastic recoil of the lungs is balanced by the elastic recoil of the chest. These opposing forces produce the subatmospheric pleural pressure of approximately 5 cm H_2O.

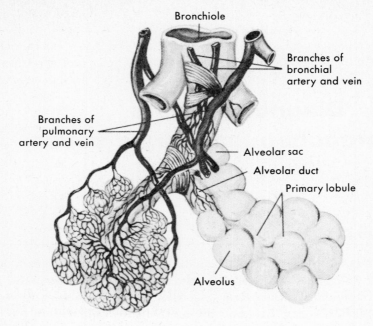

Fig. 6-1
The capillary network surrounding the alveoli. (From Schottelius, B.A., and Schottelius, D.D.: Textbook of physiology, ed. 17, St. Louis, 1973, The C.V. Mosby Co.)

The pulmonary volumes and capacities are described under "Pulmonary function tests," on pp. 151 to 155.

Partial pressure

Atmospheric air is composed of oxygen, nitrogen, carbon dioxide, and water vapor, each of which exerts a pressure proportional to its concentration. The sum of the pressures of all of the gases in the atmosphere—that is, the partial pressures—equals atmospheric pressure (760 mm Hg at sea level). Dry atmospheric air is warmed and humidified before it reaches the alveoli. Since the water vapor pressure of a saturated gas varies with temperature, this pressure at body temperature is subtracted from the barometric pressure to obtain the pressure of dry inspired tracheal air (713 mm Hg). The partial pressures of the gases in inspired tracheal air are as follows: oxygen (PI_{O_2}), 150 mm Hg; carbon dioxide (PI_{CO_2}), less than 1 mm Hg; nitrogen (PI_{N_2}), 563 mm Hg.

The partial pressure of a gas in a solution is proportional to the amount of gas that is physically dissolved (as opposed to the total concentration); the partial pressure determines the chemical reactions and the physiologic properties of the gas. For example, the concentration of physically dissolved oxygen (PaO_2) affects the rate of diffusion of O_2 into and out of capillaries and red cells, and it is one of the factors that determines how much O_2 combines with hemoglobin and the rate at which the combining occurs. The partial pressure of carbon dioxide in blood plays a major role in the regulation of alveolar ventilation. The total concentrations of O_2 and CO_2 are the amounts of these gases available for reactions.

Ventilation

Ventilation is the process in which oxygen is replenished in the alveolar gas and carbon dioxide is eliminated from that gas. The pulmonary capillary blood in turn removes the oxygen from and adds carbon dioxide to the alveolar gas. Oxygen and carbon dioxide are carried to and from from the lungs and the tissue cells by the bloodstream, oxygen being transported principally in combination with hemoglobin. Once released in the tissue capillaries, oxygen enters the tissue cells and metabolites are oxidized to obtain energy for life processes. Carbon dioxide is produced as a waste by-product of metabolism. Carbon dioxide is transported back to the lungs in combination with water, hemoglobin, and plasma protein, and as free CO_2.

Transport of oxygen and carbon dioxide in the blood
Hemoglobin

Hemoglobin is a protein found in red blood cells. Each hemoglobin molecule can carry four molecules of oxygen by means of a chemical combination that is reversible. The more hemoglobin in the blood, the more oxygen that can be carried at a given PaO_2. Oxygen physically dissolved in the plasma is in equilibrium with the oxygen physically dissolved in the intracellular fluid of red blood cells. Thus the PaO_2 of plasma equals the PaO_2 of RBC intracellular fluid, and the amount of oxygen combined with hemoglobin is directly proportional to the PaO_2 of RBC intracellular fluid.

Transport of oxygen in the blood

Only a small percentage of O_2 is carried in the blood as dissolved O_2. About 98% of all O_2 carried to tissues is transported in a reversible chemical combination with hemoglobin. The PaO_2 determines the amount of O_2 transported in each form. The O_2 bound to hemoglobin does not contribute to the PaO_2. From the capillaries oxygen diffuses down its PaO_2 gradient into the interstitial fluid and the cells. As the PaO_2 decreases, oxygen dissociates from hemoglobin to become oxygen dissolved in intracellular fluid; this oxygen diffuses more easily when the PaO_2 is low. Thus the degree of oxygen dissociation from hemoglobin is a direct function of the PaO_2. When the PaO_2 is high, as in the pulmonary capillaries, oxygen-hemoglobin binding takes place; when the PaO_2 is low, as in the tissue capillaries, oxygen is released from the hemoglobin. It should be remembered that even if both the PaO_2 and the hemoglobin concentration are normal, tissues may be hypoxic if the cardiac output is low and delivery of oxygenated blood to the tissues is inadequate.

Transport of carbon dioxide in the blood

Carbon dioxide can be transported by the blood in far greater quantities than can oxygen. Carbon dioxide is carried in three forms: physically dissolved (10%), chemically combined with amino groups on the hemoglobin molecule (25 to 30%), and converted to bicarbonate (60%).

The carbon dioxide in the blood is hydrated to form carbonic acid in red blood cells. The carbonic acid dissociates to bicarbonate (HCO_3^-) and hydrogen (H^+). Most of the HCO_3^- is produced in the red blood cells, because of the enzyme carbonic anhydrase, which is not found in the plasma. As the bicarbonate concentration increases in the intracellular fluid of red cells, it diffuses into the plasma in exchange for chloride (the chloride shift). Thus the bicarbonate is synthesized within the red cells but transported in the plasma. The hydrogen ion is retained in the red cells and is buffered by hemoglobin.

PATHOPHYSIOLOGY

Arterial hypoxia is present when the arterial PO_2 is less than expected (see Table 6-1). Major causes include (1) alveolar hypoventilation, (2) ventilation-perfusion ($\dot{V}A/\dot{Q}c$) imbalance, (3) right-to-left shunting, either intrapulmonary or intracardiac, and (4) reduced PI_{O_2} (high altitude).

Alveolar hypoventilation

Alveolar hypoventilation exists when alveolar ventilation is not sufficient for the metabolic activity of the body; this condition is reflected in increased arterial carbon dioxide tension ($PaCO_2$) (Fig. 6-2, A). If the $PaCO_2$ is normal or low, the cause of hypoxia is not hypoventilation. The adequacy of alveolar gas exchange is best evaluated by a determination of both alveolar and arterial gas tensions.

Ventilation-perfusion ($\dot{V}A/\dot{Q}c$) imbalance

The normal ratio of alveolar ventilation ($\dot{V}A$) to pulmonary arterial blood flow ($\dot{Q}c$) is approximately 0.8 when a person is in the upright position. The ratio varies from the top of the lung to the bottom of the lung, and it is affected by body position (see Table 6-1). Normally the differences in

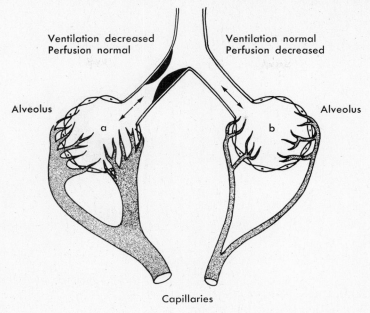

Ventilation decreased
Perfusion normal

Ventilation normal
Perfusion decreased

Alveolus

Alveolus

a

b

Capillaries

Fig. 6-2
The two possible mechanisms of altered ventilation/perfusion ratio. a, Normal or increased perfusion of poorly ventilated alveoli. b, Decreased perfusion of normally ventilated alveoli.

ventilation-perfusion relationships throughout the lung are relatively small. However, in disease, more extreme variations occur because of abnormalities in airway resistance, lung compliance, and blood vessel caliber. A diminished $\dot{V}A/\dot{Q}c$ ratio (less than 0.8) allows venous blood to flow past poorly ventilated alveoli, and arterial hypoxia results (Fig. 6-2). Ventilation-perfusion mismatch is common in asthma, chronic bronchitis, and emphysema, and it explains the hypoxia observed in these conditions.

Right-to-left shunting

Right-to-left shunting exists when venous blood, not having been exposed to oxygen, reaches the systemic circulation. This happens physiologically to about 2% to 6% of the cardiac output because of the veins (thebesian, bronchial, and pleural) that empty into the left ventricle, making the normal PaO_2 about 90 mm Hg when the $PaCO_2$ is normal. Pathologic right-to-left shunts (Fig. 6-3) are the result of alveolar filling processes, alveolar collapse (severe pneumonias, pulmonary edema) or complete obstruction of an airway.

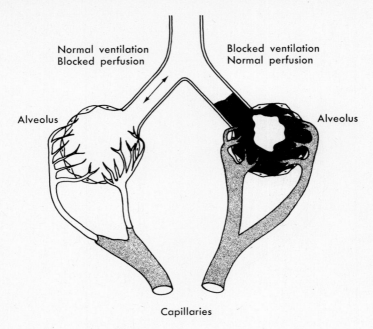

Normal ventilation
Blocked perfusion

Blocked ventilation
Normal perfusion

Alveolus

Alveolus

Capillaries

Fig. 6-3
Arteriovenous shunt (right-to-left shunt).

LABORATORY TESTS FOR BRONCHOPULMONARY DISEASE

Radiographic evaluation of lung disease

Radiographic evaluation of the lungs is a valuable extension of the physical examination. It permits visualization of the air-filled lungs and their vascular markings, easy recognition of tumors or infiltrates, and prompt diagnosis of pleural fluid, hemothorax, or pneumothorax. Enlargement of cardiac chambers and cardiac vessels can also be detected.

Routine chest radiography

The basic examination consists of two views of the chest—posterolateral and left lateral—and causes minimal radiation exposure (10 to 20 milliroentgens at the skin level).

Supplementary views can also be taken as needed:

The *"overpenetration" technique* permits better visualization of bronchi and regional cardiac structures.

Oblique views (15° or 45°) permit visualization of lung periphery without interference from breast or pectoral shadows.

Lateral decubitus views permit the detection of small amounts of pleural fluid or a small pneumothorax.

Expiratory films help detect a small pneumothorax or may demonstrate air trapping.

Apical lordotic views are sometimes used to visualize abnormalities that are superimposed on the head of the clavicle or on the first rib.

Portable chest radiographic equipment generally produces radiographs of inferior quality; thus its use should be limited to patients who cannot be safely transferred to a radiology department.

For further details of routine radiographic examination of the chest relating to the cardiovascular system, see pp. 84-89.

Tomography (laminography)

In tomography, which is an extension of the technique of plain chest radiography, a series of x-ray films is exposed, with each film visualizing a "slice of the lung" at a different depth. Radiographic shadows outside of the selected plane are blurred.

Clinical value. This radiographic technique is valuable in identifying features not seen on a routine chest radiograph, including hilar masses, calcium or a cavity in a lesion, and tracheobronchial abnormalities. Emphysema is also better evaluated with tomography.

Limitations. Tomography exposes a patient to increased radiation and cost; thus it should be used selectively.

Fluoroscopy

Fluoroscopy augments routine radiography by permitting visualization of the lungs and diaphragm during respiratory motion. Diaphragmatic function is better assessed, pleural lesions are better evaluated. Subtle nodular or parenchymal calcifications can be diagnosed even when they are not evident on plain radiographic films.

Bronchography

Bronchography is used for examining the tracheobronchial tree. A radio-opaque material is instilled into the tracheobronchial tree through a catheter introduced through the mouth, nose, or cricothyroid membrane. Regions of interest may be filled with the radio-opaque material selectively. Multiple views are obtained, including oblique views.

Clinical value. Bronchography is valuable in the diagnosis of bronchiectasis. It is generally reserved for patients who have uncontrolled and repeated infection and/or hemoptysis and in whom surgery (resection of a bronchopulmonary segment) is being considered. The usefulness of bronchography is limited, because many of the conditions for which it was done in the past (hemoptysis, carcinoma, and other abnormalities) are better evaluated with fiberoptic bronchoscopy (p. 159).

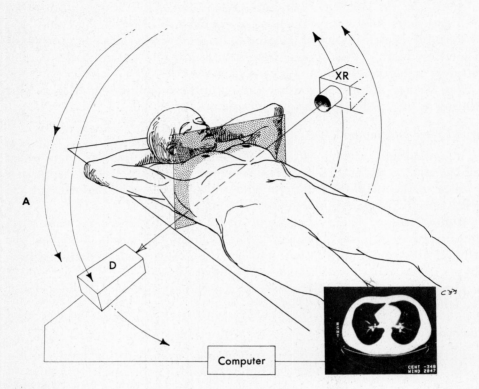

Fig. 6-4
A, Diagrammatic representation of computerized tomography of the thorax. The image of the cathode-ray tube as projected in the lower right-hand corner is shown as though the patient were being viewed from below. This is the conventional method of viewing CT scans. *XR,* X-ray. *D,* Detectors. **B** and **C,** Normal 2-second CT view of the thorax. **B,** Scan is taken at the hilar level. The pulmonary vascular markings are shown throughout the lung fields (white arrows). The descending branch of the right pulmonary artery *(RPA)* lies slightly lateral but predominantly anterior to the intermediate bronchus, which contains air (large white arrow). The esophagus (black arrow) and azygos vein (black arrowhead) are evident. The descending branch of the left pulmonary artery *(LP)* is posterior to the lower lobe bronchus at this level. *DA,* Descending aorta. **C,** By adjusting the contrast, an examiner can look within the mediastinum at the same level as the CT scan in **B** and check for normal intrapericardial structures. The course of the right pulmonary artery can be followed to the main pulmonary artery *(MPA).* The superior vena cava *(s)* is anterior to the right pulmonary artery and behind the proximal portion of the ascending aorta *(AA).* These structures are seen because of the contrast between lower-density mediastinal fat and blood-containing vessels. (From Porgatch, R.D., and Fahling, L.J.: Computed tomography of the thorax: a status report, Chest **80:**618, 1981.)

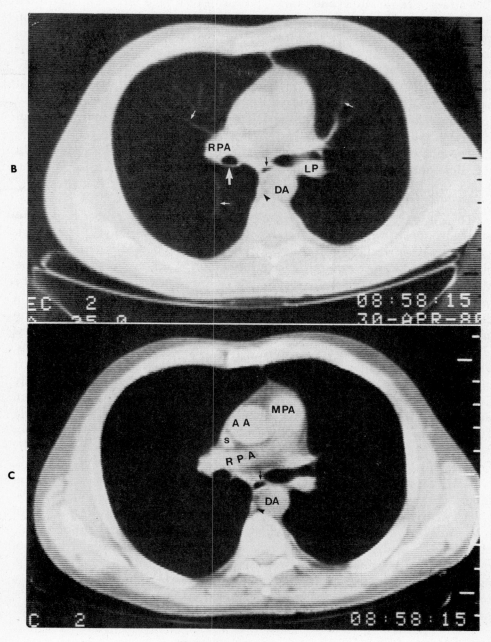

Fig. 6-4, cont'd
For legend see opposite page.

Patient preparation and care. Postural drainage may be instituted several days before the procedure if secretions are excessive. Premedication may include atropine and codeine to decrease secretions and help control cough. Light sedation is helpful, and adequate local anesthesia of the upper airways and tracheobronchial tree is essential. The patient should take nothing by mouth for 6 to 8 hours before the procedure and until cough and gag reflexes have returned after the procedure. Incentive spirometry and coughing should be encouraged, and temperature should be monitored. Informed consent is required.

Complications. Complications include allergic reaction, atelectasis, chemical and bacterial pneumonias, and bronchospasm.

Computerized tomography (CT scan)

The CT body scanner has been cited by experts as the most important breakthrough in radiology "since Roentgen discovered x-rays." It is sensitive to very fine variances in tissue density and thus provides detailed views of tissue and bone not possible through conventional x-ray techniques. Computerized tomography is accomplished quickly, with virtually no risk to the patient. The patient is placed inside the scanner, and an x-ray tube with a diametrically opposed x-ray detector (located in a fixed position on a rotating gantry) completely encircles the body or skull at a desired cross-sectional level (Fig. 6-4, A). The tube emits a tiny stream of radiation pulses as it turns. These are collected by the detector and processed by a computer, which reconstructs the image and projects it onto a screen. The image is highly detailed, since each point within the cross-sectional field is viewed from hundreds of different angles, and the density of each point can be precisely determined, permitting the imaging of mediastinal structures that cannot be visualized with conventional x-ray procedures, including tomography (Fig. 6-4, B and C).

Clinical value. In the radiographic evaluation of lung disease, CT scanning is valuable in detecting small peripheral nodules, evaluating coin lesions (solid versus cystic versus calcified), and distinguishing the chest wall from areas of pleural or parenchymal disease. Loculated and subpulmonic effusion and mediastinal and hilar masses can also be well seen. When contrast material is used, vascular structures can also be identified and a diagnosis of aortic dissection or aneurysm can be made. Future improvements in technology may permit diagnostic evaluation of cardiac chambers, masses, and infarction, as well as inspection of aortocoronary grafts.

Radioisotope techniques

Radioisotopes are used in the evaluation of pulmonary blood flow (pulmonary perfusion scan) and air distribution and flow (ventilation scan).

Pulmonary perfusion scanning (Q scan)

A pulmonary perfusion scan is obtained by injecting macroaggregates of albumin labeled with technetium or radioactive iodine into a peripheral vein. The macroaggregates are trapped in the pulmonary capillaries, blocking 0.1% of the pulmonary capillary bed and providing an indirect measure of blood flow to the lungs. In 8 hours the albumin microspheres disintegrate and clear from the circulation. Radiation exposure is limited to 1 to 2 millicuries. The Anger scintillation camera is used in obtaining images. Computers can process the data and quantitate the perfusion.

Clinical value and limitations. The Q scan is used primarily in the diagnosis of pulmonary embolism. However, since other lung disorders can also compromise pulmonary blood flow, the test is nonspecific. An abnormal result is *rarely* in itself diagnostic of pulmonary embolism; such a result must be interpreted in the context of the clinical problem, the chest x-ray film, and the ventilation scan (see following). In the correct clinical setting, with normal chest x-ray film and no abnormalities shown by ventilation scanning, a perfusion defect would indicate pulmonary embolism with a high degree of accuracy. In the presence of pulmonary infiltrates and a ventilation scan that shows abnormalities, a perfusion defect has little diagnostic value and cannot be used for the diagnosis of pulmonary embolism. When a pulmonary perfusion scan is normal, clinically significant pulmonary embolism is essentially excluded.

If, during pulmonary perfusion scanning, other organs are visualized—for example, the kidneys or spleen—one would then search for a pulmonary arteriovenous fistula, which has allowed the passage of the macroaggregates to the arterial side.

Pulmonary ventilation scanning (V scan)

In a ventilation scan, the patient inhales a mixture of air, oxygen, and radioactive gas, usually xenon (^{133}Xe or ^{127}Xe). An initial breath is taken to total lung capacity, and a scan is done (a single-breath scan). Next, the patient breathes tidally while the distribution of the radioactive gas is recorded (wash-in phase). After equilibrium has been achieved, the patient resumes breathing room air (wash-out phase).

Clinical value. The pulmonary ventilation scan is used in conjunction with the pulmonary perfusion scan. If a perfusion defect is the result of pulmonary embolism, the ventilation scan will be normal. On the other hand, if a perfusion defect is caused by airway obstruction and decreased ventilation (obstructive lung disease, pneumonia, atelectasis), the ventilation scan will reveal this situation. Thus the combined use of ventilation and perfusion scanning produces greater diagnostic accuracy than either technique used alone.

Pulmonary angiography

A catheter is introduced into the pulmonary artery from a peripheral vein, by means of a percutaneous technique or a vein cutdown. Pressures are recorded in the right atrium, the right ventricle, and the pulmonary artery, and blood samples are obtained for analysis of gases. Contrast material is injected while radiographic films are exposed in rapid sequence. Various projections may be used. Selective injection into a branch of the pulmonary artery may be done, permitting detailed visualization of the pulmonary artery and veins.

Clinical value

Pulmonary angiography permits visualization of the pulmonary vasculature; it is the most specific method of diagnosing pulmonary embolism. Pulmonary vascular malformations and pulmonary venous disorders can also be diagnosed by angiography. The hemodynamic measurements obtained during the procedure can aid in the diagnosis of pulmonary hypertension and cor pulmonale.

Selective pulmonary angiography is performed in situations in which clinical, radiologic, and isotope studies have failed to produce a specific diagnosis, or when surgical procedures (inferior vena cava interruption or embolectomy) are being considered. The patient is prepared as he would be for any cardiac catheterization procedure (p. 119). It is necessary that informed consent be obtained.

Sputum examination

A sputum examination is most helpful in the diagnosis of pneumonias and suspected malignancies. In infections of the lung, proper smearing and staining of the sputum, followed by appropriate culture techniques, are needed for a specific diagnosis of the type of infection. This stipulation applies to the various bacterial pneumonias, as well as to tuberculosis and fungal infections.

Clinical value

Cytologic evaluation of the sputum is a relatively simple method of detecting malignant disease of the lung. It is futile to perform this test on saliva. It is necessary to obtain a proper sputum specimen and to process it promptly.

Various sputum production techniques may be used by an inhalation therapist to promote a deep and productive cough. In rare instances one may resort to transtracheal aspiration to obtain a satisfactory sputum specimen.

Table 6-1

Predicted Pao_2 at various ages and body positions

Age	Seated	Supine
15	100	97
20	99	95
25	97	93
30	96	91
35	95	89
40	93	87
45	92	85
50	91	83
55	89	80
60	88	78
65	87	76
70	85	74
75	84	72
80	83	70
85	81	68

Blood gases and acid-base homeostasis
Arterial blood gases

Analysis of arterial blood gas (ABG) values has become one of the most useful tests in pulmonary medicine, providing the single best assessment of the adequacy of pulmonary gas exchange and the presence and severity of acid-base disturbances. The proper interpretation of blood gas data requires knowledge of the clinical state of the patient, and types of therapy being applied, hemoglobin content, cardiac output, and other clinical information.

Arterial oxygen tension (Pao_2)

Predicted Pao_2 at various ages and body positions. Arterial oxygen tension is that concentration of dissolved oxygen at which its partial pressure is in equilibrium with the blood. In a person who is breathing air at sea level, the Pao_2 is usually 80 to 100 mm Hg. The Pao_2 decreases with age, and it is dependent on body position, although less than 70 mm Hg is abnormal at any age or in any position (see Table 6-1).

Oxyhemoglobin dissociation curve. Oxygen is transported bound to hemoglobin, each gram of which, when fully saturated, can carry 1.34 ml of oxygen. The amount of oxygen dissolved in plasma is very small and is generally disregarded in clinical evaluation. The oxyhemoglobin dissociation curve (Fig. 6-5) represents the relationship between the Pao_2 and the amount of hemoglobin bound with oxygen. Note the progressive increase in the per-

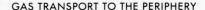

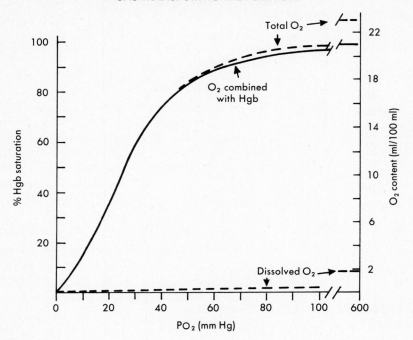

Fig. 6-5
Oxyhemoglobin dissociation curve. The solid line is the oxygen dissociation curve at pH 7.4, $Paco_2$ 40 mm Hg, and 37° C. The total blood oxygen content is also shown for a hemoglobin concentration of 15 gm/dl of blood.

centage of hemoglobin that is bound with oxygen (percent saturation of the hemoglobin) as the PaO_2 increases.

In general, hemoglobin saturation is at least 90% as long as the PaO_2 is greater than 60 mm Hg. As arterial oxygen tension drops below 60 mm Hg, oxygen saturation falls steeply, with the drops in saturation being relatively larger than the changes in oxygen tension. Temperature changes and the acid-base state will also affect the degree of the oxygen saturation of hemoglobin for a given PaO_2. The amount of oxygen that is actually delivered to the cellular (tissue) level depends on the oxygen saturation of the hemoglobin *as well as* on the hemoglobin concentration and the cardiac output. Thus in cases of severe anemia or markedly decreased cardiac output, even if the PaO_2 and the oxygen saturation of the hemoglobin are normal, delivery of oxygen to the tissue level may be inadequate.

Carboxyhemoglobin. Carboxyhemoglobin is formed when hemoglobin is exposed to carbon monoxide, as in cigarette smoking. This CO-bound hemoglobin is unable to carry oxygen. Also, the remaining hemoglobin binds oxygen more tightly and gives off less oxygen to tissue cells. Hence, even though carbon monoxide may be bound only to a certain percentage of hemoglobin, the overall consequences are more serious than the same degree of anemia. Therefore, PaO_2 should be interpreted in the context of (1) the hemoglobin concentration and whether there is abnormal hemoglobin present, such as carboxyhemoglobin or methemoglobin, (2) the status of cardiac output, and (3) other factors that affect oxygen-hemoglobin binding (temperature, pH, and drugs).

Partial pressure of carbon dioxide ($Paco_2$). The partial pressure of carbon dioxide in arterial blood reflects the balance between CO_2 production (metabolic) and CO_2 excretion through ventilation. Thus alveolar hypoventilation would cause an elevated $Paco_2$ (hypercapnia), while hyperventilation would cause a decreased $Paco_2$ (hypocapnia). The normal range for $Paco_2$ is 35 to 44 mm Hg. An arbitrary classification of the severity of changes in $Paco_2$ is as follows:

	Mild	Moderate	Severe
Hypocapnia	30-35	20-29	<20
Hypercapnia	45-55	55-65	>65

Hypocapnia and hypercapnia reflect underlying hyperventilation or hypoventilation, respectively, which may be primary or compensatory to a metabolic or other condition. In the absence of other metabolic forces (acids or alkalies) hypoventilation would lead to respiratory acidosis, while hyperventilation would cause respiratory alkalosis.

As a working rule, the sum of PaO_2 and $Paco_2$ should be less than 140 mm Hg, if a person is breathing air at sea level. A sum greater than 140 mm Hg indicates a laboratory error or the fact that a person is receiving supplemental oxygen (PI_{O_2} is greater than 21%).

Blood pH. Since the pH is the negative logarithm of the hydrogen ion (H^+) concentration, it is an expression of the degree of acidity or alkalinity. Normal values for arterial blood range from 7.37 to 7.43.

Acidemia. A low pH indicates acidemia. The source of excess acid can be respiratory, metabolic, or both. In *respiratory acidemia* an increased $Paco_2$ (hypoventilation) causes an increase in the amount of carbonic acid. In *metabolic acidemia* accumulation of various metabolic acids causes the increase in H^+ concentration.

Alkalemia. A high pH reflects alkalemia. In *respiratory alkalemia* (hyperventilation) too much carbon dioxide is lost, resulting in a decrease in the amount of carbonic acid. In *metabolic alkalemia* excessive amounts of various body acids are lost (for example, hydrochloric acid as a result of vomiting or gastric suction).

Metabolic acidosis and alkalosis. The kidneys are also intimately involved in acid-base balance; they daily excrete 50 to 100 mEq of hydrogen ions, which are formed as a result of carbohydrate and protein metabolism.

In *metabolic alkalosis* the kidneys respond by excreting bicarbonate. Respiratory compensation consists of hypoventilation, with an increase in $PaCO_2$ and the amount of carbonic acid.

In *metabolic acidosis* the kidneys reabsorb bicarbonate ions and secrete hydrogen ions. This renal process occurs gradually over several days, while the respiratory compensation of increased ventilation and hypocapnia occurs within minutes.

The term *base excess* refers to an excess of bicarbonate as well as other bases in the blood. An elevation in the bicarbonate level indicates metabolic alkalosis, while a decrease in the bicarbonate level indicates metabolic acidosis.

It is now apparent that a complete assessment of acid-base balance should include determinations of $PaCO_2$, pH, and bicarbonate concentration, as well as the levels of the other serum electrolytes (see pp. 8-18). Diagnostic possibilities include pure metabolic or respiratory acidosis, or a combination of the two, and pure respiratory or metabolic alkalosis, or a combination of the two. Respiratory and metabolic compensatory mechanisms are frequently involved, and acid-base disturbances in clinical circumstances frequently are of a mixed variety.

Specimen removal and handling. Proper sample removal and handling are important in arterial blood gas analysis. A 20-gauge or smaller needle should be used, to minimize trauma to the artery. Radial or brachial arteries are frequently used, although the femoral artery can also be used. The syringe should be precoated with a small amount of heparin. Firm pressure should be applied for 2 to 3 minutes after the puncture. If the patient is receiving anticoagulants or fibrinolytic agents, arterial puncture is relatively contraindicated and great caution should be used. Indwelling catheters may be used if multiple samples are needed. Peripheral venous sampling should be avoided. All bubbles should be expelled, exposure to air should be avoided, and samples should be "iced." Measurements should be corrected for the patient's temperature and reported in conjunction with the FI_{O_2} (fraction of inspired oxygen).

Venous blood gases

Central venous blood gas levels may also be determined for cardiopulmonary evaluation. The best "venous" sample is one obtained from the pulmonary artery, where there is complete mixing of blood; hence the term *mixed venous* sample. The oxygen saturation (and therefore the content) in pulmonary artery blood is an excellent indicator of the adequacy of oxygen delivery to the tissues.

Estimation of cardiac output. The difference between arterial oxygen content and mixed venous oxygen content (arteriovenous oxygen difference) is inversely related to the cardiac output (see Appendix C, Tables C-2 to C-4). Thus cardiac output can be estimated by concurrent measurements of arterial and mixed venous oxygen content, with an estimated value being used for oxygen consumption.

Normal blood gas values

	Arterial blood	Mixed venous blood
pH	7.40 (7.37-7.43)	7.36 (7.32-7.40)
Pao_2	80-100 mm Hg	35-40 mm Hg
O_2 saturation	95%	70%-75%
$Paco_2$	35-44 mm Hg	42-50 mm Hg
HCO_3	22-26 mEq/L	23-27 mEq/L
Base excess	−2 to +2	−2 to +2

Pulmonary function tests

Pulmonary function tests are useful in documenting the presence, type, and degree of functional impairment in various disease states. Also, when performed serially, these tests help to evaluate the response to therapy or the progression of disease.

The main types of pulmonary function tests include (1) spirometry, (2) flow-volume loop analysis, (3) determination of diffusing capacity, (4) determination of maximal inspiratory pressure, and (5) pulmonary testing during various interventions. Arterial blood gases have been discussed on p. 147. For pulmonary evaluation during sleep, see p. 335.

Spirometry

Spirometry involves the use of an instrument—a spirometer—to measure lung volumes, capacities, and flow rates. The flow of air (usually during the expiratory phase) is measured as volume per unit time. The volume of air within the lung is estimated by measuring the total volume of nitrogen a person exhales while breathing 100% oxygen or, alternatively, by having a person breathe a known quantity of helium and then measuring its concentration after equilibrium has been achieved. The commonly obtained lung volumes and capacities as seen on a spirogram are shown in Fig. 6-6. They include total lung capacity, vital capacity, residual volume, inspiratory capacity, and tidal volume. Table 6-2 lists some normal spirometric values.

Lung volumes. There are four lung volumes. Three are measured by the spirometer: tidal volume, inspiratory reserve volume, and expiratory reserve volume. The fourth, residual volume, is ascertained by subtracting expiratory reserve volume from functional reserve capacity. The sum of the four volumes is the maximum volume to which the lungs can be expanded. All

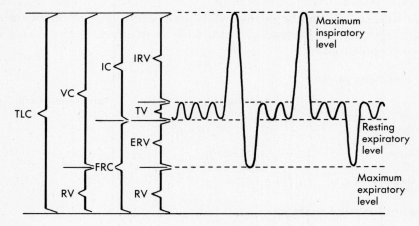

Fig. 6-6

Spirogram. *RV*, Residual volume. *FRC*, Functional residual capacity. *TV*, Tidal volume. *IRV*, Inspiratory reserve volume. *IC*, Inspiratory capacity. *ERV*, Expiratory reserve volume.

Table 6-2

Normal spirometric values

Test	Age 20-39	40-59	60+
VC (liters)			
Men	3.35-5.90	2.72-5.30	2.42-4.70
Women	2.45-4.38	2.09-4.02	1.91-3.66
FEV_1 (liters)			
Men	3.11-4.64	2.45-3.98	2.09-3.32
Women	2.16-3.65	1.60-3.09	1.30-2.53
FEV% (FEV_1/VC%)			
Men	77	70	60
Women	82	77	74
RV (liters)			
Men	1.13-2.32	1.45-2.62	1.77-2.77
Women	1.00-2.00	1.16-2.20	1.32-2.40
TLC (liters)			
Men	4.80-7.92	4.50-7.62	4.35-7.32
Women	3.61-6.18	3.41-6.02	3.31-5.86

figures for lung volumes and capacities given in this chapter are those of a normal young male adult; the figures for a female adult are about 20% to 25% lower.

Tidal volume (TV) is the volume of air inspired and expired with each normal breath (about 500 ml).

Inspiratory reserve volume (IRV) is the volume of air that can be inspired in addition to the normal tidal volume (approximately 3000 ml).

Expiratory reserve volume (ERV) is the amount of air that can still be expired, by forceful expiration, after the end of normal tidal expiration (about 1100 ml).

Residual volume (RV) is the volume of air that remains in the lung after a forced maximal expiration (about 1200 ml). This volume provides oxygen for the blood between breaths and prevents the concentrations of oxygen and carbon dioxide in the blood from rising and falling markedly with each breath.

Lung capacities. A lung capacity comprises two or more lung volumes.

Inspiratory capacity (IC) is the *tidal volume* plus the *inspiratory reserve volume* (about 3500 ml). This is the amount of air that can be inspired during a maximal inspiratory effort that starts at the normal resting expiratory level.

Functional residual capacity (FRC) is the *expiratory reserve volume* plus the *residual volume.* This is the amount of air remaining in the lungs at the end of normal expiration (about 2300 ml).

Vital capacity (VC) is the *inspiratory reserve volume* plus the *tidal volume* plus the *expiratory reserve volume.* This is the maximum amount of air that can be expelled from the lungs after maximal inspiration. The major factors affecting the measurement of vital capacity are the patient's position during the test, the strength of the muscles of respiration, and pulmonary compliance (distensibility of lungs and chest cage).

Total lung capacity (TLC) is the volume to which the lungs can be expanded with the greatest inspiratory effort (about 5800 ml).

Flow rates. Simple spirometry can usually differentiate obstructive from restrictive pulmonary disorders simply on the basis of lung volume measurements combined with expiratory flow rates. Fig. 6-7 compares a normal spirogram with those of obstructive and restrictive lung disease.

In obstructive pulmonary disorders (chronic bronchitis, emphysema, and asthma), the resistance to air flow increases and flow rates decrease. As obstruction to air flow increases, hyperinflation occurs and both residual volume and, to a lesser extent, total lung capacity increase. With the increase in residual volume, vital capacity decreases. In restrictive pulmonary disorders (pulmonary fibrosis) the lungs shrink and flow rates decrease in proportion to the decrease in lung size.

Forced expiratory volume during the first second of expiration after full inspiration (FEV₁) is the most reproducible flow rate and one of the most useful measurements of airway obstruction. It is used often in monitoring response to therapy. FEV_1 decreases linearly with time, both in normal persons and in persons with chronic obstructive lung disease (more rapidly in the latter). Thus the decline in FEV_1 with time is a very useful prognostic factor.

Maximal mid-expiratory flow (MMEF) is a more sensitive indicator of expired air flow than is FEV_1; it is obtained from the midportion of the spirogram.

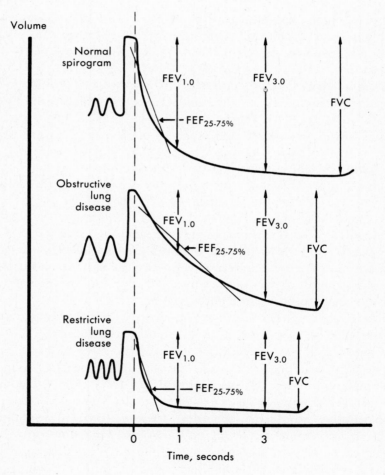

Fig. 6-7
Simple spirometry usually allows differentiation between obstructive and restrictive patterns. Note that in both, the forced vital capacity (FVC) is reduced; however, flows are reduced in obstruction and normal or "supernormal" in restriction. (From Slonim, N.B., and Hamilton, L.H.: Respiratory physiology, ed. 4, St. Louis, 1981, The C.V. Mosby Co.)

Maximal breathing capacity or *maximal voluntary ventilation (MVV)* is another useful index of overall lung mechanics. The patient breathes as deeply and as rapidly as possible for 15 seconds. The volume of exhaled air is multiplied by 4.

Flow-volume loop analysis

More and more laboratories are being equipped for recording inspiratory and expiratory flow rates and plotting these data against lung volumes to produce flow-volume loops, or curves (Fig. 6-8).

Clinical value. These flow-volume curves may be more useful than conventional spirograms in the following ways:

1. The forced expired volume in 1 second and maximum expiratory flow rates depend significantly on patient effort, while interpretation of flow volume loops is based on the shape of the down slope, an area requiring less patient effort. Hence, the diagnosis of air flow limitation may frequently be made despite poor patient cooperation.

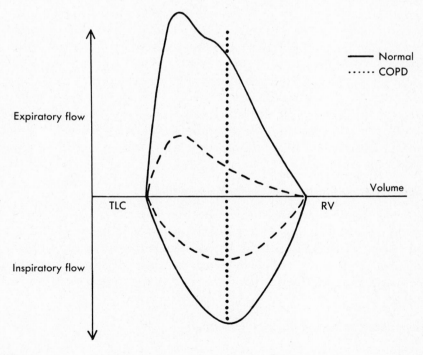

Fig. 6-8
Flow-volume loops demonstrating normal and obstructive patterns. (From Kryger, M., and others: Diagnosis of obstruction of the upper airways, Am. J. Med. **61:**86, 1976.)

2. With the possible exception of an intricate analysis of the terminal portion of the spirometric curve, a spirogram is unable to detect early stages of airway obstruction. Such mild air-flow limitation, which is believed to be caused by obstruction of small or peripheral airways, results in a reduction in flow rates at lower lung volumes. Recognition of such a situation is of great potential importance, since bronchitis and emphysema can be treated more effectively if they are diagnosed early.

3. Flow-volume loops present characteristic patterns during upper-airway obstruction. Occasionally patients are seen with obstruction at the main bronchi and carina or above. Unless flow-volume loops are analyzed, such patients may be confused with those suffering from the usual obstructive disorders, such as asthma and bronchitis.

Determination of diffusing capacity

The diffusing capacity of the lungs (DL_{CO}) is usually estimated by having a patient inhale a single breath of a carbon monoxide mixture.

Clinical value. The combination of an abnormal flow-volume loop and a reduced diffusing capacity is of value in facilitating the early diagnosis of emphysema, before x-ray and spirometric abnormalities or even symptoms appear. In the presence of normal lung mechanics, a reduced diffusing capacity in a dyspneic patient may be an important clue to pulmonary embolism, in which condition the uptake of carbon monoxide is reduced by a partially blocked pulmonary vascular bed. Finally, the diffusing capacity is frequently reduced in interstitial lung diseases such as sarcoidosis. Determination of the diffusing capacity therefore serves as a sensitive, noninvasive test for following the effects of therapeutic interventions or for following the progression of the disease.

Determination of maximal inspiratory pressure (MIP)

Maximal inspiratory pressure is the pressure generated on maximum inspiratory effort, starting at residual volume, against a closed system. Determination of MIP is a direct test of inspiratory muscle strength; it is most helpful in the evaluation of neuromuscular diseases. Assessment of patient motivation and performance is crucial to the proper interpretation of results.

Pulmonary function testing during interventions

Pulmonary function testing may be performed during various interventions, in an effort to obtain additional information. Some of the commonly used interventions include the following.

Use of bronchodilators. The pulmonary function tests discussed thus far are done in the resting state. If abnormal flow rates or volumes are noticed, bronchodilators may be given by inhalation and the studies repeated. A significant improvement in flow rates and volumes would indicate *reversible* bronchial obstruction—that is, bronchospasm. Such information is useful in selecting appropriate treatment.

Bronchodilators should be used with caution in patients with coronary artery disease, angina pectoris, or arrhythmias.

Bronchial provocative testing. If resting flow rates and volumes are normal and the clinical presentation suggests episodic bronchospasm, provocative tests may be done to identify the triggering agent. Bronchospasm can be induced in the pulmonary laboratory by inhalation of a suspected agent (for example, smog, cold air, atmospheric pollutants, or specific drugs or antigens). Whether the response is positive or negative is determined from spirograms produced before and after the provocative test.

Exercise pulmonary function evaluation. This test is valuable in patients who complain of effort dyspnea or fatigue or who have cardiopulmonary disease or exercise-induced bronchospasm.

During graded levels of exercise (using a bicycle or a treadmill), heart rate, blood pressure, respiratory rate and volume, and volumes of expired gases are measured, electrocardiographic data are recorded, and samples are taken for arterial blood gas determinations. The functional capacity of the oxygen transport system may be evaluated by measuring maximal oxygen consumption. During exercise, hypoxemia or hypercapnia that is not apparent from the resting data may be recognized, limitations to exercise (cardiac or pulmonary) can be assessed, the need for supplemental oxygen can be evaluated, and the degree of improvement achieved through treatment or rehabilitative efforts can be measured.

Although physiologists for years appreciated the value of exercise testing in pulmonary function evaluation, the techniques were difficult. The ear oximeter, however, has been a major breakthrough in technology, permitting reliable measurement of oxygen saturation during exercise. Breath-by-breath analysis of expired gas in real time is now possible. The use of computers and microprocessors, which permit rapid analysis of this large amount of information, has brought exercise testing to the level of clinical usefulness. Information obtained during exercise pulmonary testing is helpful in answering these two important questions: (1) What is the extent of exercise limitation? (2) what is the cause of exercise limitation—psychological factors (poor motivation, anxiety), prolonged physical inactivity (poor conditioning), or organic disease (cardiovascular, pulmonary, other)?

Pleural fluid examination and biopsy

Normally the pleural cavity is only a potential space; it has moist membranes and contains only a few millimeters of fluid, which acts as a lubricant between the visceral and parietal portions of the pleura. Pleural effusion is an abnormal accumulation of fluid within this pleural space.

Diagnostic thoracentesis

Numerous systemic and intrathoracic diseases can cause pleural effusion, a sample of which may be obtained by means of *diagnostic thoracentesis*. In this technique a small volume of fluid is removed by means of a needle that has been introduced into the pleural space at the appropriate intercostal level. The fluid is sent to a laboratory for chemical, cytologic, and bacteriologic evaluation.

Therapeutic thoracentesis

Up to 1 liter of pleural effusion may be removed to improve a patient's respiratory status. (Note that when volumes much larger than 1 liter are rapidly removed, hypotension and pulmonary edema may occur.) A complete bacteriologic evaluation of the fluid is done, including evaluations for tuberculosis and fungal diseases. A cell count and a differential count help in the diagnosis of empyema. Malignant effusions are diagnosed by means of cytologic and cell-block evaluations.

Clinical value. If acute pancreatitis is the cause of the pleural effusion, an elevated amylase level in the pleural fluid will be diagnostic. Other subdiaphragmatic inflammatory processes can also cause effusions. Meigs' syndrome, which is associated with tumors of the ovaries, may cause a pleural transudate, which disappears when the tumor is removed.

If the effusion has a milky appearance, the presence of chyle should be suspected, along with obstruction or rupture of the thoracic duct.

Pleural fluid collected in an arterial blood gas syringe and promptly analyzed in a blood gas machine provides an accurate pH measurement, which may be of diagnostic help:
1. A very low pH (<6.00) is most likely caused by a ruptured esophagus.
2. A pH of 6.00 to 7.00 is very likely a consequence of infection (empyema); this diagnosis should be carefully pursued, even in the absence of positive pleural fluid cultures. Such cultures are frequently negative, especially if the patient was given a course of antibiotics prior to hospitalization.
3. Tuberculous effusions are usually characterized by pH values of less than 7.20.
4. Malignant effusions frequently exhibit pH values of 7.40 or above.

Following thoracentesis or pleural biopsy, chest x-ray film should be obtained to check for the possibility of pneumothorax induced by the pleural tap. Informed consent is necessary.

Bronchoscopy and endobronchial biopsy

A tube with a light source and biopsy forceps is introduced into the tracheobronchial tree. Originally a rigid bronchoscope was used, which required general anesthesia and permitted only a limited view of the tracheobronchial tree. The technique has been much improved with the introduction of the *flexible fiberoptic bronchoscope (FFB)*, which has almost replaced the rigid scope. With the FFB, general anesthesia is not required; local (topical) anesthetics are used. The bronchoscope may be introduced through the mouth or the nose, or through an endotracheal tube. An endotracheal tube may be used if airway control is desirable and if multiple biopsy specimens are to be taken. A systematic inspection of the nasopharynx, the oropharynx, and the larynx is done. The trachea, the carina, and all segmental branches and orifices are inspected. Suction is applied if secretions are encountered. Abnormal masses or lesions are brushed and biopsied, and all specimens are sent for complete bacteriologic, cytologic, and histologic evaluation.

Clinical value

The FFB is valuable in the evaluation of cases involving suspected neoplasms, as well as in the evaluation of hemoptysis of unknown cause. The instrument can be used to remove tenacious secretions from the tracheobronchial tree, to improve ventilation, and to treat atelectasis. It is also valuable in the removal of small foreign bodies and can be used for lung lavage. Transbronchial biopsy by means of a bronchoscope is used in the diagnosis of diffuse pulmonary disorders.

Risk

In trained hands the procedure is very safe. Minor morbidity is seen in 1 in 1000 cases (0.1%), and mortality is as low as 1 in 10,000 (0.01%).

Complications

Complications include the side effects of the anesthetic, as well as bleeding (in patients in whom biopsies are done). Hypoxia, arrhythmias, bronchospasms, bacteremia, and postbronchoscopic pneumonias can also occur.

Patient care

Careful attention to technique and patient oxygenation is necessary during the procedure. Heart rhythm monitoring also contributes to safety.

Following a biopsy, a minor amount of hemoptysis is expected. Vital signs are monitored until they are stable. Informed consent is necessary.

Mediastinoscopy

Mediastinoscopy is an operative procedure used for the diagnosis of mediastinal disease. A 3- to 5-cm incision is made in the suprasternal notch, and blunt dissection is done, with the finger anterior to the trachea. Lymph nodes around the trachea and the right main stem bronchus are evaluated with a mediastinoscope introduced through the incision. Blunt dissection is carried out. The technique permits visualization and biopsy of paratracheal and subcarinal lymph nodes.

Clinical value

Mediastinoscopy is valuable in the diagnosis and evaluation of pulmonary malignancies. Other mediastinal diseases (sarcoidosis, lymphoma, and tuberculosis) can also be diagnosed.

Complications

Complications include hemorrhage, pneumothorax, damage to the left recurrent laryngeal nerve, and infection.

The death of a patient as a result of the procedure, which is very rare, is almost always secondary to biopsy of a major intrathoracic vessel. Informed consent is required, and patient preparation is similar to that for any operative procedure.

Lung biopsy

A lung biopsy may be a necessity for a specific diagnosis. If at all possible, closed-chest techniques are used. In diffuse involvement of the lung, a biopsy specimen obtained through a fiberoptic bronchoscope may yield satisfactory results. In focal or nodular lesions, needle-aspiration biopsy may be used.

There are infrequent instances in which *all* diagnostic attempts, including biopsy by means of a bronchoscope and needle-aspiration biopsy are unsuccessful. In such a situation, a limited thoracotomy is performed and *open-lung biopsy* is done. The tissue is sent to a laboratory for pathologic evaluation and culturing. Open-lung biopsy is an operative procedure, requiring appropriate patient preparation and informed consent.

Alpha₁-antitrypsin determination

When there is evidence of a family history of emphysema, a serum alpha₁-antitrypsin level should be obtained. Two results are significant: a severe deficiency, associated with a homozygous genotype, and an intermediate deficiency, associated with a heterozygous genotype. The heterozygous state is suspected of being a risk factor for emphysema, and the homozygous state clearly predisposes a person to the early development of emphysema, particularly a cigarette smoker.

CLINICAL APPLICATION OF LABORATORY TESTS

Chronic obstructive lung disease

Several disease entities may, during their natural histories, have a component of air-flow limitation—that is, a reduction in expiratory flow rate. The three major obstructive disorders are chronic bronchitis, emphysema, and asthma; frequently these three conditions overlap. Other, less frequently encountered obstructive processes include cystic fibrosis and diffuse bronchiectasis.

Chronic bronchitis

Chronic bronchitis is primarily related to cigarette smoking; it is clinically diagnosed on the basis of cough and sputum production in association with characteristic mucous gland changes shown by pathologic examination. Air-flow limitation is variable in this condition, and at times there may be little or no evidence of a significant reduction in flow rate.

Emphysema

Emphysema may demonstrate little spirometric change, despite relatively extensive pathologic changes; it may be diagnosable only on the basis of a reduction in flow rates at low lung volumes (flow-volume loop) combined with a reduced diffusing capacity.

Asthma

Although asthma defies absolute definition, it is characterized by air-flow limitation at some time in its course. The airway obstruction may be minimal or quite severe, transient or prolonged (lasting even for years).

Differential diagnosis

Asthma is differentiated from fixed obstructive processes, such as emphysema, in that it improves with the use of conventional bronchodilators and/or with steroid therapy and may be exacerbated by various stimuli, both specific (inhaled pollens, fungi, chemical fumes) and nonspecific (cold air, dust, cigarette smoke, exercise). In some cases of asthma, a history of intermittent dyspnea and wheezing may not be apparent from preliminary spirometric tests, although flow-volume loops may show abnormally reduced flow rates at low lung volumes, in association with normal carbon monoxide diffusing capacity.

As the degree of air-flow limitation increases, pulmonary hyperinflation occurs. Characteristically, lung-volume measurements show an increased residual volume and, to a lesser extent, an increased total lung capacity. Also, the matching between ventilated and perfused areas becomes deranged, and arterial hypoxia ensues, with a reduction in the arterial oxygen tension.

Finally, in the most severe cases, with increasing air-flow obstruction, ventilation does not keep up with carbon dioxide production; arterial carbon dioxide tensions increase (hypercapnia), and respiratory failure may be diagnosed.

Exercise testing may demonstrate significant reductions in arterial oxygen tensions, resulting in oxygen desaturation, as well as in hypercapnia, considerably before these changes are demonstrable in resting blood samples. Likewise, exercise testing documents the degree to which maximal oxygen consumption is limited; exercise testing may suggest the need for pulmonary rehabilitation.

Chest x-ray films are of little value in diagnosing any of these disorders, with the exception of the more severe degrees of emphysema and perhaps of bronchiectasis.

Full-lung tomograms are of value in demonstrating the vascular disruption attendant to the more advanced stages of emphysema.

Restrictive lung disease

Many diseases elicit a fibrosing or scarring reaction within the lungs. When this reaction is diffuse, such as in sarcoidosis or in the not uncommon idiopathic form of interstitial fibrosis, the physiologic consequences can be extensive.

Lung volumes and flow rates

In the initial stages of restrictive lung diseases, all lung volumes diminish. Flow rates, however, do not necessarily fall at first, and may in fact increase (particularly at larger lung volumes—for example, peak flow). This is because the fibrosis increases the traction on airways, tending to pull them open, thus reducing airway resistance. The fibrosis eliminates alveoli, decreasing the surface area for diffusion, and the carbon monoxide diffusing capacity falls. In the later stages of restrictive lung diseases, lung volumes fall even more dramatically, and flow rates decrease proportionately.

Blood gas levels

Characteristically, some degree of arterial hypoxia exists because of ventilation-perfusion mismatching, and arterial oxygen tension falls. In the early stages of restrictive disease, however, resting PaO_2 may be normal, but arterial blood gas tests carried out with exercise frequently demonstrate abnormally low oxygen tensions. For reasons that are not entirely clear, some patients with restrictive interstitial diseases hyperventilate, producing a primary, chronic, hypocapnea (respiratory alkalosis). In the later stages of disease, resting oxygen desaturation may be present, but hypercapnia is not usually seen except as a terminal or very late event.

X-ray studies

X-ray studies are of great importance in diagnosing restrictive lung diseases. X-ray films may be diagnostic at a time when, perhaps partially because of a low level of activity on the part of the patient, symptoms are minimal or nonexistent. On the other hand, some patients who complain of shortness of breath and coughing have normal x-ray film, and yet have unequivocal, extensive, pathologic changes as shown by biopsy. Thus relatively extensive emphysema may exist in spite of normal x-ray film, and so may relatively extensive interstitial disease. One must have a high index of suspicion and look at clinical, physiologic, and radiologic information together.

Lung biopsy

Confirmation of the diagnosis and classification of an interstitial process usually requires a lung biopsy. In sarcoidosis the diagnosis is usually readily achieved with a transbronchial lung biopsy, while in the usual form of interstitial fibrosis, open biopsy is preferred because transbronchial specimens may be too small to allow pathologic diagnosis.

Causes

The following are some of the many causes of restrictive lung disease:
1. Infections such as those caused by bacteria, fungi, and parasites, and the viruses of influenza, chickenpox, and measles
2. Neoplasm
3. Metabolic disorders (for example, uremic pneumonitis)
4. Physical agents or processes, such as blast or heat injury, oxygen toxicity, or postirradiation fibrosis
5. Hereditary infiltrative diseases, such as cystic fibrosis, familial idiopathic pulmonary fibrosis, and neurofibromatosis
6. Circulatory disorders, such as multiple pulmonary emboli, fat embolism, sickle cell anemia, foreign body vasculitis from parasites or drug addiction, pulmonary edema, and chronic passive congestion with fibrosis
7. Immunologic disorders, such as occur in hypersensitivity pneumonias, collagen diseases, and Goodpasture's syndrome

8. Occupational factors, such as mineral dusts and chemical fumes
9. Sarcoidosis
10. Histiocytosis X
11. Idiopathic pulmonary hemosiderosis
12. Pulmonary alveolar proteinosis
13. Desquamative interstitial pneumonia

Pulmonary embolism

Pulmonary embolism is commonly diagnosed under the dramatic circumstances of pulmonary infarction with pleuritic chest pain and hemoptysis, or in the setting of acute dyspnea, tachypnea, and tachycardia in a patient who has an obvious predisposition to this disorder (postoperative, obese, heart failure). Occasionally, patients who have had dyspnea for a long time—even many months—are ultimately diagnosed as having chronic multiple pulmonary emboli.

In the absence of cor pulmonale, chest x-ray film and resting electrocardiographic data are frequently normal. Pulmonary function studies result in normal spirograms or flow-volume loops and normal lung volumes. The carbon monoxide diffusing capacity, however, is reduced, and the resting PaO_2 is normal or decreased.

With exercise there are frequently characteristic changes, depending on the degree of pulmonary vascular obstruction, including decreased arterial oxygen tension, decreased maximal oxygen consumption, an unusually high pulse rate for actual oxygen consumed, and the generation of an unusually high base deficit (metabolic acidosis, presumably resulting from poor cardiac output, tissue hypoxia, and anaerobic metabolism with lactic acid production).

In the absence of obvious cardiac disease, pulmonary vascular disease must be carefully ruled out; ventilation scanning, perfusion scanning, and even catheterization of the right side of the heart, with pulmonary angiography, should be considered.

Perfusion lung scanning is helpful if used correctly. A normal scan practically excludes a clinically significant pulmonary embolus. On the other hand, an abnormal scan should not be equated with a pulmonary embolus. Numerous other disorders, all of which could be confused with the clinical picture of pulmonary embolism, can produce an abnormal or "positive" perfusion lung scan.

Ventilation lung scanning may help exclude some of these other causes.

Pulmonary angiography is the most specific diagnostic test for pulmonary embolism. It is used when the less specific tests have not yielded a clear picture, or when surgical intervention (inferior vena cava ligation, possible pulmonary embolectomy) is being considered. Pressures on the right side of the heart may be obtained during angiography to provide a hemodynamic assessment. In major vascular occlusion there is increased pulmonary artery pressure and possibly secondary tricuspid regurgitation.

Pulmonary edema

Pulmonary edema may have cardiac causes (left ventricular failure, mitral stenosis) or noncardiac causes (drug hypersensitivity, trauma and shock, sepsis, and others). It can mimic bronchial asthma or interstitial lung disease. The differential diagnosis is made by means of clinical history, cardiac examination, and response to therapy. Pulmonary function tests are generally not used.

Carcinoma of the lung

X-ray examination of the chest is the most important initial diagnostic tool in carcinoma of the lung. Frequently the patient is completely asymptomatic while the routine x-ray film reveals a nodule. After identification of the nodule, tomograms are obtained to visualize possible calcification, which helps in the diagnosis of granuloma versus carcinoma but does not necessarily rule out either.

CT scanning of the chest is used in the detection of peripheral nodules.

Bronchoscopy, with bronchoscopic biopsy and, if possible, bronchoscopic aspiration for cytologic studies, is of help, particularly in medially located lesions. Bronchial brushings are used for more distal lesions.

Scalene node biopsy is helpful when lung cancer is inaccessible by bronchoscopy. The scalene fat pad contains lymph nodes that receive lymphatic drainage from the lungs. Thus, a biopsy specimen from this area often discloses carcinoma of the lungs, granulomatous infections, or sarcoidosis.

Sputum cytology studies can be helpful, but the yield is low in peripheral lesions. The positive yield in cases of lung carcinoma ranges between 30% and 70%, depending on the eagerness and expertise of the pathologist and the adequacy of the specimen.

Needle biopsy is useful when a lesion is peripheral and nonresectable. The biopsy provides a tissue diagnosis before the institution of radiation therapy and/or chemotherapy.

Thoracentesis and *needle biopsy of the pleura* should be performed when pleural fluid is present. The pleural fluid exudate is usually bloody. Fluid cytologic studies may yield the diagnosis.

Mediastinoscopy is a very good method for visualizing the lymph nodes and obtaining a biopsy of the accessible ones.

Pulmonary function tests are frequently performed before a thoracotomy. These tests are valuable in evaluating the feasibility of pulmonary resection, either lobectomy or pneumonectomy.

SEVEN Diagnostic tests for renal disorders

ANATOMY AND PHYSIOLOGY

Each kidney contains over 1 million nephrons, which are the functioning units of the kidney. Each is capable of forming urine. Each nephron is composed of two major units, the *glomerulus*, through which the blood is filtered, and a long *tubule* where the filtered blood is modified by the processes of reabsorption and secretion and converted into urine. The nephron and its blood supply are shown in Fig. 7-2. The tubule has a blind end that begins in the cortex of the kidney (Fig. 7-1). From there its path is tortuous, bending back on itself, in a section called the *first* or *proximal convoluted tubule*. The tubule then plunges down into the medulla, where its course is smooth, and then bends back to return to the cortex. The loop thus formed is called the *loop of Henle*. Within the cortex again, the tubule twists and turns in a section known as the *second* or *distal convoluted tubule* (Fig. 7-2). It finally joins the *collecting tubule*, which ends in the pelvis of the kidney.

The glomerulus is a tuft of up to 50 capillaries that begin with an afferent arteriole and end with an efferent arteriole (Fig. 7-2). The glomerulus is invaginated into the blind upper end of the tubule. The little sac thus formed is *Bowman's capsule*. The pressure of the blood within the glomerular capillaries causes the blood to be filtered into Bowman's capsule, where it begins to pass down the tubule. As the blood filtrate passes through the tubules, all substances useful to the body are reabsorbed while the end products of metabolism are cleared.

Because of their size, red blood cells and protein do not normally pass through the glomerular filter. Thus the fluid in Bowman's capsule is a protein-free filtrate of blood plasma. Capillary permeability is increased in many renal diseases, permitting plasma proteins to pass into the urine. Also, the glomerular membrane may be so injured by disease that it fails to function as a filter, permitting blood cells and plasma protein to leak through the injured capillary to be excreted in the urine.

The glomerulus is not the only capillary bed supplying the nephron. The efferent arteriole leaving Bowman's capsule goes on to form another capillary bed, this time a low-pressure bed that supplies the tubules (Fig. 7-2). This low pressure in the peritubular capillary system causes it to function in much the same way as the venous ends of the tissue capillaries, with fluid being absorbed continually into the capillaries.

Laboratory tests for renal function are related chiefly to the three main functions of the nephron—glomerular filtration, tubular reabsorption, and tubular secretion. It is through these three mechanisms that the kidney clears the blood of unwanted substances.

The fluid that filters through the glomerular membrane into Bowman's capsule is called glomerular filtrate. The rate at which glomerular filtrate is formed in all nephrons is called the *glomerular filtration rate*. Normally, this averages about 125 ml/min. However, the normal rate may be as high as

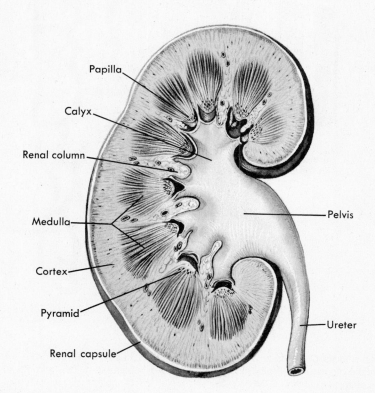

Papilla

Calyx

Renal column

Medulla

Cortex

Pyramid

Renal capsule

Pelvis

Ureter

Fig. 7-1
Coronal section of the right kidney. (From Anthony, C.P., and Kolthoff, N.J.: Textbook of anatomy and physiology, ed. 9, St. Louis, 1975, The C.V. Mosby Co.)

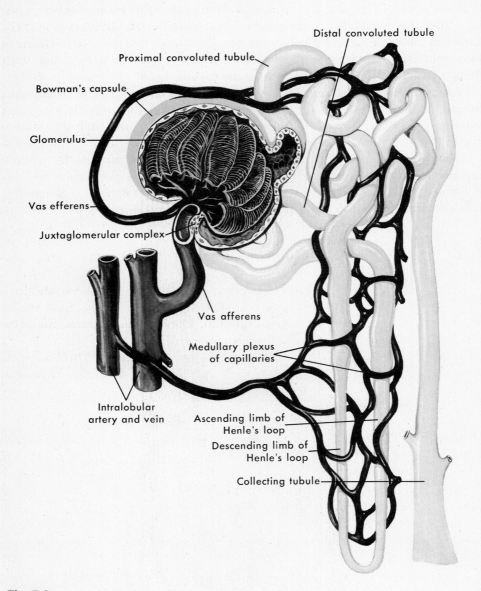

Fig. 7-2
The nephron and its blood supply. The wall of Bowman's capsule has been cut away to reveal the detail of the glomerulus. (From Schottelius, B.A., and Schottelius, D.D.: Textbook of physiology, ed. 17, St. Louis, 1973, The C.V. Mosby Co.)

200 ml/min. Usually, over 99% of the glomberular filtrate is reabsorbed in the tubules. The remainder passes into the urinary bladder.

Tubular reabsorption is accomplished by active and passive transport across the membranes of the tubular system into the peritubular capillaries and interstitial tissue. Substances actively reabsorbed through the tubular epithelial cells include glucose and amino acids, as well as sodium calcium, potassium, phosphate, urate, chloride, and other ions.

Some solutes, such as urea, are *passively* diffused from the tubular fluid into the peritubular fluid in response to the concentration difference across the membrane and the permeability of the tubular membrane to the solute. Some substances, especially hydrogen, potassium, and urate ions, are *actively* secreted into the tubules.

Aldosterone

The adrenal cortex secretes a group of hormones called corticosteroids, of which there are two major types: mineralocorticoids and glucocorticoids. Mineralocorticoids are so called because of their effect on electrolytes. Glucocorticoids are so named because they increase blood glucose concentration, although they also have an effect on protein and fat metabolism. Of the 30 different steroids isolated from the adrenal cortex, two have major importance in endocrine and renal function. They are *aldosterone*, the principal mineralocorticoid, and *cortisol*, the principal glucocorticoid.

Aldosterone is secreted by a very thin layer of cells located on the adrenal cortex just beneath the capsule. The basic effect of aldosterone is to increase the rate of tubular reabsorption of sodium, with a concomitant loss of potassium.

Large amounts of aldosterone may cause only a few milligrams per day of sodium to be lost in the urine. In such a case, although total-body sodium may be increased, the plasma sodium concentration is not abnormal, because the individual will become thirsty and dilute the sodium with water.

Conversely, a lack of aldosterone causes loss of as much as 20 gm of sodium per day into the urine.

The extracellular potassium concentration is one of the main factors regulating the rate of aldosterone secretion. When the potassium concentration increases, so does the aldosterone concentration, which in turn produces an increase in potassium excretion and sodium retention by the kidneys.

Another factor controlling the rate of aldosterone secretion is the *renin-angiotensin* system. This system is one of the main intermediaries by which sodium depletion exerts its effect upon aldosterone secretion. Renin is an enzyme secreted by the juxtaglomerular cells in the walls of the renal afferent arterioles in response to decreased intravascular volume secondary to sodium depletion or to a change from the supine to the upright position.

Renin then acts as a catalyst on one of the plasma proteins to produce angiotensin I and angiotensin II, which are potent stimulators of aldosterone secretion. Water and salt retention is thus promoted in an effort to return the arterial pressure to normal.

PATHOPHYSIOLOGY

The functioning nephron is made of glomerular, tubular, and interstitial tissue. Therefore, even though a disease state may begin in one spot, if it progresses it ultimately involves the whole kidney, because the processes in the tubular system are dependent upon the production of a filtrate by the glomerulus. If the glomerulus is involved initially in a disease and becomes grossly abnormal with decreased perfusion and filtration, the tubules ultimately show varying degrees of atrophy or fibrosis. This is why end-stage glomerular nephritis can result from an acute poststreptococcal proliferative lesion originally involving solely the glomerulus.

Oversecretion of aldosterone, commonly caused by a benign adrenocortical tumor, may result in hypertension because of excessive sodium reabsorption with a concomitant hypokalemia. Aldosterone may also be elevated as a result of congestive heart failure, renovascular hypertension, malignant hypertension, nephrosis, or cirrhosis with ascites.

LABORATORY TESTS FOR RENAL FUNCTION

Urinalysis

A complete urinalysis, with careful attention being paid to microscopic examination of the sediment, remains one of the most important tests in the diagnosis of renal diseases (see pp. 46-49).

Glomerular filtration tests

Glomerular filtration is evaluated through clearance tests, which measure the rate at which certain substances are cleared from the plasma. The tested substance must be freely filtered and neither reabsorbed nor secreted by the tubules, for a true picture of glomerular filtration rate (GFR), which is usually 105 to 135 ml/min.

Inulin clearance test

Inulin is a polysaccharide that is neither reabsorbed nor secreted by the renal tubular cells. It is completely cleared by the kidney and is, therefore, the best indicator of glomerular function. However, an inulin clearance test is cumbersome and not suitable for routine clinical work. It involves the intravenous injection of a priming dose of inulin, followed by continuous infusion in an attempt to keep a uniform blood level. Urine flow during the test must be accurately measured. Plasma and urine inulin concentrations are measured and the glomerular filtration rate is estimated by means of this formula:

$$\text{GFR} = \frac{\text{Urine inulin concentration} \times \text{Urine volume}}{\text{Plasma inulin concentration}}$$

▶ Normal inulin clearance
(corrected to 1.73 sq m of body surface)

Males: 124 ± 25.8 ml/min
Females: 119 ± 12.8 ml/min

The inulin clearance test, although valid, is too cumbersome for routine clinical use. Simpler ways of accurately assessing GFR including measurement of the serum concentration of creatinine and the clearance of endogenous creatinine.

Serum creatinine level and creatinine clearance test

Creatinine is an endogenous waste product originating from the creatine and phosphocreatine of skeletal muscle. Creatinine clearance is a reliable indicator of glomerular filtration rate, since creatinine is excreted by means of glomerular filtration and is not appreciably reabsorbed or secreted by the tubule cells. The serum creatinine level, therefore, rises when the glomerular filtration rate falls. At the same time the creatinine clearance rate, determined on a 24-hour urine specimen, is low.

This test is similar to the inulin clearance test, except that instead of infusing inulin, the body's own sustained production of creatinine provides the test agent. Urine and plasma concentrations of creatinine are measured, and a timed urine specimen is collected and measured for volume (at 2, 12, or 24 hours). Thus:

$$\text{Creatinine clearance} = \frac{\text{Urine creatinine concentration} \times \text{Urine volume}}{\text{Plasma creatinine concentration}}$$

▶ Normal creatinine clearance
115 ± 20 ml/min

▶ Normal serum creatinine
0.6-1.2 mg/dl

Use of radioisotopes

The glomerular filtration rate can also be measured by means of radioisotopes. Iothalamate labeled with iodine 125 is injected subcutaneously or intravenously. There is no protein binding, and the renal clearance of ^{125}I remains independent of variations in the plasma level. By measuring the ^{125}I levels in the urine and the plasma, a person can calculate ^{125}I clearance, which accurately reflects the GFR.

Blood urea nitrogen (BUN) and urea clearance test (see also p. 28)

Urea is the end product of protein metabolism; it is similar to creatinine in that nitrogen is an endogenous waste product cleared by the kidneys. An elevated BUN level reflects a decreased glomerular filtration rate. Two factors make the BUN and urea clearance test less reliable than the creatinine clearance test: (1) urea, after being filtered, tends to diffuse back into the renal tubular cells and thus its clearance is dependent on the *rate* of urine formation, and (2) urea production varies according to the state of liver function and protein intake and breakdown. Thus urea clearance is infrequently used and BUN, although routinely used, must be interpreted with these limitations in mind.

Tests of renal plasma flow (RPF)

Renal plasma flow is measured by means of substances that are completely cleared, through glomerular filtration and tubular secretion, in a single passage through the kidney.

Para-aminohippurate (PAH) clearance test

One such substance is the exogenous agent para-aminohippurate. Thus the clearance of PAH is a direct measurement of RPF. The test is cumbersome and involves a procedure similar to that of the inulin clearance test. Iodohippurate sodium I 131 can be used as a substitute for PAH; its clearance will correlate well with renal plasma flow, simplifying the test.

Phenolsulfonphthalein (PSP) excretion test

Intravenously injected PSP is excreted by active transport at the proximal tubules at a rate proportional to renal blood flow. If renal blood flow and proximal tubular function are normal, 28% to 35% of the PSP will be excreted in the first 15 minutes after the IV injection.

Many factors can interfere with the accurate estimation of PSP excretion; incomplete emptying of the bladder, low urine volume, liver disease, congestive heart failure, low serum albumin levels, and various drugs can invalidate the test. Recent modifications of this test have tried to overcome these limitations by correlating the PSP dose to body size and limiting the collection time to 15 minutes. Since even kidneys with markedly diminished renal blood flow will excrete a relatively normal amount of PSP in 1 or 2 hours, the amount excreted in the first 15 minutes is the most sensitive measure of renal blood flow.

Indications and contraindications for the measurement of GFR and RPF

Measurements of GFR and RPF are essential in the evaluation of any kidney dysfunction. They also are used in the evaluation of kidney donors, and in the follow-up care of patients who have had kidney transplants. The severity and rate of progression of glomerular nephritis and other renal disorders can be assessed further through serial GFR and RPF measurements. Serial measurements also help in the decision to delay or initiate long-term hemodialysis.

Determination of GFR and RPF should not be done during periods of *changing* renal function. Changing renal function suggests osmotic diuresis, dehydration, or overhydration. The data will be misleading, possibly resulting in the overestimation or underestimation of renal function.

The presence of radioisotopes other than those used in the clearance tests just discussed may interfere with the measurement of levels of ^{125}I or ^{131}I in blood and urine. Therefore, a renogram (p. 177) should not be performed within 24 hours of determination of GFR and PRF if radioactive methods are used. Radioisotope studies should not be performed in pregnant women, because of the risk to the fetus posed by radiation exposure.

When it is important to measure the GFR of each kidney separately (differential renal function), catheters can be introduced into each ureter and the clearance of each kidney can be measured separately. This test is invasive and not frequently used.

Tubular function tests

Clinically, tubular function is best measured by tests that determine the ability of the tubules to concentrate and dilute the urine. Tests of urinary dilution are not as sensitive in the detection of renal disease as are tests of urinary concentration. This fact is especially valuable because the first function to be lost in renal disease is the ability of the kidney to concentrate urine.

Since the concentration of urine occurs in the renal medulla (interstitial fluids, loops of Henle, capillaries of the medulla, and collecting tubules), the disease processes that disturb the function or structure of the medulla produce early impairment of the concentrating ability of the kidney. Such disorders are acute tubular necrosis, obstructive uropathy, pyelonephritis, papillary necrosis, medullary cysts, hypokalemic and hypercalcemic nephropathy, and sickle cell disease.

In azotemic patients, because of disturbed glomerular and tubular function, subjection to prolonged dehydration and/or being challenged with an excess amount of water may be hazardous.

Specific gravity

Determinations of specific gravity is a relatively simple and inexpensive method of estimating the concentration of all solids in the urine (p. 46). As routinely performed, it is not an accurate test and would reflect only major deviations from the normal. This test is being replaced by the more accurate test of urine osmolality.

Urine and serum osmolality

The measurement of urine osmolality is a more refined and accurate method than specific gravity for determining the diluting and concentrating ability of the kidneys. Osmolality is an expression of the total number of particles in a solution. Plasma osmolality is the main regulator of the release of antidiuretic hormone (ADH). When sufficient water is not being taken in, the osmolality of the plasma rises, ADH is released from the pituitary gland, and the kidneys respond by reabsorbing water from the distal tubules and producing a more concentrated urine. The converse occurs with excessive water ingestion. With the decrease in plasma osmolality, ADH is not released, more water is lost, and the urine becomes more dilute. A change in plasma osmolality of as little as 1% to 2% will either suppress or stimulate thirst and ADH secretion.

The normal urine osmolality depends upon the clinical setting. With maximal ADH stimulation, the normal can be as much as 1200 mOsm/kg of body weight; with maximum ADH suppression, the normal can be as little as 50 mOsm/kg. Thus urine osmolality should be interpreted in the light of what is known about the patient's hydration status and plasma osmolality.

In normal kidney function this mechanism allows tremendous flexibility in the volume of water that can be ingested—as little as 500 ml or as much as 25 liters per day. Abnormalities in urine diluting or concentrating capacity markedly reduce this flexibility. When the limits just mentioned are exceeded, an abnormality in body fluid osmolality occurs. Since sodium is the most abundant plasma electrolyte (p. 16), such an abnormality is reflected in changes in plasma sodium concentration.

Simultaneous determination of serum and urine osmolality is often valuable in assessing the distal tubular response to circulating ADH. For example, if a patient's serum is hyperosmolar or in the upper limits of normal ranges and the patient's urine osmolality measured at the same time is much lower, inadequate ADH secretion or a decreased responsiveness of the distal tubules to circulating ADH should be suspected.

In advanced renal medullary disease, the ability to concentrate urine is lost, and, irrespectively of the state of hydration or fluid intake, a dilute urine of *fixed* specific gravity or osmolality is excreted (hyposthenuria).

◆ **Normal urine osmolality**

50-1400 mOsm/L (range)
500-800 mOsm/L (random specimen)

◆ **Normal serum osmolality**

280-295 mOsm/L (range)

Urinary sodium concentration

The excretion of sodium is very sensitive to plasma volume and sodium intake. Thus the presence of large amounts of sodium in the urine would be expected in the setting of expanded intravascular volume and increased sodium intake. When the urinary sodium concentration is high in a setting of hypovolemia and decreased sodium intake, the following possibilities need to be explored:

1. The presence of diuretic medications or osmotic agents
2. Adrenal insufficiency
3. Renal diseases of various types

Determinations of the urinary levels of potassium, magnesium, calcium, phosphorus, and other elements, in the context of plasma measurements and intake amounts, can give additional information about renal handling of cations. A detailed discussion is beyond the scope of this chapter.

◆ **Normal urinary sodium**

80-180 mEq/24 hr (varies with dietary ingestion of sodium)

Measurement of plasma renin activity (PRA)

The release of renin is controlled by several factors, including the sympathetic nervous system, the systemic blood pressure, and the composition of fluid that enters the distal tubule of the macula densa. The plasma levels of potassium, ADH, catecholamines, and various drugs, as well as the plasma osmolality, influence the rate of renin release. The determination of plasma renin activity is important in the diagnosis of renal vascular hypertension as well as primary hyperaldosteronism. Selective renal vein sampling may be necessary. Radioimmunoassay techniques are used in the determination of PRA.

◆ **Normal plasma renin activity**

Na-depleted, upright (peripheral vein specimen):
    Ages 20-39: 2.9-24 ng/ml/hr
    Ages 40 and up: 2.9-10.8 ng/ml/hr
Na-replete, upright (peripheral vein specimen):
    Ages 20-39: <0.6-4.3 ng/ml/hr
    Ages 40 and up: <0.6-3.0 ng/ml/hr

Measurement of serum level of angiotensin-converting enzyme (SACE)

Angiotensin-converting enzyme is involved in the terminal step in the generation of angiotensin II, a very potent vasoconstrictor. Thus the determination of the SACE level is of some use in the evaluation of special cases of hypertension.

◆ Normal serum angiotensin-converting enzyme

23-57 U/ml (U = nanomoles/min; patients >20 years old: 2 SD)

Determinations of aldosterone levels (plasma and urinary)

Aldosterone, the most potent natural mineralocorticoid, is instrumental in sodium and potassium homeostasis and in maintenance of blood pressure. Elevated levels of aldosterone can result from increased secretion because of an adenoma (primary aldosteronism) or from increased levels of angiotensin II. When aldosterone levels are elevated, sodium excretion is decreased, potassium wasting occurs, and usually there is hypertension. The reverse can occur in conditions of low aldosterone secretion. Radioimmunoassay techniques are used in measurements of plasma and urinary aldosterone levels.

◆ Normal serum aldosterone

1-21 ng/dl (morning peripheral vein specimen)

◆ Normal urine aldosterone

2-16 µg/24 hr

Determination of urinary protein levels

Proteinuria is a frequent occurrence in glomerular disease. Twenty-four hour protein quantitation is necessary for the detection of proteinuria. The protein excreted in the urine may be composed of albumin or immunoglobulins. In some types of glomerular disease, large amounts of albumin may be excreted, causing hypoalbuminemia and edema. Electrophoresis and immunoelectrophoresis of the protein in the urine make possible the recognition of various immunoglobulins seen in disease states, such as multiple myeloma, lymphoma, and amyloidosis.

Urine culture

A urine culture and a test of antimicrobial sensitivity of any organism detected should be ordered in cases of suspected genitourinary infection. In a urine culture the colony count is important. The presence of fewer than 10,000 viable bacterial units per milliliter of urine is probably of no significance. If 10,000 to 100,000 colonies are cultured, no positive conclusion can be drawn. There should be over 100,000 colonies before an infection is considered significant. However, samples of urine from the ureters and renal pelvis might contain fewer bacteria and still indicate infection, because bacteria multiply while urine is being held in the bladder.

In the absence of symptoms, a positive urine culture should elicit an inquiry into how the specimen was collected. Unless a catheter was used or the sample is a midstream voided specimen obtained after proper cleansing of the genitalia, contamination will occur.

It should also be remembered that a negative urine culture does not necessarily rule out chronic low-grade pyelonephritis.

Radioisotope renography

A radioactive material that is rapidly excreted is injected intravenously. The amount of radioactivity over each kidney is measured with a gamma camera or a probe. The amount of radioactivity in each kidney rises rapidly (within minutes) and then declines as the radioactive tracer leaves the kidney via the ureters. The curve describing these changes as a function of time is called a renogram. It makes possible a composite evaluation of renal plasma flow, glomerular filtration, and tubular secretion, as well as excretory function. Any process that interferes with these functions will produce an abnormal renogram. The data is usually evaluated in a qualitative manner. Recent computer processing of the data has made possible the semiquantitation of renal function. Various patterns in abnormal renograms can be recognized and equated with specific conditions, such as renal vascular hypertension, tubular disease, urinary obstruction, pyelonephritis, or absence of kidney function.

Initially, this test was important as a diagnostic tool in the evaluation of hypertension, particularly unilateral renal vascular hypertension. However, at the present time, timed-sequence IVP is the preferred screening test.

Methods of imaging the kidney
KUB (kidney, ureter, bladder) film

Simple KUB x-ray film gives an estimate of kidney position, size, and calcifications. It should be reviewed before more extensive radiologic studies are performed.

Tomography

Tomography provides improved resolution at a desired level of the body and thus builds on the information available from plain films. It is helpful when the gastrointestinal tract or other organs blur the renal outlines.

Computerized tomography

CT scanning of the abdomen provides excellent visualization of the kidney. Kidney size can be evaluated, and tumors and suprarenal masses (adrenal tumors, pheochromocytoma) can be detected. The injection of contrast material further improves image quality. (See also p. 148.)

Intravenous pyelography (IVP)

An intravenous pyelogram is obtained by injecting intravenously a contrast medium that, because it is cleared from the blood by glomerular filtration, can visualize the renal parenchyma and collecting system (calyses, renal pelvis, ureters, and urinary bladder) on multiple x-ray films.

This is a very valuable test because it provides visualization of the entire urinary tract. The test is helpful in the diagnosis of renal masses and cysts, ureteral obstruction, retroperitoneal tumors, renal trauma, bladder abnormalities, and so on. It also gives an estimate of renal function based on the appearance time and concentration of the contrast medium in each kidney. In the presence of moderate to severe renal disease with a compromised glomerular filtration rate, visualization may be poor. If improved images are needed, drip-infusion IVP may be performed; in this procedure a larger volume of contrast medium is injected rapidly.

In IVP there is a slight risk of an allergic reaction to the contrast material. The most severe reaction is anaphylaxis, which can be lethal.

Patient preparation and care. The patient remains fasting after midnight prior to IVP, in order to produce the moderate dehydration necessary for better concentration of the contrast medium. When drip-infusion IVP is to be performed, this fast is not necessary. In order that the films not be obscured by intestinal contents, a strong cathartic is administered the afternoon prior to the test. Dilution of the contrast medium in the bladder is prevented by having the patient void immediately prior to the test.

Nephrotomography

Nephrotomography combines tomography and intravenous pyelography, providing a more detailed visualization of the specific level of the body under study.

Timed-sequence IVP

Timed-sequence IVP is a modification of standard IVP. Films are made every minute for 5 minutes after injection of the contrast medium. A difference between the times of excretion of the dye from the two kidneys indicates unilateral kidney disease. In such a case, the normal kidney shows some concentration of the dye before the abnormal one does.

It should be noted, however, that although this test is the best screening test for hypertension secondary to unilateral kidney disease, it does not differentiate between renal artery stenosis and chronic pyelonephritis or nephrosclerosis. If the patient has hypertension, the test does not differentiate between hypertension resulting from renal parenchymal disease or diffuse small-vessel disease and that caused by obstruction of a major renal artery.

Patient preparation and care are the same as in standard IVP.

Retrograde pyelography

Retrograde pyelography is performed by passing a catheter from the urethra to the urinary bladder, then to the right or left ureter, and injecting a contrast medium. This test is more involved than regular IVP, but it provides detailed visualization of the urinary collecting system, independent of the status of renal function. It is very helpful in the diagnosis of ureteral obstruction.

Risks include the trauma of manipulation and the attendant risk of infection.

Patient preparation and care. The contents of the bowel should be cleared in order to avoid obscuring shadows on the x-ray films. Whether the patient remains fasting depends upon the type of anesthesia to be used.

Following the procedure the urine of the patient should be observed for amount, hematuria, and signs of urinary sepsis. Drainage from a ureteral catheter should be noted separately from that of the urethral catheter. Failure of the ureteral catheter to drain should be reported immediately.

Renal angiography

Renal angiography provides visualization of the entire renal arterial, capillary, and venous systems. This test is performed by introducing a catheter into the renal artery (selective angiography), or into the aorta proximal to the origin of the renal arteries (aortorenal angiography), and injecting contrast material while rapid x-ray filming is performed.

This test is most helpful in the diagnosis of renal artery stenosis (renal vascular hypertension), renal masses, trauma, venous thrombosis, or obstructive uropathy.

Risks of the test are the same as in any selective angiographic study; they include the possibilities of bleeding, thrombosis, damage to the vessel, and allergic reactions.

Informed written consent is necessary before the test is performed.

Patient preparation and care. Patient preparation may include administration of vitamin K or protamine sulfate if the patient has been taking Coumadin or heparin, respectively. Cathartics may be administered as needed. The skin is prepared in the usual manner. The contrast medium is an osmotic diuretic. Therefore, in order to avoid an overdistended bladder during the procedure, the patient should void immediately prior to the test. In patients with multiple myeloma or diabetes with dehydration, special care is necessary to avoid renal shutdown; the volume of contrast medium injected may have to be limited.

Bed rest is necessary for 12 to 24 hours after the procedure. The arterial puncture site should be checked for hematoma formation (manifested by swelling and bleeding). If this occurs, manual pressure should be applied cephalad to the puncture and the physician should be notified.

Vital signs and peripheral pulses should be frequently evaluated. Baseline values should have been established prior to the procedure.

Ultrasound

Ultrasonic examination of the kidney is part of an abdominal ultrasonic examination. This test is most valuable in detecting renal or perirenal masses and in the differential diagnosis of renal cysts versus solid masses. It is also valuable for the evaluation of ureteral obstruction.

Renal scans (nuclear imaging)

Radioactive material is injected intravenously and its distribution in the kidney is scanned or mapped. Various agents are used. This technique is useful in showing the location, size, and shape of the kidneys and generally assessing blood perfusion and ability to secrete urine. Abscesses, cysts, and tumors may appear as "cold spots" because of the presence of nonfunctioning tissue.

Renal biopsy

Percutaneous biopsy of the kidney under fluoroscopic or ultrasonic guidance yields histologic information about both the glomeruli and the tubules, and thus may permit a precise diagnosis. The tissue is processed for light and electron microscopy as well as immunofluorescent studies and cultures when indicated. The precise histologic diagnosis thus made may be useful in the treatment of the patient and may also prove of prognostic value.

Risks include uncontrolled bleeding and hematuria and loss of the kidney. Informed consent is necessary.

Patient preparation and care

Since uncontrolled bleeding is a major risk, a complete coagulation evaluation is necessary. Preventive care consists of bed rest for 24 hours following the procedure and increased intake of fluids. Vital signs are monitored and hematocrit is determined frequently.

CLINICAL APPLICATION OF LABORATORY TESTS

Diseases primarily affecting glomerular structure and function
Acute glomerulonephritis

Acute glomerulonephritis is an acute inflammation that primarily involves the glomerulus, although some minor changes are noted in the tubules.

Diagnostic laboratory tests. Creatinine clearance studies are helpful in initially evaluating the extent of glomerular damage and following the progression of the disease. Further laboratory tests are usually needed to arrive at a definite diagnosis.

Characteristic urine findings are mild to moderate proteinuria (albumin), hematuria, RBC casts, granular casts, and, depending on the diffuseness and extent of involvement, blood urea nitrogen and creatinine retention, indicating significant diminution of glomerular function.

Differential diagnosis. Previously, glomerulonephritis was immediately equated with poststreptococcal nephritis. However, many other diseases are known to have renal involvement and the typical picture of glomerulonephritis. Thus in the following discussion the other diseases will be mentioned and a differential diagnosis discussed.

Acute poststreptococcal glomerulonephritis. This is seen more frequently in children but also occurs in adults. It is an inflammatory reaction of the kidney glomerulus to deposition of immune complexes composed of antigen from the streptococcal organism and the body's own antibodies—thus the name "immune complex disease." For an etiologic diagnosis, necessary tests include a throat culture for group A β-hemolytic streptococci, and determination of the serum antistreptolysin-O titer to confirm the presence of the infecting organism.

Systemic lupus erythematosus nephritis. Kidney involvement in this systemic disease may present as acute glomerulonephritis. The diagnosis should be suspected when many organs are involved in the disease process; a diagnosis can be confirmed by characteristic results of serologic tests, including fluorescent antinuclear antibodies, anti-DNA antibodies, and serum complement measurement. (See Chapter 12.)

Other diseases. The list of other diseases that may present as acute glomerulonephritis is long. Among the important ones are bacterial endocarditis, which is diagnosed by means of the clinical picture and blood cultures (see p. 312); viral hepatitis, diagnosed by the presence of the Australia antigen and by antibody tests; and malaria or syphilis, which are suggested by the clinical picture and blood smears or serologic tests.

In many cases renal biopsy is needed for a specific diagnosis (for example, membranous glomerulonephritis, focal glomerulonephritis, Goodpasture's syndrome). Light and electron microscopy as well as immunofluorescent studies may be necessary.

Chronic glomerulonephritis

Many of the disease processes presenting as acute glomerulonephritis may not resolve completely and may progress into a subacute or chronic phase involving progressive destruction of glomerular function, the end-stage of which is called chronic renal failure.

Diagnostic laboratory tests. Persistent hematuria or proteinuria should lead the examiner to suspect latent chronic glomerulonephritis. As the disease progresses, there will be a decrease in creatinine clearance and, after the loss of approximately 50% of glomerular function, serum creatinine and blood urea nitrogen levels may start rising. The urinary specific gravity is usually low (around 1.010) and fixed. A lower serum complement level may be seen in active immunologic processes. In the early stages of chronic glomerulonephritis, renal biopsy may be of help in diagnosis.

As the disease progresses and end-stage renal failure is present, even kidney biopsy may not yield a definite diagnosis. Hypertension frequently accompanies this stage. Anemia may appear in the far-advanced cases, and there would be an elevation of the serum potassium level, a decrease in the serum sodium level, and onset of metabolic acidosis.

Differential diagnosis. When chronic glomerulonephritis progresses to end-stage kidney disease with persistent azotemia and elevated creatinine levels, it is sometimes impossible to differentiate among the following conditions: the chronic stage of acute glomerulonephritis, end-stage pyelonephritis, and end-stage nephrosclerosis.

Nephrotic syndrome

The hallmark of the nephrotic syndrome is massive proteinuria (over 3.5 gm per day) resulting from increased permeability of the glomerular membranes to protein.

Various disease processes may lead to this syndrome, including various types of glomerulonephritis, diabetes mellitus, amyloidosis, renal vein thrombosis, allergic reactions, drugs, and tumors. Edema, ascites, and pleural effusion are commonly present.

Diagnostic laboratory tests. The diagnosis of nephrotic syndrome is made when a 24-hour urine specimen contains 3.5 gm or more of protein; the protein is usually the albumin fraction of the serum proteins.

In addition to the massive proteinuria, the serum cholesterol level increases, the serum albumin level decreases, and fat bodies and fat casts appear in the urine.

In searching for a specific cause for the nephrotic syndrome, one may utilize all the diagnostic tests discussed earlier in this chapter, as well as other tests as indicated. Frequently, a renal biopsy is performed, the findings of which may guide treatment and indicate a prognosis.

Differential diagnosis. More than fifty specific disease entities are characterized by the nephrotic syndrome at one stage or another in their natural histories. The more common ones include the following:

1. Acute glomerulonephritis, usually acute poststreptococcal, or any of the other acute glomerulonephritides
2. Metabolic disorders, such as diabetic nephropathy or amyloid kidney disease
3. Systemic disease, such as systemic lupus erythematosus and certain malignancies (multiple myeloma)
4. Circulatory disease, such as renal vein thrombosis or right-sided congestive heart failure
5. Ingestion of nephrotoxins, such as heavy metals, and lead poisoning
6. Infections and reactions to certain allergens and drugs

Diseases affecting tubular structure and function
Acute tubular necrosis

Acute tubular necrosis, also known as lower nephron nephrosis, may follow renal circulatory impairment (shock of various types), or be the result of toxic damage to the kidney. There is also involvement of the glomeruli. However, the main pathologic condition is at the tubular level.

Since acute tubular necrosis is reversible if properly managed and treated, it is important to make the correct diagnosis. The condition usually follows a state of shock, be it cardiogenic, toxic, or bacteremic, and it is usually the result of impaired circulation to the tubules.

The disease presents with a sudden onset of oliguria (urine volume less than 300 ml per day) associated with signs and symptoms of uremia.

Diagnostic laboratory tests. The urine volume and the specific gravity are low. Blood urea nitrogen and serum creatinine levels are elevated. Urinalysis may reveal proteinuria and hematuria. Serum potassium, phosphate, and sulfate levels may be elevated, while sodium, calcium, and CO_2 levels will be decreased. Metabolic acidosis may be present. Evaluation of urinary electrolyte levels may show increased sodium excretion during the diuretic phase.

Spontaneous recovery is frequent; it most commonly occurs in 1 to 2 weeks but may be delayed for 5 to 6 weeks. During the recovery stage a polyuric phase may occur, with urine volumes of 5 to 20 liters per day. This state requires careful management of fluid and electrolyte levels.

When the diagnosis is not clear, further evaluation—by renography, intravenous pyelography, retrograde pyelography, or renal angiography—

may be needed. It is important to exclude ureteral obstruction. A renal biopsy is generally not indicated.

Polyuric states

When polyuria exists, the following possibilities should be considered. (The polyuric phase of acute tubular necrosis has already been mentioned.)

Diabetes insipidus. This is not a renal disease, but because of the absence of ADH, which is responsible for the reabsorption of water from the distal tubules, there is a massive polyuria, with urine production sometimes approaching 15 to 20 liters per day. Although ADH is absent, the renal response to ADH is normal. An injection of ADH corrects the polyuria of diabetes insipidus, while polyuria secondary to renal tubular disease (nephrogenic diabetes insipidus) does not respond to ADH.

Chlorpropamide (Diabinese) has an action similar to that of ADH on the distal tubular cells and partially corrects the polyuria of diabetes insipidus. This fact is helpful in the differential diagnosis of diabetes insipidus versus renal tubular disease.

Renal tubular diseases. Like diabetes insipidus, this group of diseases is associated with polyuria because of the impairment of the reabsorption of water and electrolytes. Polyuric states can be seen in hypercalcemic nephropathy, hypokalemic nephropathy, and in certain kinds of renal tubular acidosis of hereditary conditions.

Renal tubular disease also is usually associated with abnormal excretion of amino acids, such as in cystinuria and Fanconi's syndrome.

Analgesic nephropathy. This disease simulates renal tubular acidosis; it is characterized by polyuria and azotemia, with a more or less fixed specific gravity. This is because of tubular involvement secondary to the use of analgesics, which impair absorption. The most common of the analgesic nephropathies is phenacetin nephropathy.

Congenital anomalies

Recognition of congenital anomalies is important because of the predisposition of patients with these conditions to repeated urinary tract infection.

Diagnostic laboratory tests. The patient should be checked frequently through urinalysis and urine culture, which will identify an infecting organism. Intravenous pyelography can be used to define the anatomic or structural anomaly.

Differential diagnosis. Horseshoe kidney, ectopic kidney, or an unusually mobile kidney may be associated with ureteral obstruction and infection. Polycystic kidney may also predispose a person to infections. In addition, polycystic kidney may cause hematuria and may ultimately lead to chronic renal failure.

Diseases associated with pure hematuria

Pure hematuria usually indicates a disease process below the nephron, which can be anywhere from the collecting ducts to the bladder. In this situation there is usually no RBC casts, and the microscopic examination of the urine shows gross RBCs.

Painless hematuria

If there is no pain associated with the hematuria, an examiner should suspect renal tumors, renal tuberculosis, or inflammatory or malignant disease involving the structures below the nephron—that is, the collecting ducts, the kidney pelvises, the ureters, or the bladder.

Intravenous pyelography, retrograde pyelography, nephrotomography, renal tomography, and computerized tomography are the diagnostic tests frequently used.

Painful hematuria

Nephrolithiasis is usually painful, particularly when calculi obstruct the urinary tract or move in the ureters. However, a big staghorn calculus located in the pelvis of the kidney may be asymptomatic and a cause of intermittent pure hematuria.

Pure pyuria and bacteruria

In an acute case of fever, chills, and pyuria, the diagnosis is acute pyelonephritis. This disorder usually affects the renal parenchyma as well as the tubules and collecting ducts in the renal pelvis, and eventually the bladder. Under such circumstances it is imperative that a urine culture be obtained to identify the organism involved. The most common organism in an otherwise uncomplicated case is *Escherichia coli*.

When there are repeated episodes of acute pyelonephritis, an examiner should investigate the kidney for any correctable structural conditions that may predispose the patient to repeated episodes of pyelonephritis. Unless this is done and the condition is corrected, the patient may develop chronic pyelonephritis. Under such circumstances an IV pyelogram and an excretory cystourogram are usually done to rule out reflux at the cystourethral junction. Any indication of chronicity warrants a thorough investigation of the genitourinary tract for partial obstructive uropathy.

Renal vascular hypertension

The hypertension associated with renal vascular disease may be the result of a pathologic state at the level of the major renal vessels (obstructive vascular disease) or at the level of the smaller arteries and arterioles (nephrosclerosis). The pathologic finding of nephrosclerosis in an elderly person's kidney is quite common; it is found in generalized atherosclerosis. In addition to the general atherosclerotic process involving the smaller arteries, there are several curious conditions in which there is unilateral or bilateral involvement of the renal artery. Significant narrowing of the renal arteries can result from either fibromuscular hyperplasia, which is common in women between 35 and 45 years of age, or an atherosclerotic plaque that narrows the renal artery to such a degree that an appreciable pressure gradient is created on either side of the obstruction. The narrowing triggers a hormone system called the renin-angiotensin system, which causes hypertension by means of the mechanism described on p. 169. The hypertension thus produced eventually affects the kidneys further by causing more nephrosclerotic changes in the renal arteries, thus establishing a self-perpetuating cycle. It is imperative that patients with this disease be identified—particularly those in the younger age group, for whom surgical correction is possible.

Diagnostic laboratory tests

Renal vascular hypertension may be manifested as minor, nonspecific urinary findings such as a few red blood cells with some RBC casts and a slight diminution of glomerular filtration rate (as shown by creatinine clearance).

Differential diagnosis

The tests employed for differentiating renal vascular hypertension from other hypertensions, as well as for presurgical evaluation, are as follows (in the order of their importance and yield):

1. Timed (rapid)-sequence IVP. This test should be done if renal function is not significantly decreased. The early appearance of the contrast medium in one kidney as compared with the other suggests stenosis of the arteries of the kidney in which the appearance was delayed. Timed-sequence IVP is also helpful in evaluating kidney size, which is another indication of renal vascular hypertension; an abnormally small kidney may have a compromised blood supply. These, and other, more subtle changes, detectable through timed-sequence IVP, may identify 70% to 75% of patients with renal vascular hypertension.

2. Radioisotope renography. The clearance rate of the radioisotope will approximate renal plasma flow. The examiner analyzes time-activity curves for each kidney, looking for delayed appearance of the radioisotope. Radioisotope renography is the initial study of choice in patients who have a history of allergy to contrast material. The sensitivity of this test is similar to that of rapid-sequence IVP.

3. Renal arteriography. This definitive test should be considered when the results of the two preceding screening studies are abnormal. The

test is invasive and involves slightly more risk than timed-sequence IVP.

Demonstration of renal artery stenosis by arteriography does not complete an evaluation. The stenosis has to be severe (at least 75%) to cause hemodynamic compromise of the kidney. More important, biochemical evidence of "ischemia," in the form of increased plasma renin activity in the renal vein, should be documented on the side of the narrowed artery. After these evaluations, a decision about surgery (vein or graft bypass of the stenosed artery) can be made. In some cases, balloon-catheter dilation of the narrowed segment may be done at the time of arteriography, obviating the need for surgery.

Renal artery stenosis is one of the commonest causes of reversible or "curable" hypertension. Other causes include:

1. Pheochromocytoma—a catecholamine-secreting tumor of the adrenal medulla or other areas. The laboratory diagnosis of this type of hypertension involves measurement of plasma levels of catecholamines, epinephrine, and norepinephrine, as well as 24-hour urinary measurement of the total levels of the catecholamines and their metabolites—metanephrine, vanillylmandelic acid (VMA), and homovanillylmandelic acid (HVA). Scanning of the perirenal areas by means of intravenous pyelography, nephrotomography, and computerized tomography helps in the anatomic localization of the tumor. Arteriography may also be a necessity. Once a tumor has been identified, it is removed surgically.

2. Primary aldosteronism, which results from the secretion of aldosterone by small adrenocortical tumors. The laboratory diagnosis is difficult. Hypokalemia is frequently a clue. Plasma renin activity and serum and urine levels of aldosterone are measured. In primary aldosteronism one would expect to find elevated urinary and plasma levels of aldosterone and decreased (suppressed) plasma renin activity. Anatomic confirmation of an adrenocortical tumor is difficult because of its small size.

The majority of cases of hypertension in adults involve no clearly defined cause; hence the diagnostic label "idiopathic" or "essential" hypertension. In such a setting, after completion of screening studies, drug therapy is instituted.

EIGHT Diagnostic tests for gastrointestinal disorders

ANATOMY AND PHYSIOLOGY

The gastrointestinal (GI) system begins in the oral cavity and ends in the anal orifice. Accessory organs, either located in the main digestive tract or opening into it, including the salivary glands, the liver, the gallbladder, the pancreas, and the appendix, as shown in Fig. 8-1.

The digestive system forms a tube that runs through the ventral cavities of the body. It is, therefore, possible with fiberoptic endoscopes to directly visualize a good portion of the GI tract. In addition, laboratory studies can be directed toward the GI functions: propelling the nutritional items from the oral cavity to the different parts of the digestive tract and breaking down these nutritional items into absorbable units through the secretion of digestive enzymes.

The anatomy and physiology of each major accessory organ will be discussed separately in this chapter.

LABORATORY TESTS FOR GASTROINTESTINAL DISEASES (GENERAL OBSERVATIONS)

A study of the gastrointestinal system involves not only the main digestive tract but the accessory organs as well. In this chapter diagnostic laboratory tests are discussed under each division of the digestive tract and under each major accessory organ. A few general observations follow.

Radiologic examination

Radiologic examination involves the introduction of a contrast medium into the gastrointestinal tract (barium enema, barium swallow, oral cholecystography) or into the circulatory system (selective angiography) so that the outlines of structures or pathologic conditions can be observed on x-ray film.

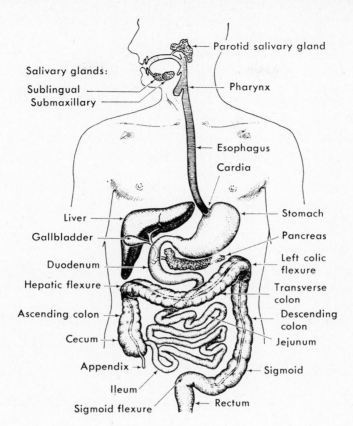

Salivary glands:

Sublingual

Submaxillary

Parotid salivary gland

Pharynx

Esophagus

Cardia

Liver

Gallbladder

Duodenum

Hepatic flexure

Ascending colon

Cecum

Appendix

Ileum

Sigmoid flexure

Stomach

Pancreas

Left colic flexure

Transverse colon

Descending colon

Jejunum

Sigmoid

Rectum

Fig. 8-1

The gastrointestinal system and its accessory organs. (From Schottelius, B.A., and Schottelius, D.D.: Textbook of physiology, ed. 17, St. Louis, 1973, The C.V. Mosby Co.)

If a thorough study of the GI tract is necessary, the most convenient procedure is to perform an oral cholecystogram first, followed by a barium enema and then an upper GI radiographic series.

The upper GI series is performed for the purpose of visualizing the esophagus, stomach, and duodenum. A small-bowel examination may be performed at the same session by requiring the patient to drink additional barium. The barium swallow is specific for visualization of the esophagus and involves various techniques to study the cardioesophageal junction and the mucosal pattern of the esophagus, and to demonstrate the presence of foreign bodies, hiatal hernia, or gastroesophageal reflux.

Before any radiologic studies are performed, the dangers of introducing barium into the GI tract should be considered as well as the risks involved in preparing a patient for the procedure. The use of strong cathartics in the presence of obstructing lesions of the colon or small intestine or in the presence of active ulcerative colitis may be hazardous or life threatening. The preparation of the patient or the introduction of the barium may aggravate acute ulcerative colitis or cause a partial obstruction to become complete.

A major disadvantage of contrast barium studies in the presence of gastrointestinal bleeding is that it does not allow a physician to associate an observed lesion with the bleeding site. If lesions are multiple, then the bleeding site should be established by endoscopy. Two other disadvantages are that barium contrast material in the GI tract may interfere with other tests until the barium has been passed out and that, in cases of obstruction, the barium may be difficult to get rid of.

Study of various gastrointestinal secretions

Examination of the contents and secretions of the various digestive organs can provide valuable information about how well they are functioning. Gastric analysis, for example, provides information about the secretory output of the stomach. Duodenal drainage with stimulation of the gallbladder or the pancreas evaluates secretions from these organs. Fecal examination helps a physician to evaluate the absorptive function of the gastrointestinal tract, by determining the amount of fecal fat and the levels of electrolytes, and to check for the presence of bacteria and parasites.

Such tests will be discussed in detail under each organ heading in this chapter.

Direct visualization (endoscopy)

The fiberoptic endoscope allows direct visualization of otherwise inaccessible structures, and the usual endoscopic procedures can be performed easily and with little hazard and discomfort to the patient.

The fiberoptic endoscope consists of bundles of thin, flexible, transparent fibers through which light can be transmitted to different regions of the gastrointestinal tract. The light from a light source is transmitted down some of the fibers; from the illuminated area the light is then reflected back up the remaining fibers to produce an image. The modern endoscope has a tip deflection of 180 degrees and is equipped with channels to permit the passage of biopsy forceps, cytology brushes, irrigating or injecting cannulas, snares, and/or cauteries, which help a physician to perform the following procedures:

1. Biopsies of various organs
2. Collection of cytologic specimens

3. Polypectomy by snaring and electrocauterization
4. Cannulation of the ampule of Vater for retrograde cholangiography to visualize the bile duct or for pancreatography, which involves the injection of contrast material to visualize the pancreatic ducts
5. Sphincterotomy—that is, the widening of a sphincter. For example, the sphincter of Oddi (the common opening of the pancreatic and biliary ducts to the duodenum) could be widened to allow passage of biliary calculi.
6. Retrieval of ingested foreign objects
7. Cauterization of sites of internal bleeding, either in the usual way or, in the near future, by means of laser beams

Motility and pressure studies

Manometric studies are particularly valuable in evaluating esophageal function. An esophageal manometer is an instrument used to measure the pressure gradients generated by peristalsis as the peristaltic wave progresses from the hypopharynx to the stomach. Abnormal pressure determinations can be helpful in diagnosing a number of disease entities, such as achalasia, esophageal spasm, or collagen vascular diseases (scleroderma or dermatomyositis), that involve the esophagus.

Colonic motility studies are still in the experimental stages.

Pressure recordings of the sphincter of Oddi may be helpful in diagnosing biliary spasm.

THE ESOPHAGUS

Anatomy and physiology

The esophagus (Fig. 8-1) extends from the pharynx to the stomach and has no secretory function. It is a flexible, muscular tube, about 10 inches long, through which a bolus of food is propelled after having been swallowed. An initial peristaltic wave originates in the pharynx, and secondary peristaltic waves originate in the esophagus if food still remains there. The lower end of the esophagus acts as a physiologic sphincter to prevent the reflux of food from the stomach.

Pathophysiology

One of the more common causes of esophageal pain is acid reflux, which leads to irritation of the lower esophagus. This condition results from weakness of the cardioesophageal sphincter. Persistent reflux produces an irritated, inflamed, and friable esophagus. Bleeding, esophagitis, and ulceration may result. Often, a hiatal hernia coexists with the reflux.

Laboratory tests for esophageal disease

The barium swallow, motility tests, and upper-GI endoscopy have already been described on p. 190. By far the majority of esophageal problems are diagnosed by these methods. Esophageal manometry helps evaluate motor abnormalities of the esophagus. Cytologic examination is a helpful diagnostic adjunct, provided it is done skillfully, with proper collection of specimens, and by an experienced examiner.

The sequence of tests used to examine the esophagus usually begins with the barium swallow. If that is not diagnostic, the examiner proceeds to endoscopy and, if necessary, to the tests described below.

Bernstein test (acid perfusion test)

The Bernstein test demonstrates reflux esophagitis. Hydrochloric acid (HCl) 0.1% is started as a drip into the esophagus after normal saline has first been used. The production of symptoms in the patient within a half-hour after the HCl drip starts is indicative of esophagitis.

In order to verify whether or not the HCl is causing the esophageal symptoms, the drip should be switched to saline without the patient's knowledge as soon as pain develops. The distress should disappear after a few minutes and reappear again when the HCl drip is reinstated (again, without the patient's knowledge).

Test for esophageal acidity

A pH electrode attached to a manometric catheter and placed in the esophagus provides the most accurate way of measuring esophageal acidity.

When the lower esophageal sphincter has been located manometrically, the pH catheter and the manometer are withdrawn to a level 2 cm above the sphincter. The patient is then asked to perform a Valsalva maneuver, to lift his legs, or to sniff vigorously. If no reflux is demonstrated, approximately 300 ml of HCl 0.1% is introduced into the stomach via cannula. Then the maneuvers just described for the production of reflux are repeated, and the pH of the esophagus is determined. Normally, the pH is 5 to 6; it drops to 1.5 to 2 with acid reflux.

Clinical application of laboratory tests
Esophagitis

Esophagitis usually results from the irritating effect of reflux of gastric juice from the stomach into the lower part of the esophagus.

Laboratory tests. The most common laboratory tests employed in the diagnosis of reflux esophagitis are radiologic studies demonstrating reflux of a contrast material, the Bernstein acid perfusion test, and the demonstration of esophageal acidity.

Differential diagnosis. Coronary heart disease is important in the differential diagnosis of reflux esophagitis, with the clinical history being the most helpful. In reflux esophagitis a radiologic diagnosis of hiatal hernia is frequently made. However, the mere demonstration of hiatal hernia is not necessarily an indication that reflux exists; nor does it necessarily indicate that the symptoms produced are a result of the hiatal hernia, since hiatal hernia can be found in asymptomatic individuals.

Esophagoscopy and biopsy are important in studying chronic esophagitis, since this condition is not always the result of chronic acid reflux. It may be caused by a fungal or viral disease or even by a neoplastic process. Therefore, esophageal biopsy is mandatory.

Diffuse esophageal spasm

Diffuse esophageal spasm is probably the second most common of the esophageal diseases. A disorder of esophageal motility, it has various causes, including reflux esophagitis.

Laboratory tests. The diagnosis is usually made radiologically, with a cine-esophagogram that shows the disturbed segmental contractions without a peristaltic wave in the distal esophagus. The disorder can be confirmed with manometric pressure studies of the various parts of the esophagus.

Differential diagnosis. Diffuse esophageal spasm is commonly associated with aging (presbyesophagus), ganglion degeneration (seen in the early stages of achalasia), mucosal irritation (usually secondary to gastroesophageal reflux), obstruction of the cardia, and neuromuscular disorders (diabetic neuropathy and amyotrophic lateral sclerosis). Or the condition may be idiopathic.

Achalasia

Achalasia is a motor disorder, the symptoms of which appear to reflect impaired cholineric innervation of the esophagus.

Laboratory tests. The diagnosis is made by means of radiologic contrast studies, showing abnormal esophageal motor function caused by a characteristic beaklike narrowing of the distal esophageal segment, and by means of esophageal manometry, showing markedly increased lower esophageal sphincter pressure.

Differential diagnosis. Carcinoma of the lower esophagus and adenocarcinoma of the stomach with extension to the esophagus are sometimes difficult to differentiate radiologically from achalasia. Endoscopic study with biopsy is most helpful in the differential diagnosis.

Scleroderma (progressive systemic sclerosis)

Scleroderma involves the esophagus in approximately 80% of cases; it is characterized by decreased esophageal peristalsis, mainly in the lower third of the esophagus.

Dermatomyositis

Dermatomyositis is characterized by oropharyngeal dysphagia (including difficulty in propelling the bolus from the mouth to the esophagus) and decreased pressures of the upper esophageal sphincter, as shown by manometry.

Neurologic conditions

Neurologic conditions may possibly affect deglutition. One must be aware of the possibility of myasthenia gravis in deglutition problems. Edrophonium chloride (Tensilon) can be used for diagnostic testing. If the muscular weakness is caused by myasthenia gravis, the edrophonium injection will produce prompt relief.

Carcinoma of the esophagus

Carcinoma of the esophagus is mainly squamous cell carcinoma when it occurs in the upper or middle portion of the esophagus; in the lower portion, it can also be adenocarcinoma. The incidence of carcinoma of the esophagus is increased in smokers and heavy alcohol drinkers. The most common symptom is dysphagia.

The diagnosis is usually made by barium examination and by endoscopy and biopsy.

THE STOMACH

Anatomy and physiology

The relationship of the stomach to the rest of the digestive tract, the liver, and the pancreas is shown in Fig. 8-1. After food enters the stomach, it is stored, mixed with gastric juice, and then slowly emptied into the small intestine through the pyloric sphincter.

The gastric juice is secreted by the gastric glands in the walls of the stomach. Gastric juice is normally clear, pale yellow, and of high acidity, with a pH of about 1.0. It is 97% to 99% water, 0.2% to 0.5% hydrochloric acid, with the remainder consisting of mucin, electrolytes, and pepsin.

The stimulation of gastric secretion is divided into three phases: cephalic (psychic), gastric, and intestinal. When no stimuli are present, gastric secretion still occurs and is termed "basal."

Cephalic stimulation results from the sight, smell, taste, or thought of food. Vagal impulses will then directly stimulate the parietal cells to secrete HCl and the mucosa of the antrum to secrete the hormone gastrin.

In the gastric phase partially digested protein and the distention of the antrum stimulate the release of gastrin. Gastrin is absorbed into the blood and carried back to the stomach to potently stimulate gastric acid secretion. It also moderately stimulates pepsinogen secretion and gastric and intestinal motility, as well as enhances sphincter mechanisms of the esophagus. When the pH of the gastric juice reaches 2.0, gastrin secretion usually stops.

The intestinal phase appears to be a more complex mechanism, involving the release of intestinal gastrin and the inhibition of gastric secretion by various other hormones, which interrelate with gastrin or directly inhibit or stimulate gastric acid secretion.

Pathophysiology

The total gastric HCl secretion is determined by the parietal cell mass—the number of parietal cells present and functioning. It has been shown that patients with duodenal ulcer have a secretion of HCl that is almost twice normal. Gastric ulcer patients secrete less acid than normal, and gastric cancer patients secrete less still.

Laboratory tests
Tests for gastric acid analysis

Gastric acid studies are done for the following reasons:
1. To determine whether a patient is able to secrete acid. Such a determination is done to establish the differential diagnosis of pernicious anemia and gastric ulcer. In these conditions very little gastric acid is secreted.
2. To determine how much acid a patient secretes. Such a determination is indicated in rare conditions in which the clinical diagnosis strongly suggests peptic ulcer disease in spite of an equivocal upper GI series. A high basal secretion (10 mEq/hr or more) is suggestive of active peptic ulcer disease. Very high secretory rates of acid are seen in tumors that secrete gastrin (as in Zollinger-Ellison syndrome).
3. To determine the type of surgery necessary. In hypersecretors, there is increased risk of stomal ulcer following ordinary gastric resection without vagotomy. If the patient is still having symptoms after a vagotomy for peptic ulcer, the completeness of the vagotomy should be ascertained by means of a Hollander test, which is explained below.

Determination of basal secretion rate. The basal secretion rate is determined to ascertain how much acid a patient secretes without stimulation to do so. The patient is intubated under fluoroscopic visualization. The gastric contents are then aspirated continuously for 2 hours, with the aspirate being titrated at half-hour intervals. A secretion rate of 6 mEq/hr or more is indicative of hypersecretion. A secretion rate of 15 mEq/hr or more should lead one to suspect a hormonal abnormality affecting the parietal cells.

♦ Normal basal acid output (BAO)

0-6 mEq/hr

Augmented gastric secretion test. A gastric secretion stimulation test should immediately follow the basal secretion test, since the capacity of the gastric cells to secrete, on a particular occasion, may not be significant in the basal state. In this test, gastric secretion is stimulated by means of an injection of histamine or Histalog (or pentagastrin, which is safer than Histalog). A secretion rate of 50 mEq/hr or more indicates hypersecretion. The specimens are collected as in the basal state. This is a useful test to confirm the achlorhydria of pernicious anemia and in the diagnosis of Zollinger-Ellison syndrome.

Diagnex blue test. By means of a Diagnex blue test, the presence or absence of acid can be determined without intubation. This test involves the ingestion of a tablet of caffeine followed by a dye (Diagnex blue) and an exchange resin. If the gastric contents have a pH of 3.0 or less, dye is released from the resin and excreted in the urine. If the results of this test are negative or inconclusive, a gastric stimulation test is indicated.

Saline load test. This is a test to evaluate gastric outlet obstruction. A nasogastric Levin tube is inserted into the stomach. The gastric residue is aspirated and measured. Then 750 ml of 0.9% (normal) saline is instilled. After 30 minutes the gastric contents are again aspirated and measured. If more than 400 ml of fluid is still present in the stomach, gastric outlet obstruction should be suspected.

Hollander insulin test. This test is performed in order to determine whether a complete vagotomy has been performed or not. The test is based on the fact that insulin-induced hypoglycemia stimulates vagal centers because of their direct communication with the anterior hypothalamus. A 2-hour basal gastric analysis is performed, and a blood glucose analysis is done. The patient is then given an intravenous injection of insulin to produce hypoglycemia, and specimens of gastric juice are collected every 15 minutes for the next 2 hours. When symptoms of hypoglycemia appear, a second blood glucose analysis is done. The level should fall to 50% of the initial, fasting level. If any measurement of the gastric secretion in the first two postinsulin hours exceeds that of the higher of the 2 basal hours (pre-insulin fasting stage, two determinations) the vagotomy is incomplete.

The safety of the Hollander test is in question; risk factors should be considered before patients are selected for this kind of stimulation.

Gastric analysis using calcium infusion. The differential diagnosis between hypersecretory states with and without inappropriate gastrin production can be made by performing the gastric analysis while the patient is receiving a calcium infusion. In this procedure serum gastrin levels are measured in the basal state and then again during calcium infusion. If the secretion of gastric acid approaches maximal levels and the serum gastrin levels rise appreciably with the calcium infusion, ectopic gastrin production, such as is seen in Zollinger-Ellison syndrome, should be suspected.

Gastric analysis using secretin. This is another test performed to differentiate Zollinger-Ellison syndrome from hypersecretory states that do not involve inappropriate secretion of gastrin. Secretin is given intravenously and should cause a decrease in acid secretion. However, in Zollinger-Ellison syndrome the acid secretion is increased and the serum gastrin level rises.

Determination of serum gastrin level. Gastrin is a polypeptide secreted by the gastric antrum; the secretion of gastrin in turn stimulates acid secretion by the parietal cells of the stomach. In the normal situation gastric acid inhibits further secretion of gastrin, by means of a feedback mechanism.

A marked elevation of the serum gastrin level occurs in pernicious anemia. This elevation reflects the characteristic failure of patients with this disorder to secrete gastric hydrochloric acid.

There is significant diminution of the secretion of gastric acid in gastric carcinoma. Thus, because of the mechanism of feedback already mentioned, there is increased gastrin secretion.

In Zollinger-Ellison syndrome there is a characteristically severe gastrinemia. In this syndrome excessive amounts of gastrin are secreted by tumors of the gastrointestinal tract. These tumors produce gastrin independently of the normal feedback mechanism. So, although there is high gastric acidity, which would normally suppress gastrin secretion, there is an extremely high serum gastrin level, which indicates an autonomous production of gastrin.

In Zollinger-Ellison syndrome, stimulation of gastrin production can be accomplished by means of intravenous infusions of calcium and secretin. The response to the calcium infusion is a markedly elevated serum gastrin level. The response to secretin infusion in normal situations is a diminution of the serum gastrin level, but in Zollinger-Ellison syndrome there is a paradoxical rise in serum gastrin level.

♦ Normal serum gastrin

20-100 pg/ml

Endoscopy of the upper gastrointestinal tract

The general principle of endoscopy has been discussed on p. 190.

Endoscopy is one of the most effective ways of examining the upper gastrointestinal tract when a physician is looking for bleeding sites or when a histologic diagnosis of lesions of the stomach or duodenum is needed.

Patient preparation. Prior to most elective upper GI endoscopic examinations, the patient should take nothing by mouth for a 6- to 8-hour period. In emergency procedures, particularly in patients with upper GI bleeding, gastric lavage becomes necessary to aid in visualization.

Prior to endoscopy, a local anesthetic is frequently administered to the pharynx, and the patient is frequently sedated with intravenously administered diazepam (Valium) and/or meperidine (Demerol). After endoscopy it is advisable that the patient eat nothing until the anesthetic wears off and that his condition be monitored closely, with particular attention being given to respiratory function.

Clinical application of laboratory tests
Gastritis

The most common disorder of the stomach is probably superficial gastritis resulting from ingestion of irritants such as aspirin and/or alcohol, stress, or acid hypersecretion.

The diagnosis of gastritis is usually made by endoscopy, since superficial gastritis may not be visualized by barium studies. The acutely inflamed, edematous mucosa can easily be seen with a gastroscope, and the condition can be confirmed by gastric biopsy.

Gastric ulcer disease

Gastric ulcer disease is probably less common than gastritis.

Laboratory tests. The diagnosis depends on radiologic and endoscopic examinations. The combination of these two tests brings the diagnostic accuracy up to approximately 90% or 95%.

Differential diagnosis. In the differentiation between benign and malignant gastric ulcer, radiologic examination of the stomach is an important diagnostic aid.

The diagnostic value of cytologic examination of the gastric juice depends on the expertise of the pathologist. Accuracy varies from 30% to 80%. The yield is greater when the specimen is obtained during endoscopy.

Gastric acid examination is of some help. If true histamine-fast achlorhydria is present, there is no good, reassuring way of ruling out the diagnosis of carcinoma. However, the presence of acid does not necessarily rule out carcinoma either.

The most accurate way of diagnosing gastric ulcer is to perform an endoscopic examination of the upper gastrointestinal tract. Biopsy specimens and brushings for cytologic studies should be obtained, so that the examiner can differentiate a benign ulcer from a malignant ulcer.

Duodenal peptic ulcer

X-ray contrast barium study is very helpful in diagnosing duodenal ulcer. The demonstration of a crater on the films is the main characteristic of peptic ulcer disease. Endoscopy, however, is the most definitive way of making the diagnosis.

Gastric analysis is usually not important in ordinary ulcer disease, with two possible exceptions: (1) The presence of histamine-fast achlorhydria makes peptic ulcer disease very unlikely. (2) In severe peptic ulcer disease the gastric acid secretion rate may be important, particularly to differentiate it from Zollinger-Ellison syndrome, which causes severe gastric acid hypersecretion.

Stomal or gastrojejunal ulceration

Because of the altered anatomy after gastric surgery, a large proportion of stomal ulcers cannot be visualized radiographically. However, the stoma and the ulceration can be visualized quite easily with the aid of a gastroscope.

Zollinger-Ellison syndrome

Zollinger-Ellison syndrome is caused by the hypersecretion of gastrin by adenomas of the gastrointestinal tract, usually non-beta islet cell tumors of the pancreas (gastrin-producing adenomas). The syndrome is characterized by profound gastric acid hypersecretion that typically causes severe, malignant peptic ulceration.

An inappropriately high output of gastric acid, both in the basal and in the Histalog-stimulated states, is seen in this condition. If equivocal rises are seen, gastric acid measurements and serum gastrin determinations should be performed following calcium or secretin stimulation (as described on p. 197).

Complications of peptic ulcer

Hemorrhage. In hemorrhage of the upper gastrointestinal tract, it is essential to locate the site of bleeding. Thus a vigorous, aggressive diagnostic approach is recommended. It is negligent to assume that the bleeding is from esophageal varices when the patient has cirrhosis of the liver. The bleeding might be a result of a gastric ulcer or a duodenal ulcer.

Intubation of the stomach should be performed for every patient with GI bleeding. This will help determine whether the bleeding is from the upper part of the intestinal tract. If blood or "coffee ground" material is noted on aspiration, the stomach should be lavaged with iced saline. Following this, an attempt should be made to locate the source of the bleeding, preferably by endoscopy. If endoscopy is not possible, an emergency GI radiographic series should be performed.

Perforation. Of patients with perforated ulcers, 85% have free air under the diaphragm that can be detected by x-ray examination of the abdomen both when the patient is in a reclining position and when he is in an upright position. It should be noted, however, that the absence of free air under the diaphragm does not necessarily rule out perforation.

An elevated serum amylase level correlating with the clinical picture is extremely suggestive of perforation.

Occasionally, in equivocal cases, a perforation may be identified through the use of water-soluble contrast material (Gastrografin).

Gastric outlet obstruction. Obstruction of the gastric outlet may result from any of a number of conditions. Ulceration and edema near the pylorus, scarring of the pyloric channel, and tumors are the most common ones.

Symptoms commonly seen are vomiting, abdominal distention, and (occasionally) pain. During physical examination a succussion splash and visible peristalsis are helpful diagnostic clues.

Diagnosis is made by nasogastric aspiration and measurement of gastric residue. If, 4 hours after eating, the gastric residue is greater than 300 ml, or if the overnight gastric residue is greater than 200 ml, a saline load test is performed.

X-ray film frequently shows the stomach to be large and distended. Endoscopic and/or barium contrast studies should then be considered. However, before any of these diagnostic studies are performed, it is always advisable to decompress and cleanse the stomach.

Gastric carcinoma

Adenocarcinoma of the stomach presents either as an ulcer or as a mass lesion. For unknown reasons, the incidence of this cancer is on the decline.

An upper GI series, with barium, and endoscopy, with biopsy and cytologic studies, are the means of making the diagnosis. Hyposecretion of gastric acid is frequently seen, though not diagnostic, and elevations in the serum level of carcinoembryonic antigen may be seen in this type of cancer, as in other carcinomas of the GI tract.

THE SMALL INTESTINE

Anatomy and physiology

The small intestine is a tube approximately 1 inch in diameter and 20 feet in length. The duodenum, the first segment of the small intestine, begins at the pyloric end of the stomach; it can be seen in Fig. 8-1, in the shape of a C around the pancreas. The jejunum and the ileum constitute the rest of the small bowel.

The chyme is propelled through the small bowel by segmentation contractions and peristalsis, and digestion is completed by the action of the intestinal juices.

Through the process of digestion nutrients are reduced to simple components for transport across the intestinal mucosa to the portal blood system. Fingerlike projections called villi and microvilli on the surface of the intestine increase the area of the absorbing surface to about 600 times that of an ordinary tube of equal length and circumference.

Only the salient features of fat, protein, and carbohydrate digestion and absorption will be mentioned here.

The principal lipid, triglyceride, is digested in the duodenum and jejunum in the presence of bile salts and lipase (a pancreatic enzyme).

Protein digestion and absorption require a pH of about 6.5. In the duodenum, protein stimulates the release of secretin and pancreozymin, which in turn causes the release of bicarbonate and the pancreatic proteases.

Carbohydrate digestion takes place (1) in the duodenum, by reaction with amylase from the pancreas, and (2) on the brush border of the cells of the intestinal mucosa, by the action of disaccharidase.

Absorption of the hematopoietic factors—iron, folate, and vitamin B_{12}—also requires specialized processes.

Pathophysiology

Intrinsic intestinal disease will cause malabsorption syndrome, and so will any failure of the liver and gallbladder to secrete bile acid or the pancreas to secrete its enzymes. For example, inadequate levels of bile salts or lipase will cause maldigestion of lipid and an acid pH. Malabsorption of protein may result from inadequate secretion of pancreatic enzymes. Carbohydrate malabsorption can be the result of a deficiency of brush-border disaccharidase.

Laboratory tests
Stool examination

Stool examination for ova, parasites, and occult blood is very helpful. Cultures will determine the presence of bacterial infection or overgrowth, and microscopic examination for meat fibers and fat aids in the diagnosis of malabsorption.

Determination of fecal fat content

Determination of fecal fat content is the best screening test for overall malabsorption syndrome. The total 24-hour fecal fat content should be less than 6 gm, given a daily intake of 75 to 100 gm of fat. If it is more than 6 gm, malabsorption is indicated. However, this test does not differentiate between true malabsorption and maldigestion.

Inadequate specimen collection should be suspected if a 3-day stool weight is less than 300 gm.

Serum carotene level and prothrombin time

Since absorption of the fat-soluble vitamins is impaired in fat-malabsorptive states, serum carotene levels and prothrombin time are diminished. The abnormal bleeding time results from vitamin K deficiency.

D-Xylose absorption test

The D-xylose absorption test is a useful one; a positive result usually indicates intrinsic intestinal disease. D-xylose is normally not metabolized; it is absorbed intact and excreted via the kidneys. This compound is given orally, after which urine is collected for a 5-hour period. Provided the patient has good renal function, a decreased amount of D-xylose in the urine implies malabsorption of the compound. It is important to hydrate the patient well during the test, to get an adequate urinary output and thus minimize error.

Lactose tolerance test

A lactose tolerance test will identify persons who are unable to digest lactose because of insufficient levels of intestinal lactase. A fasting blood glucose level is determined, and 100 gm of lactose is given orally. Normally there is a rise in the blood glucose level of at least 20 mg/dl within a 2-hour period. Failure of the level to rise suggests low levels of intestinal lactase.

X-ray films

Barium studies of the small bowel are extremely helpful in providing clues to the diagnosis of celiac disease, regional enteritis, lymphomas, fistulas, and so on.

Biopsy

Biopsy of the small intestine is done by having the patient swallow a biopsy capsule attached to a tube; the capsule is eventually passed, under fluoroscopic control, into the jejunum. At this point a biopsy specimen of the jejunal mucosa is obtained by suctioning the mucosa against the biopsy capsule and moving the cutting blade of the capsule to sever a piece of tissue.

Clinical value. This test is most important in diagnosing malabsorption resulting from celiac sprue; diseases of the small bowel that affect the shape, size, and configuration of the villi; and infiltrative diseases of the bowel, such as amyloidosis, lymphomas, and mastocytosis.

In addition to tissue examination of the biopsy specimens, the intestinal cells can be assayed for disaccharidase activity. This would help a physician determine if there are deficiencies of lactase, sucrase, or isomaltase. These deficiencies may be either congenital or secondary to intrinsic small bowel disease.

Secretin test

The secretin test can be helpful in differentiating between malabsorption secondary to pancreatic disease and that resulting from intrinsic intestinal disease. Secretin is a polypeptide that stimulates the production of pancreatic fluid that is high in bicarbonate content but low in enzyme content. After the passage of a double-lumen tube for separate gastric and duodenal aspiration, secretin is given intravenously. The gastric and duodenal contents are collected separately, with the latter being analyzed for volume, bicarbonate content, and amylase activity. A volume of less than 1.5 ml/kg body weight per 30 minutes, or a bicarbonate concentration less than 70 mEq/L after stimulation indicates subnormal pancreatic function. Cytologic examination of the aspirate may be helpful in the diagnosis of carcinoma.

Flat film of the abdomen

In addition to the secretin test, a flat film of the abdomen that permits visualization of pancreatic calcification is extremely helpful in differentiating chronic pancreatitis from intrinsic intestinal disease as a possible cause of steatorrhea and malabsorption.

Celiac angiogram

A celiac angiogram often shows a pancreatic tumor or a pancreatic cyst secondary to pancreatitis to be the cause of malabsorption.

Schilling test for vitamin B$_{12}$ absorption

Ingested vitamin B$_{12}$ combines with intrinsic factor, secreted by the stomach, to pass into the distal portion of the ileum, where it is absorbed.

In the conventional Schilling test the patient is first given 1000 mg of vitamin B$_{12}$ intramuscularly to saturate the body stores and then is given a test dose of radioactive vitamin B_{12} orally. Assuming the patient has normal renal function (which should be checked prior to this test), at least 7% of the radioactive B_{12} will be excreted in the urine within 24 hours of its injection. An excretion of less than that amount indicates decreased absorption.

Pitfalls. Deficiencies of intrinsic factor may produce low test results. Thus the same procedure just described, with the addition of the administration of intrinsic factor, is necessary in patients who have pernicious anemia or who have had gastric resections. The results of the Schilling test may also be misleadingly abnormal in conditions of bacterial overgrowth of the small bowel, because of binding of the B_{12} by bacteria. In such a situation antibiotic treatment before the test corrects the problem.

Once these conditions have been compensated for, the examiner will be able to tell whether the patient is actually absorbing the vitamin B_{12}.

Bile acid breath test

The bile acid breath test is a sensitive, relatively new method of detecting malabsorption and/or small bowel bacterial overgrowth.

Most of the bile acids secreted in bile are reabsorbed in the distal portion of the small bowel and recirculated. Bile acids not absorbed enter the colon, where bacteria deconjugate and metabolize different portions of the bile acid molecules, eventually producing CO_2.

If a small tracer amount of radioactive (^{14}C) bile salt is given by mouth, it should, under normal circumstances, be absorbed in the small bowel and enter the bile salt pool. If small bowel disease exists or bacterial overgrowth of the small bowel is present, then the radioactive bile salt will be metabolized by the bacteria and $^{14}CO_2$ will be produced. Eventually the $^{14}CO_2$ will be extracted by the lungs. Thus by assaying the breath for radioactivity one can determine whether small bowel disease or bacterial overgrowth is present.

Under normal conditions practically no $^{14}CO_2$ should be present in the breath.

Tissue typing

A large number of patients who have inflammatory bowel disease, particularly in association with joint disorders such as arthralgias and arthritis, have tissue type HLA-B27. Thus, tissue typing may identify members of certain genetic subgroups that are susceptible to inflammatory bowel disease.

Clinical application of laboratory tests
Malabsorption syndrome

The motility of the small intestine and its total surface area are factors in its absorptive capabilities, as are adequate pancreatic and biliary secretions.

Thus, malabsorption syndromes are divided into two major categories: (1) those resulting from intrinsic disease of the wall of the small intestine, with normal digestion but abnormal absorption because of the lesions of the bowel wall, and (2) those caused by digestive problems related to pancreatic insufficiency or to bile acid secretory problems, either of which can lead to delayed or inadequate absorption.

The initial screening test is a peripheral blood film to check for early folate deficiency. Low serum levels of iron, vitamin B_{12}, and folate will confirm the deficiency. The absorption of vitamin D and calcium may be evaluated through an estimation of serum calcium, phosphorus, and alkaline phosphatase levels. Vitamin K absorption is evaluated by determination of the prothrombin time. A low level of serum albumin may reflect malabsorption of protein or protein-losing enteropathy. A low serum carotene level may indicate malabsorption of fat if dietary intake of carotene is adequate.

All of the more specific tests of malabsorption are described on pp. 202-204.

Inflammatory intestinal disease (regional enteritis, or Crohn's disease)

Initial suspicion of this disease occurs as a result of chronic intermittent diarrhea, fever, crampy abdominal pain, joint pains, and abdominal masses revealed by physical examination. Perianal ulceration and stricture are quite common.

Nonspecific laboratory findings are leukocytosis, blood loss, anemia, undernutrition, hypoalbuminemia, hypocalcemia, hypokalemia, elevated erythrocyte sedimentation rate, elevated serum alkaline phosphatase level, hypoprothrombinemia, and macrocytic anemia.

The radiologic picture, along with the clinical suspicion, usually establishes the diagnosis. It can be definitely established histologically. Fistulous tracts are common, particularly in the ileocecal region, and are virtually pathognomonic.

Biopsies of the small intestine and lymph nodes, obtained surgically, can provide adequate bases for microscopic diagnosis and can be used to rule out tuberculosis, various lymphomas, sarcoidosis, and fungous diseases. When the disease process involves the colon along with the small bowel, biopsies can also be obtained from the colon, by sigmoidoscopy or colonoscopy.

Acute intestinal obstruction

The causes of intestinal obstruction are numerous, but they can be divided into three categories:

1. Intrinsic bowel lesions, such as congenital abnormalities, atresia, stenosis, or benign or malignant tumors

2. Obturation obstruction, caused by bezoars, parasites, gallstones, meconium, or intussusception
3. Extrinsic bowel lesions, such as adhesions, volvulus, or hernias

Laboratory tests. Taking flat films of the abdomen is the single most important examination method in suspected cases of intestinal obstruction. From the type of lumen pattern, the level of obstruction can more or less be determined: air-fluid levels are a hallmark of obstruction. If the symptoms are acute and the obstruction is suspected to be low in the intestine, barium should not be given orally. If the obstruction is thought to be in the colon, then a carefully administered barium enema may be used to demonstrate the obstructive lesion.

The other laboratory findings in cases of intestinal obstruction are nonspecific signs of inflammation, such as leukocytosis, elevation of the lactic dehydrogenase level, mild elevation of the amylase level, and electrolyte abnormalities.

Differential diagnosis. The differential diagnosis includes paralytic ileus and intestinal pseudo-obstruction. Laboratory tests are usually not helpful in differentiating these conditions from mechanical obstruction. One helpful clue can be found, however, during physical examination. In both of the first two conditions bowel sounds are significantly diminished, while in mechanical obstruction one can hear high-pitched bowel sounds that come in rushes.

Mesenteric arterial insufficiency

The mesenteric arteries supply the splanchnic area. Atherosclerotic or other degenerative changes in these arteries or in the celiac axis can produce pain that is steady and agonizing. Mucosal changes and mural deterioration lead to malabsorption, causing weight loss and other symptoms of malabsorption.

Vascular insufficiency in elderly patients may contribute significantly to malabsorption. The syndrome in these patients may be at the subclinical level and thus be undetected if it is not looked for particularly.

To evaluate the vascular integrity of the gastrointestinal tract, celiac angiograms and superior and inferior mesenteric angiograms are quite helpful in certain cases.

THE COLON

Anatomy and physiology

The large intestine is 5 to 6 feet in length and 2½ inches in diameter. It begins as the cecum and proceeds in turn as the ascending colon, the transverse colon, the descending colon, the sigmoid colon, the rectum and the anal canal (Fig. 8-1). The functions of the colon are the absorption of water and electrolytes from the chyme and the storage and elimination of the waste products of digestion.

Laboratory tests for diseases of the large intestine
Radiologic examination —barium enema

Radiologic examination of the colon is a most important diagnostic tool. It should be noted, however, that acutely ill patients do not tolerate well the necessary preparation for a barium enema. If a patient is not acutely ill, a diagnosis can be determined by a simple barium enema or by an air-contrast barium enema, which is even more diagnostic. The barium enema is employed for the possible diagnosis of malignancies, benign growths, diverticular disease, and inflammatory disease of the lower gastrointestinal tract, such as ulcerative colitis. Also included in this list are the bacterial granulomatous diseases, such as tuberculous enteritis, tuberculous colitis, and amebic colitis.

In some of these conditions, a specific diagnosis can be made fairly well by means of the barium enema alone. However, a more direct visual examination and a biopsy are often necessary. Therefore, the second most important test in the examination of the colon is sigmoidoscopy, with or without colonoscopy.

Patient preparation and care. The colon is thoroughly cleansed by means of diet, cathartics, and/or enemas. If gas or feces are still present in the large intestine at the time of the examination, the procedure may have to be repeated. Hence all care should be taken to adequately prepare the patient.

Because of the danger of an impaction caused by the barium in the large bowel, cleansing enemas or laxatives may be ordered to evacuate the residual barium.

The extensive preparation may have produced dehydration. Therefore, the patient should be encouraged to take fluids, unless medically contraindicated.

Sigmoidoscopy

The rectum and sigmoid colon can be inspected by means of the conventional, rigid-tube sigmoidoscope or by means of the new fiberoptic proctosigmoidoscope. Sigmoidoscopy is used for two major reasons: (1) The lower 15 to 18 cm of the colon is difficult to visualize radiologically, particularly the sigmoid region, but is easily seen through a sigmoidoscope. (2) A definitive diagnosis in certain conditions can be achieved through biopsy under direct visualization, which is possible with sigmoidoscopy. Ulceration is seen easily, and a biopsy is the determining factor in the differential diagnosis of many bowel disorders, particularly the different types of inflammatory bowel diseases.

Colonoscopy

Recently, with the advent of the fiberoptic endoscopes, it has been possible to visualize the whole colon. Thus colonoscopy, in experienced hands, is another means by which the colon can be visualized directly and a biopsy can be taken. It may also be used therapeutically, for the removal of polyps of the large bowel.

Patient preparation for colonoscopy is similar to that for a barium enema, except that the patient is also frequently kept on a liquid diet for 2 days prior to the test, to ensure appropriate cleansing of the bowel.

Rectal biopsy

A rectal biopsy is of significant importance in certain conditions, such as inflammatory bowel diseases, amyloidosis, and some parasitic diseases (such as schistosomiasis). The specimen can be obtained by a punch technique at the time of sigmoidoscopy or by suction via a biopsy capsule.

Carcinoembryonic antigen (CEA) test

When it was first discovered, the carcinoembryonic antigen was thought to be relatively specific for carcinoma of the gastrointestinal tract, including the liver and pancreas. However, later it was found that this antigen is relatively nonspecific. In clinical practice at the present time, the role of the carcinoembryonic antigen test is restricted mainly to follow-up studies. If a patient with known carcinoma has an elevated carcinoembryonic antigen level before surgery or other therapy, and if this level rises during subsequent care, recurrence or growth of the carcinoma has probably occurred. However, since so many factors will cause an elevation, the CEA test is considered nonspecific and is not used for a definitive diagnosis of carcinoma of the gastrointestinal tract. Highest titers of this antigen are found in carcinoma of the colon and pancreas.

Clinical application of laboratory tests
Ulcerative colitis

Ulcerative colitis is a disease of unknown etiology that causes ulceration of the mucosa of the colon. It is a chronic disease, with remissions and exacerbations. Manifestations include loose bowel movements, rectal bleeding, and passage of mucus. The disease can have serious local and systemic complications, including cholangitis, arthritis, and skin manifestations.

The diagnosis is made via sigmoidoscopy and colonoscopy, by visualizing the colonic mucosa. The diagnosis can be confirmed by biopsy. A barium enema can be helpful in establishing the diagnosis. However, if ulcerative colitis is suspected before the enema, it is important to prepare the patient without laxatives, since they may exacerbate the manifestations of the disease.

Granulomatous colitis (Crohn's disease of the colon)

Granulomatous colitis is a disease of unknown etiology that can involve the entire colon; it differs from ulcerative colitis in that it also frequently involves the small bowel.

The disease is characterized by segments of inflammation, with microscopic granulomas and lymphoid hyperplasia shown by biopsy. Manifestations frequently include diarrhea, abdominal pain, weight loss, and fever; rectal bleeding is not a frequent manifestation.

The diagnosis is made radiologically, by demonstrating areas of inflammation; these areas are frequently separated by normal segments of bowel. Further documentation of the presence of the disease can be made by biopsy, with the specimen being obtained by either sigmoidoscopy or colonoscopy, depending on the accessibility of the inflamed areas.

Neoplastic diseases of the colon

Neoplastic diseases of the colon may be benign, such as polyps, or malignant. The presenting symptoms are usually a change in bowel habits, rectal bleeding, and abdominal pain.

The diagnosis is usually made radiologically with a barium enema or by endoscopy (sigmoidoscopy or colonoscopy).

THE GALLBLADDER

Anatomy and physiology

The gallbladder is a pear-shaped sac lying on the underside of the liver. Bile produced by the liver enters the gallbladder via the hepatic and cystic ducts to be concentrated and stored until needed.

During digestion, the gallbladder contracts and rapidly supplies bile to the small intestine through the common bile duct (Fig. 8-2). This contraction of the gallbladder, and also the relaxation of the sphincter muscle, occurs in response to a hormone (cholecystokinin) that is secreted by the intestine, mainly in the presence of fats.

The most common disorders of the gallbladder are gallstone disease and cholecystitis.

Laboratory tests for biliary tract disease
Flat film of the abdomen

If gallstones are calcified, they are easily seen in flat films of the abdomen. Unfortunately, most gallbladder stones are composed of cholesterol, with less than 50% being calcified; therefore, contrast studies of the gallbladder are necessary.

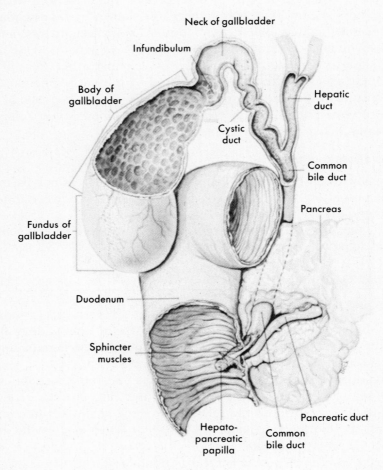

Fig. 8-2
The gallbladder and its divisions: fundus, body, infundibulum, and neck. Obstruction of either the hepatic duct or the common bile duct by stone or spasm blocks the exit of bile from the liver, where it is formed, and prevents bile from being ejected into the duodenum. (From Anthony, C.P., and Kolthoff, N.J.: Textbook of anatomy and physiology, ed. 9, St. Louis, 1975, The C.V. Mosby Co.)

Oral cholecystography

The night before oral cholecystography is to be performed, an iodine dye is given orally in order to allow time for absorption and concentration of the dye in the gallbladder, assuming normal gastrointestinal absorption and hepatic handling of the dye.

On x-ray film, calculi will frequently be demonstrated. If they are not, then a second dose of the contrast material is given. If the gallbladder still is not visualized, then, given normal absorption and hepatic function, one assumes that the gallbladder is diseased and that the lack of concentration is the result of inflammation, which is frequently associated with gallstones.

Intravenous cholangiography (IVC)

When an iodine contrast medium is given intravenously, both the biliary tree and the gallbladder can be visualized. However, since the visualization is much poorer than with oral cholecystography, tomography must frequently be used as well.

Intravenous cholangiography cannot be performed if hepatocellular disease or high-grade obstruction of the biliary tree is present. In general, visualization is extremely poor if the serum bilirubin level is over 3 mg/dl.

Abdominal ultrasonography

A noninvasive method of imaging the abdomen is the use of sound waves. Cystic lesions can be well delineated, and this method is particularly helpful in demonstrating gallstones.

Advantage. This test requires no contrast material and involves no radiation exposure, making it particularly valuable in pregnant patients.

Patient preparation. The patient should eat or drink nothing for 6 to 8 hours before the test, for best visualization of the gallbladder.

Percutaneous transhepatic cholangiography

The visualization of the biliary tree achieved with percutaneous transhepatic cholangiography helps to differentiate major obstructive jaundice from hepatocellular jaundice.

The liver is entered percutaneously with a thin needle; once the bile duct is entered, contrast material is injected and the biliary tree and gallbladder are radiologically visualized.

Sensitivity to iodine is a contraindication to the test, as is severe coagulopathy.

Operative cholangiography

Cholangiography may also be performed during surgery. Dye is injected into the common bile duct or the gallbladder. If a T tube is left in, it can be utilized postoperatively for the injection of dye and thus cholangiography.

Endoscopic retrograde cholangiography

Fiberoptic endoscopy permits cannulation of the ampulla of Vater and retrograde injection of contrast material. Approximately 85% of obstructive lesions of the biliary tree can be visualized by this method when it is used by skilled endoscopists.

Retrograde cholangiography and percutaneous cholangiography have become very helpful in visualizing the biliary tree in obstructive jaundice.

Angiography

Selective hepatic angiography can result in visualization of the cystic artery and the gallbladder walls. However, this visualization cannot be accomplished in all cases; therefore, the diagnostic value of the procedure is restricted to very select situations.

Computerized tomography

Computerized tomography is described in more detail on p. 288. Briefly, this radiologic technique, applied to the right upper quadrant, permits visualization of the liver, biliary tree, and gallbladder. Thus an obstruction resulting in a distended gallbladder may be documented, as well as dilated bile ducts and gallstones in the gallbladder or biliary tree.

Radioisotope visualization of the biliary tree

Technetium 99–labeled HIDA is injected intravenously. This substance, with its tracer isotope, is normally excreted in the bile, thus visualizing the biliary tree.

This test is helpful in demonstrating biliary or cystic duct obstruction, since the excretion of the isotope is blocked if there is an obstruction, resulting in accumulation of the isotope above the obstruction.

THE LIVER

Anatomy and physiology

The liver is the largest gland and the major metabolic factory in the human body. It lies immediately under the diaphragm, occupying most of the right upper quadrant (Fig. 8-1). The liver is involved in protein synthesis and other metabolic functions, regulation of blood volume, immune mechanisms, formation and excretion of bile, and detoxification and excretion of toxic elements. The liver is also important in the synthesis, esterification, and excretion of cholesterol.

Liver function tests

The routine screening tests for liver disorders have already been discussed in Chapter 1.

Serum bilirubin level

Bilirubin is the chief bile pigment in humans. It is derived principally from the breakdown of hemoglobin, and is normally bound to albumin in the circulation. Bilirubin is then carried to the liver, where it is conjugated with glucuronic acid. This *conjugated* bilirubin is more water soluble than the *free* bilirubin, and therefore is secreted more easily into the bile. Once within the intestine, the bilirubin is reduced to *urobilinogen* by the action of intestinal bacteria. Some of this urobilinogen is absorbed into the circulation and is either excreted in the urine or reexcreted in the bile. The rest of the intestinal urobilinogen is excreted in the stool as *fecal urobilinogen*.

◆ Normal serum bilirubin

Direct or conjugated:	up to 0.3 mg/dl
Indirect or unconjugated:	0.1-1.0 mg/dl
Total:	0.1-1.2 mg/dl

◆ Normal urine urobilinogen

2 hr:	0.3-1.0 Ehrlich units
24 hr:	0.05-2.5 mg/24 hr or
	0.5-4.0 Ehrlich units/24 hr

◆ Normal fecal urobilinogen

75-350 mg/100 gm of stool

Serum enzyme assays

The transaminases, glutamic-oxaloacetic transaminase (GOT) and glutamic-pyruvic transaminase (GPT), are liberated from destroyed cells. GOT is found particularly in skeletal muscles, cardiac muscle, and the liver, while GPT is found mainly in liver tissue. In the absence of cardiac or other muscle injury, elevated serum levels of these enzymes (SGOT AND SGPT) are suggestive of hepatocellular damage.

The serum alkaline phosphatase level (see p. 18) is one of the most important tools in the differential diagnosis of obstructive jaundice. For all practical purposes, a normal alkaline phosphatase level strongly suggests liver disease other than obstruction. Normal values are listed in Chapter 1 and Appendix A.

The serum levels of 5'-nucleotidase and serum leucine aminopeptidase are measured in conjunction with the alkaline phosphatase level because they are not related to bone destruction, as is the alkaline phosphatase level, and they are not elevated in bone disease. However, they are not as sensitive as the alkaline phosphatase level in diagnosing obstructive jaundice.

The lactic dehydrogenase (LDH) level is not very helpful in the diagnosis of liver disease because this enzyme is found in all organs and it is released into the circulation after a variety of tissue injuries. See p. 357 or Appendix A for normal values.

◆ **Normal SGPT**

1-36 U/ml

◆ **Normal SGOT**

8-33 U/ml

◆ **Normal serum 5'-nucleotidase**

0.3-3.2 Bodansky units

◆ **Normal serum leucine aminopeptidase**

50-220 U/ml

Serum protein level

Determination of the serum protein level is important because albumin is synthesized in the liver and because serum globulins are produced by Kupffer cells. Therefore, in typical chronic liver disease, the albumin/globulin ratio is reversed, with diminution of the albumin level and elevation of the globulin level, which is a broad gamma type of elevation.

Neoplastic and inflammatory diseases of the liver produce elevation of the $alpha_2$ globulin fraction, and sometimes biliary obstruction results in elevation in the beta globulin levels. Elevation of the gamma globulin level is noted frequently in chronic active liver disease. See Appendix A for normal values.

Although the determination of serum protein level is a good overall screening test for extensive liver disease, the influence of nonhepatic factors on protein metabolism should be remembered.

Prothrombin time and vitamin K administration test

The increase in prothrombin time in liver disease may be the result of either malabsorption of fat-soluble vitamin K or a deficiency in the formation of one of the clotting factors (I, II, V, VII or X, all of which are produced in the liver). The prolongation of prothrombin time would be manifested by bleeding tendencies.

The differential diagnosis of obstructive problems versus hepatocellular damage is made by giving an intramuscular injection of vitamin K. If the prothrombin time returns to a normal level or rises at least 30%, the implication is that the patient has obstructive problems rather than hepatocellular damage. However, continued prolongation of prothrombin time indicates severe hepatocellular damage.

◆ **Normal prothrombin time**

12-14 sec

Blood lipid and cholesterol levels

Blood lipid and cholesterol levels are usually elevated in obstructive jaundice and particularly in Zieve's syndrome (fatty liver), in which case there is extreme elevation of cholesterol and triglyceride levels. In chronic liver disease cholesterol levels are diminished. In both obstructive and chronic liver disease the percentage of esterified cholesterol is diminished. See p. 7 or Appendix A for normal values.

Other tests helpful in evaluating liver function
Blood ammonia levels

Blood ammonia levels are elevated in severe liver cirrhosis, especially following gastrointestinal bleeding. This occurs because ammonia is usually metabolized to urea in the liver and is then excreted by the kidney. However, in the presence of marked liver disease, ammonia levels would be elevated. (It has been suspected that some hepatic encephalopathy is probably a result of a high ammonia level in the cerebrospinal fluid, which interferes with the normal function of the central nervous system.) In association with an elevated blood ammonia level, the BUN level will be diminished.

Sulfobromophthalein (Bromsulphalein, BSP) excretion test

This is a general screening test of overall liver function. It is a relatively simple test that can be done mainly on patients who are not jaundiced. The test provides an index to the extent of parenchymal disease in that it gives some indication of hepatocellular damage and cell loss. The serum BSP levels are, however, also elevated in obstructive disease and are therefore not helpful in differentiating the causes of jaundice.

BSP dye is administered intravenously; it is almost completely cleared from the blood in approximately 45 minutes by the normal liver. Hepatocellular disease results in a delay in BSP clearance, causing the serum level to remain high beyond the 45-minute period.

Hepatic scanning

This is a means of visualizing the liver by giving a tracer dose of technetium sulfur colloid and by imaging its uptake by the reticuloendothelial system of the liver.

Under normal conditions a homogenous uptake is seen. This test can be helpful in diagnosing masses, abscesses, or cysts of the liver, which would appear as "cold" spots—that is, as areas of decreased isotope uptake.

Percutaneous needle biopsy

Percutaneous biopsy is a method of establishing the pathologic and microscopic picture of the liver cells. It is most useful in the diagnosis of diffuse parenchymal disorders of the liver. It is also helpful in differentiating disseminated granulomatous disease from tumors.

The major indications for needle biopsy are:
1. Unexplained hepatomegaly and hepatosplenomegaly
2. Persistently abnormal results of liver function tests
3. Suspected systemic or infiltrative disease
4. Sarcoidosis or miliary tuberculosis
5. Suspected primary or metastatic liver malignancy

Needle biopsy should not be performed if the prothrombin time is significantly prolonged, if there is tense ascites, or if the patient cannot hold his breath or is uncooperative. All of these situations increase the risk of severe bleeding as a complication of the procedure. Needle biopsy is also contraindicated in obstructive jaundice, since bile leakage and bile peritonitis might ensue.

Patient preparation and care. The patient is given nothing by mouth prior to the test. A bleeding tendency or a clotting defect is a contraindication for the procedure. Blood is kept ready on call. Because hemorrhage is the most serious, though uncommon, complication of this procedure, the patient should lie on his right side for 2 to 4 hours following the biopsy. In general, ambulation is not permitted for 24 hours.

Peritoneoscopy

This is a useful but not a routinely employed way of studying cases of liver disease. The procedure is performed by introducing a peritoneoscope into the peritoneal cavity and thus directly visualizing the gallbladder, liver, and serosal lining with a minimum of discomfort and hazard to the patient. The procedure is additionally helpful in determining the site for a liver biopsy; the biopsy specimen can be obtained under peritoneoscopy.

Alpha fetoprotein ("fetal" alpha₁ globulin) level

This fetal antigen is found in elevated levels in patients with hepatocellular carcinoma. Normally, in an adult only trace amounts are detected by radioimmunoassay.

Ultrasonography

This is a helpful means of identifying cystic lesions and abscesses of the liver.

Computerized tomography

This can be helpful in imaging masses or cysts of the liver (see pp. 212 and 288).

Selective hepatic angiography

Hepatic angiography permits visualization of the arteries supplying the liver and is helpful in delineating neoplastic lesions.

Hepatitis B surface antigen (HBsAg) test

This antigen was previously known as the Australia antigen; it is an antigenic marker for hepatitis B virus, which causes long-incubation hepatitis (previously known as serum hepatitis).

The most sensitive way of assaying for HBsAg is by radioimmunoassay. The presence of this antigen is diagnostic of hepatitis B infection.

Hepatitis B surface antibody (anti-HBs) test

Anti-HBs can also be assayed for; its presence is indicative of previous infection with hepatitis B virus.

Hepatitis B core antibody (anti-HBc) test

This antibody is a marker that represents past infection, as well as active infection of either the acute or the chronic form. In the absence of HBsAG and anti-HBs, the presence of anti-HBc is an indication of recent infection with hepatitis B virus.

e antigen

This antigen is frequently found in sera of patients who have chronic active liver disease associated with hepatitis B surface antigenemia. Its presence suggests that persisting liver enzymes could be indicative of chronic active hepatitis, the diagnosis of which is made by liver biopsy.

Hepatitis A antibody (anti-HAV) test

The presence of this antibody indicates previous infection with hepatitis A virus (previously called infectious hepatitis). The presence of an antibody of the IgM type implies very recent or current infection, while the presence of an antibody of the IgG type implies infection at least 6 to 8 weeks prior to the test. The IgG-type antibody is present for years in the serum of a person exposed to hepatitis A and confers life-long protection against reinfection.

Clinical application of laboratory tests
Viral hepatitis

The term "viral hepatitis" is given to at least three diseases; these diseases are clinically similar but etiologically and epidemiologically different. All of these conditions are characterized by malaise, low-grade temperature elevation, jaundice, and anorexia, along with markedly elevated SGOT and SGPT levels. The bilirubin and alkaline phosphatase levels are also elevated.

Hepatitis A (formerly infectious hepatitis) is caused by hepatitis A virus, an RNA virus. This disease is characterized in the acute phase by elevation of the liver enzyme levels and the presence of the IgM type of anti–hepatitis A virus antibody; subsequently, after convalescence, IgG type of anti–hepatitis A virus antibody is present.

Hepatitis B (formerly serum hepatitis) is caused by hepatitis B virus, a DNA virus. Hepatitis B has a longer incubation period than hepatitis A and is frequently more severe. It may become chronic and end in cirrhosis. Besides the elevation of liver enzyme levels, one will be able to detect the presence of a hepatitis B surface antigen during the acute phase and an antibody to the surface antigen during the convalescent phase.

Non-A, non-B hepatitis is a term given to viral hepatitis in which liver enzyme level elevations and a clinical picture of viral hepatitis are noted and yet none of the antigenic markers that are used to identify hepatitis A or B are present. This entity may be caused by more than one virus. It is usually seen in people who have received blood transfusions.

A liver biopsy is helpful in demonstrating viral hepatitis in any of the three clinical forms; however, it does not help to identify the etiology.

Obstructive jaundice

Obstructive jaundice results from obstruction of the flow of bile from the liver to the duodenum. The condition is manifested mainly by elevations of serum bilirubin and alkaline phosphatase levels and to a lesser extent by elevations of SGOT and SGPT levels. The most common cause is the presence of calculi in the biliary tree; the second most common cause is neoplastic obstruction between the ampulla of Vater and the hepatic ducts.

Tests to identify these conditions are discussed on pp. 212-215.

Hepatocellular carcinoma (hepatoma)

A hepatoma is a primary tumor of the liver (as opposed to a metastatic tumor). It is associated frequently with an elevated alkaline phosphatase level, occasionally with jaundice or an elevated CEA level, and perhaps with an elevated alpha fetoprotein level. The tumor can be visualized by isotopic liver scanning, angiography, or computerized tomography.

THE PANCREAS

Anatomy and physiology

The pancreas is composed of two major types of tissues: the acini, which secrete digestive juices into the duodenum, and the islets of Langerhans, which secrete insulin and glucagon into the bloodstream.

In response to the entry of food into the small intestine and to the hormones secretin and cholecystokinin, the pancreas secretes pancreatic juice into the intestinal tract.

Pancreatic juice contains bicarbonate and water, which neutralize the acidic chyme, and enzymes for digesting proteins, carbohydrates, and fats.

Laboratory tests of pancreatic function

Serum amylase and lipase levels

Amylase is the digestive enzyme for carbohydrate. In pancreatitis the serum amylase level is usually elevated in the early phase. Amylase is also excreted by the kidneys, and so its level can also be elevated in renal disease. Amylase is also excreted by the salivary glands; its level can therefore also be elevated in salivary gland diseases.

Serum lipase levels parallel the amylase levels, though the latter rise slightly later and lipase persists in the serum longer than amylase.

Determination of the serum amylase and lipase levels is indicated in patients with upper abdominal pain.

◗ Normal serum amylase

4-25 U/ml

◗ Normal serum lipase

0-1.5 U/ml (Cherry-Crandall technique)
2 U/ml or less

Urine amylase level

The usefulness of a determination of the urinary amylase level is limited because of the wide range in the normal value. In pancreatitis there is usually an increased excretion.

A more useful test is to measure a 2-hour urinary amylase excretion and correlate this finding with the serum amylase and lipase levels.

The ratio of urinary amylase clearance to creatinine clearance is helpful in correcting for variations in renal function.

Hypotonic duodenography

Hypotonic duodenography is another barium study performed for the purpose of detecting pancreatic disease. Barium is introduced by nasal catheter into the duodenum, which has been rendered atonic through the injection of an anticholinergic drug, such as propantheline bromide (Pro-Banthine). Pancreatic masses may then be seen impinging upon the flaccid duodenal wall. Men with prostatism should void immediately prior to the procedure, restrict their intake of fluids for several hours following the procedure, and be checked for voiding, because transient urinary retention is a side effect of anticholinergic drugs.

Endoscopic retrograde pancreatography

Endoscopic retrograde pancreatography is performed by cannulating the ampulla of Vater by fiberoptic endoscopy and then entering the pancreatic duct for the purpose of injecting contrast material. The visualization of the pancreatic duct is helpful in studying chronic pancreatitis and neoplasia of the pancreas.

Abdominal ultrasonography

Abdominal ultrasonography helps to visualize cystic or solid lesions of the pancreas. It is particularly helpful in diagnosing pseudocyts.

Abdominal angiography

Angiography can help visualize the arterial blood supply of the pancreas and thus can help to delineate mass lesions of this organ.

Computerized tomography

Computerized tomography is described on p. 212. It permits visualization of the pancreas, helps to delineate masses and cysts, and demonstrates calcification.

Other specific tests of pancreatic function

The secretin test, described on p. 203, is indicated when pancreatic insufficiency is a possibility. Intestinal malabsorption tests have already been described and should be used when pancreatic insufficiency is suspected.

Clinical application of laboratory tests

Acute or chronic pancreatitis and pancreatic carcinoma are usually accompanied by abdominal pain, while pancreatic insufficiency is usually manifested more by malabsorption and malnutrition than by abdominal pain.

Acute pancreatitis

In acute pancreatitis, which has various causes, the locally released enzymes destroy the pancreas.

Since amylase and lipase are released from the pancreas, their levels will rise in acute pancreatitis. The hematocrit, probably reflecting intravascular volume contraction, also rises. Serum triglyceride levels may also be elevated. Methemalbumin may be found in the serum if the pancreatitis is hemorrhagic. If the common bile duct has been obstructed by an edematous pancreas, the serum bilirubin level will be elevated.

Chronic pancreatitis

Chronic pancreatitis is usually the result of repeated injury of the pancreas. The cause is frequently alcohol.

Amylase and lipase levels show variable elevations. Pancreatic calcification is common. Results of the secretin test are usually abnormal, and endoscopic retrograde pancreatography shows diagnostic changes.

Cystic fibrosis

The clinical features of cystic fibrosis, which is a genetic illness, are chronic pulmonary disease, pancreatic dysfunction, and high concentrations of sodium and chloride in the sweat. Mucus plugs the pancreatic ducts, the intestinal mucous glands, and the bronchial tree. The pulmonary symptoms are usually more significant than the pancreatic symptoms.

The electrolyte concentration of the sweat will be elevated to 60 mEq/L or more. The normal concentration is less than 40 mEq/L. There will also be evidence of malabsorption, mainly because of maldigestion, with resultant steatorrhea. In addition, the results of a secretin test will be abnormal.

NINE Diagnostic tests
for endocrine disorders

The organs of the endocrine system all produce small amounts of hormones, each of which is manufactured by one particular organ and secreted into the bloodstream to exert its influence on other organs or tissues ("target tissues").

The established endocrine system, shown in Fig. 9-1, is composed of the following organs: hypothalamus, anterior and posterior pituitary, thyroid, parathyroids, adrenals, pancreatic islets of Langerhans, ovaries, testes, and placenta. Fig. 9-2 shows the interrelationships between the pituitary gland, the hypothalamus, and the target organs.

Since the endocrine system contains inherent checks and balances, the results of most of the endocrine function tests depend not only on overproduction or underproduction of a particular hormone but also on the reciprocal effects such overproduction or underproduction has on other endocrine organs. For example, excess cortisone production by the adrenal glands suppresses production of ACTH by the pituitary gland. A differential diagnosis is therefore required to determine the location of the main pathologic process.

THE THYROID GLAND

Anatomy and physiology

The thyroid gland (Fig. 9-3) consists of two lobes and a connecting portion (isthmus), giving the gland an H-shaped appearance. There is one lobe on each side of the trachea. This gland is unique among the endocrine glands because of its large amounts of stored hormones and the slow rate at which they are excreted.

The principal hormones secreted by the thyroid are *thyroxine* (T_4) and *triiodothyronine* (T_3). These hormones stimulate the oxidative reactions of most of the cells of the body, help to regulate lipid and carbohydrate metab-

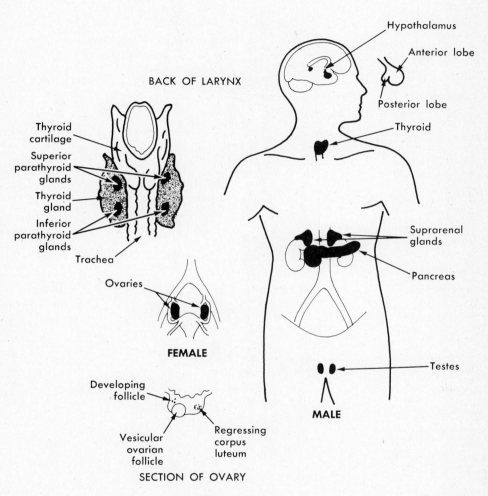

BACK OF LARYNX

Hypothalamus

Anterior lobe

Posterior lobe

Thyroid

Thyroid
cartilage

Superior
parathyroid
glands

Thyroid
gland

Inferior
parathyroid
glands

Trachea

Suprarenal
glands

Pancreas

Ovaries

FEMALE

Testes

MALE

Developing
follicle

Vesicular
ovarian
follicle

Regressing
corpus
luteum

SECTION OF OVARY

Fig. 9-1
The endocrine system.

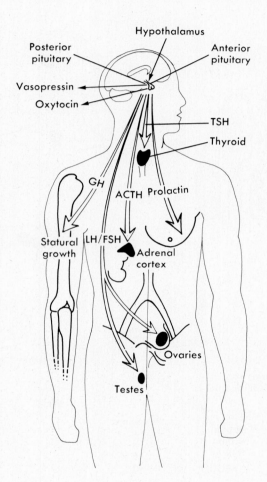

Fig. 9-2
The interrelationships between the pituitary gland, the hypothalamus, and the target organs.

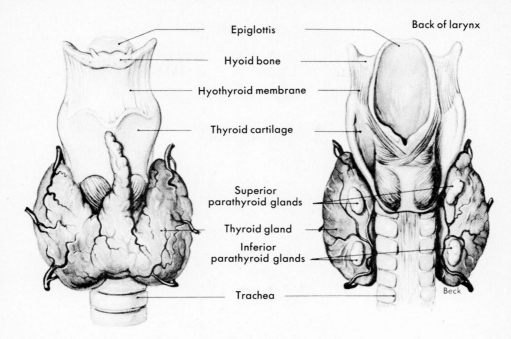

Epiglottis — Back of larynx

Hyoid bone

Hyothyroid membrane

Thyroid cartilage

Superior parathyroid glands

Thyroid gland

Inferior parathyroid glands

Trachea

Beck

Fig. 9-3
The thyroid and parathyroid glands. (From Anthony, C.P., and Kolthoff, N.J.: Textbook of anatomy and physiology, ed. 9, St. Louis, 1975, The C.V. Mosby Co.)

olism, and are necessary for the normal growth and development of the human organism. Most of the action of the thyroid hormones is mediated through the sympathetic nervous system. This is why beta adrenergic blockers are effective in controlling the symptoms of hyperthyroidism.

The first step in the synthesis of the thyroid hormones is absorption of dietary iodide from the small intestine into the circulation. The circulating iodide that is not taken up by the thyroid gland is cleared by the kidneys through glomerular filtration. After entering the thyroid, iodide is oxidized and combines with the amino acid tyrosine within the protein molecule thyroglobulin, where the thyroid hormones triiodothyronine and thyroxine are formed and stored.

The next step is the release of T_3 and T_4 from the thyroid gland. Under the influence of thyroid-stimulating hormone (TSH), secreted by the anterior pituitary gland, thyroglobulin is hydrolyzed and T_3 and T_4 are released into the circulation. Of the circulating thyroid hormones, 99.95% of the T_4 and 99.5% of the T_3 are bound to serum proteins, particularly to thyroxine-binding globulin (TBG). These hormones are inactive when bound to serum proteins. Therefore, only very small amounts of unbound thyroid hormone circulate to provide biologic activity.

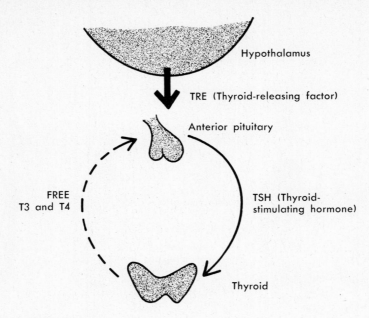

Fig. 9-4
The regulation of the thyroid gland through a feedback system.

The regulation of the thyroid gland occurs through a feedback system (Fig. 9-4) consisting of three main components: (1) the thyroid gland, which secretes T_3 and T_4, (2) the anterior pituitary gland, which secretes thyroid-stimulating hormone, and (3) the hypothalamus, which secretes thyrotropin-releasing factor (TRF). TRF stimulates the release of TSH and causes the synthesis of new TSH in the pituitary gland.

Normal levels of unbound T_3 and T_4 are maintained by a negative feedback effect. Increased levels of free hormones cause decreased TSH secretion, and decreased levels of free hormones cause increased TSH secretion.

Thyroid function tests

The most useful and accurate tests for evaluating thyroid function are determinations of the serum levels of thyroxine and triiodothyronine, by radioimmunoassay (RIA), and determination of the free thyroxine index, which is calculated from the T_4 and T_3 resin uptake (RU). Radioactive iodine (RAI) uptake and thyroid-stimulating hormone assay are also employed in situations in which the T_3 and T_4 results are borderline or do not fit into the clinical picture. The TSH assay is the most important test for the diagnosis of hypothyroidism.

To evaluate homeostatic controls, thyroid reserve, and feedback mechanisms, additional tests are employed: the TSH stimulation test, the thyrotropin-releasing hormone (TRH) stimulation test, and the TSH suppression test.

With the development of methods for directly measuring the levels of the thyroid hormones, measurement of the basal metabolic rate (BMR) and the level of butanol-extractable iodine (BEI) has become obsolete. The BMR test was a way of measuring metabolic activity, not thyroid hormone level, and was affected by many nonthyroidal factors; the BEI test was time-consuming and technically difficult, and its results were influenced by organic iodides and thyroxine-binding globulin.

Serum thyroxine (T_4) level

The most dramatic improvement in thyroid function tests occurred between 1960 and 1966 with the development of a direct way of determining the thyroxine level.

The serum T_4 concentration is determined either by competitive protein-binding assay or by radioimmunoassay.

A competitive protein-binding assay evaluates the ability of stable T_4 to displace radioactive thyroxine from a protein mixture containing thyroxine-binding globulin.

A radioimmunoassay is an elaborate antigen-antibody reaction requiring special reagents. The T_4 RIA measures the serum concentration of T_4 by indicating the ability of stable T_4 to displace radioactive T_4 from a specific anti-T_4 antibody.

Clinical value. The total T_4 level is a good index of thyroid function when the TBG level is normal. The T_4 determination is used to screen for thyroid dysfunction or to monitor hyperthyroid patients. Elevated levels are seen in hyperthyroidism and acute thyroiditis. Low levels are seen in hypothyroidism, myxedema, cretinism, chronic thyroiditis, and occasionally in subacute thyroiditis.

Limitations. If the TBG level increases or decreases, so does the T_4 level, in which case the T_4 level does not provide a valid estimate of thyroid function. The TBG level increases in pregnancy and in patients who are receiving estrogen medication; it decreases in patients who are taking anabolic steroids, in chronic liver disease, and in nephrosis.

◆ Normal serum T_4

5-11.0 μg/dl

Serum triiodothyronine (T_3) level

T_3 occurs in very small quantities in the active form. It is more active metabolically and less stable than T_4, and it has a shorter duration of effect than T_4.

The serum T_3 level is measured by one of two methods: the T_3 resin uptake test and radioimmunoassay.

The *T_3 resin uptake test* does not measure the concentration of T_3 in the patient's blood; instead it provides an indirect assessment of thyroid function. The test measures the availability of binding sites present in thyroid hormone–binding proteins.

The T_3 resin uptake test is an in vitro procedure in which T_3 labeled with ^{125}I is added to the patient's serum and incubated. This labeled T_3 will then become bound to the available binding sites in the thyroid hormone–binding proteins. Because the amount of labeled T_3 is excessive, a certain amount will normally remain unbound. In order to measure the amount of unbound radioactive T_3, a resin is added to the test tube and the unbound labeled T_3 is taken up by the resin.

In patients with thyroid dysfunction the concentration of thyroid-binding proteins is normal. In *hyperthyroidism* there are fewer binding sites available because they are occupied as a result of high levels of circulating thyroxine; thus less labeled T_3 is bound, and there is a high T_3 resin uptake. In *hypothyroidism* fewer binding sites are occupied, because of low levels of circulating thyroxine; thus more labeled T_3 is bound, and there is a low T_3 resin uptake. Normal values, which vary considerably in different laboratories, are expressed as percentages of the labeled T_3 that was taken up by the resin.

The *radioimmunoassay test* is a direct measurement of the actual T_3 concentration in the serum.

Clinical value. The T_3 determination by RIA is the preferred test for the diagnosis of T_3 thyrotoxicosis. When a patient has all of the symptoms of hyperthyroidism but a normal serum level of T_4, T_3 measurements (by RIA) may identify a T_3 thyrotoxicosis, a very rare clinical entity (seen in less than 5% of persons with hyperthyroidism).

Limitations. Some patients with clinical hypothyroidism have normal T_3 levels.

♦ **Normal serum T_3**

RIA: 80-160 ng/dl
RU: 25%-35% relative uptake

Free thyroxine level and free thyroxine index

Free T_4 is only a fraction of total T_4. It is the free, unbound thyroxine that enters the cell; it is metabolically active, and it is not affected by TBG abnormalities. This is, therefore, the substance whose measurement would be of most diagnostic value. However, the serum concentration of free thyroxine is difficult to measure clinically. Instead, the T_3 in vitro uptake is measured, and the product of this and the total serum T_4 concentration is the *free thy-*

roxine index, which varies directly with changes in the serum concentration of free thyroxine.

Advantages. The free thyroxine index is unaffected by changes in the level of TBG and thus more closely correlates with the true hormonal status than do T_3 or T_4 determinations.

‣ **Normal free thyroxine index**

0.9-2.3 ng/dl

Thyroid-stimulating hormone (TSH) assay

Thyroid-stimulating hormone is secreted by the anterior pituitary gland in response to stimulation by thyrotropin-releasing hormone (TRH), which is secreted by the hypothalamus. When the circulating thyroid hormone concentration is too high, TSH secretion falls; when it is too low, TSH secretion increases. The TSH level is measured by means of radioimmunoassay.

Clinical value. The serum TSH level is an indication of thyroid reserve. Determining this level is thus the most reliable and accurate test for primary hypothyroidism, which can be excluded when the TSH level is normal. The TSH assay is also used to evaluate and monitor exogenous thyroid replacement in persons with primary hypothyroidism.

‣ **Normal serum TSH**

$<5 \mu U/ml$

Radioactive iodine (RAI) uptake test

A small tracer dose of ^{125}I is given intravenously; it provides an indirect measure of thyroid activity, as reflected by the ability of the thyroid gland to concentrate iodide from blood plasma. The test has lost some of its specificity because of the increased use of iodinized food, which results in the RAI uptake being suppressed.

An elevated RAI uptake usually indicates hyperthyroidism. When the RAI uptake is low, in conjunction with elevated T_3, T_4, and free thyroxin levels, the following diagnostic possibilities should be considered:

1. Hyperthyroidism induced by excessive amounts of iodine in the diet (Jod-Basedow phenomenon)
2. Thyrotoxicosis factitia
3. Painless subacute thyroiditis
4. Certain forms of chronic thyroiditis

‣ **Normal RAI uptake**

1%-13% absorbed after 2 hr
2%-25% absorbed after 6 hr
15%-45% absorbed after 24 hr

Serum level of protein-bound iodine (PBI)

This test is much less specific than the test for the serum level of T_4, which has replaced it. It measures all the iodine that is bound to protein in the serum.

Limitations. The levels of thyroid-formed iodoproteins other than thyroxine are also measured by this test; the results may therefore be grossly elevated in subacute thyroiditis. In addition, exogenous iodine preparations interfere extensively with the test.

▶ **Normal value**

4-8 μg/dl

TSH stimulation test

In the TSH stimulation test, the radioactive iodine uptake is measured before and after an injection of thyroid-stimulating hormone.

Clinical value. This test is helpful in differentiating between primary and secondary hypothyroidism (intrinsic disease versus insufficient stimulation by the pituitary) and in assessing thyroid reserve.

If there is no response to the injection of TSH, primary hypothyroidism is suggested; if the thyroid reserve is significantly diminished, the thyroid gland will already be under maximal stimulation by endogenous TSH, and thus will show no further response to the injected TSH, and there will be very minimal increases in T_4 level and RAI uptake.

TRH stimulation test

The hypothalamus produces thyrotropin-releasing hormone, which stimulates the release of thyroid-stimulating hormone and causes the synthesis of new TSH in the pituitary gland. The TRH stimulation test is performed by injecting intravenous TRH and measuring the TSH response.

Fig. 9-5 shows the normal serum TSH response to administration of TRH and the responses that occur in primary hypothyroidism, decreased pituitary TSH reserve, thyrotoxicosis, pituitary hypothyroidism, and hypothalamic hypothyroidism.

A supranormal response occurs in patients with primary hypothyroidism (that is, hypothyroidism of thyroid origin).

A subnormal response usually indicates decreased pituitary TSH reserve.

If there is no response, thyrotoxicosis or pituitary hypothyroidism, as opposed to hypothalamic hypothyroidism, is indicated.

The TSH response to TRH is increased during pregnancy. In addition, the response is modified by the presence of thyroxine, antithyroid drugs, corticosteroids, estrogens, or levodopa.

Normal response. There is a significant rise from the basal level at 20 minutes (see Fig. 9-5); the TSH concentration returns to normal by 120 minutes. This response is usually greater in women than in men.

TSH suppression test (thyroid suppression test)

The patient is given an oral dose of T_3, the most active thyroid hormone. If the administration of T_3 is followed by suppression of TSH secretion, reflected by at least a 50% decrease in the RAI uptake and/or a significant decrease in the level of T_4, hyperthyroidism is ruled out. However, an abnormal test result is not diagnostic of hyperthyroidism; it merely indicates that thyroid hormone production is not under the normal homeostatic control mechanism and that it is being stimulated by unsuppressible TSH and/or by some factor not related to TSH, such as long-acting thyroid stimulator (LATS). An abnormal result may also indicate autonomous thyroid function.

Normal response. Decrease in the RAI uptake to less than half the control; decline of the serum T_4 level (to low normal or subnormal).

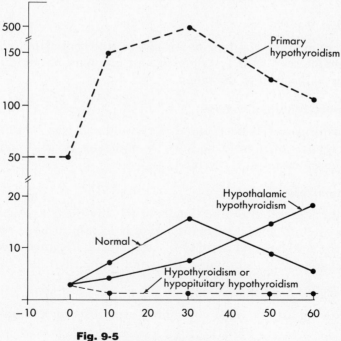

Fig. 9-5
TSH response to administration of TRH.

Thyroid scanning

A thyroid scan measures the thyroid uptake of RAI. During this test the overall pattern of thyroid gland radioactivity can be visualized by means of a scintillation scanning camera. The gland is outlined on film and paper.

Clinical value. This test is of greatest value in studying solitary thyroid nodules. Hyperactive and hypoactive areas can be localized, and the size of the gland can be determined. Hyperactive areas indicate a hyperfunctioning nodule ("hot nodule"), thus allowing differentiation between diffuse hyperplasia and toxic nodule as a cause of thyrotoxicosis. Hypoactive areas indicate a hypofunctioning nodule ("cold nodule") and thus increase the suspicion of carcinoma. A hot nodule is seldom malignant.

Tests for circulating antibodies

Antithyroglobulin and antimicrosomal antibodies. Moderate to high titers of these antibodies are found in the serum of patients with Hashimoto's thyroiditis, indicating that this condition is an autoimmune thyroid disease.

Long-acting thyroid stimulator (LATS). This antibody is an immunoglobulin that is directed against some component of the thyroid cell plasma membrane. This abnormal thyroid stimulator is found in approximately 50% of patients in the active phase of Graves' disease.

Thyroid sonography

Thyroid sonography is used as an aid in differentiating between solid and cystic nodules. It is the test of choice for pregnant patients, since radioactive iodine is harmful to the fetus.

Needle aspiration of thyroid nodules

Needle aspiration has been found fairly safe and very helpful in the differential diagnosis of thyroid nodules (hypoplastic thyroid nodules versus adenomas, carcinomas, and thyroid cysts).

Serum calcitonin level

Calcitonin is secreted by the C cells of the thyroid gland in response to high serum calcium levels. Its main action is to inhibit bone resorption by regulating the number and activity of osteoblasts. Elevated levels of calcitonin are diagnostic of medullary carcinoma of the thyroid.

Summary of thyroid function tests

The following are the most commonly used tests for evaluating thyroid function:
1. T_4 determination
2. T_3 determination
3. Free thyroxine index

4. TSH assay
5. RAI uptake

The following tests are employed to further test homeostatic controls and feedback mechanisms:

1. TSH stimulation
2. TSH suppression
3. TRH stimulation

The following tests provide information of historical interest:

1. PBI
2. BEI
3. BMR

Clinical application of thyroid function tests
Simple diffuse nontoxic goiter

A patient with a simple goiter will have a normal metabolic state, which should be demonstrated. In addition, this condition must be differentiated from Hashimoto's disease.

Laboratory tests. A normal metabolic state is demonstrated by a T_4 level that is low normal or slightly below normal; a radioimmunoassay shows the T_3 level to be just within the upper limits of normal.

Differential diagnosis. Simple diffuse nontoxic goiter versus Hashimoto's thyroiditis: Besides the palpation of a tender mass in Hashimoto's thyroiditis, the levels of antithyroglobulins and antimicrosomal antibodies will be elevated in Hashimoto's thyroiditis and normal in a case of simple goiter. Sometimes a needle-aspiration biopsy may help in the differential diagnosis. Also, the T_3, T_4, and free thyroxine levels are valuable in evaluating Hashimoto's thyroiditis; these values will be normal, high, or low, depending upon the time sequence of the disease.

Hypothyroidism

In hypothyroidism the T_4 level and the free thyroxine index are decreased.

An elevated TSH level in a patient with symptoms of hypothyroidism is nearly diagnostic of hypothyroidism. Because of the decrease in serum thyroxine level, the feedback suppression of TSH is not present; thus the TSH level is markedly increased.

The Achilles tendon reflex is another test used in the evaluation of thyroid function. In hypothyroidism, there is a delay in the relaxation phase of the reflex.

In a patient with documented hypothyroidism, if the TSH level is normal or low, a TRH stimulation test will make possible the differential diagnosis. A subnormal response of serum TSH to administered TRH will confirm the diagnosis of pituitary hypothyroidism.

Diffuse toxic goiter (Graves' disease)

In accordance with the clinically unique hypermetabolic picture, the T_3 and T_4 levels will be elevated and the free thyroxine index will be increased.

The TSH level is normal or low normal.

Differential diagnosis. A thyroid scan will distinguish a diffuse goiter from a nodular goiter or a toxic nodular goiter. In a case of diffuse toxic goiter there will be a uniform increase in the uptake of radioactive iodine, while in a case of toxic nodule there will be one area of excessive uptake of radioactive iodine. In such a case the surrounding tissue will show diminished uptake.

In mild cases of hyperthyroidism the T_3 and T_4 levels and the thyroxine index may be slightly elevated but within the normal ranges, perhaps at the upper limits of normal. In such cases the thyroid suppression test or the TRH stimulation test becomes crucial in the diagnosis.

Neoplasms of the thyroid

Thyroid neoplasms may be either adenomas or carcinomas. Both usually present as a solitary nodule and the patient is usually euthyroid. If the neoplasm is functioning antonomously it will accumulate ^{131}I, and the thyroid scan will show a hot nodule. If this is associated with frank thyrotoxicosis it is called toxic adenoma.

Carcinoma of the thyroid is very similar in appearance and consistency to a nodular goiter. ^{131}I uptake will most frequently demonstrate a cold nodule. However, a hot nodule does not rule out the possibility of carcinoma. Microscopic examination of a biopsy specimen is necessary to make a definitive diagnosis.

In medullary carcinoma of the thyroid, elevation of the calcitonin level is the hallmark of the diagnosis. In recent years thyroid ultrasound has been of some help in differentiating cystic benign tumors from solid thyroid tumors, and needle-aspiration biopsy in experienced hands has been found to be useful in the differential diagnosis of thyroid nodules and in the cytologic diagnosis of neoplasms.

THE PARATHYROID GLANDS

Anatomy and physiology

The four, small parathyroid glands (Fig. 9-3) are so closely associated with the thyroid that in the past they were often removed during thyroidectomy. The parathyroid hormone is essential for life; it is responsible for the maintenance of ionized calcium in the blood as well as for the renal reabsorption of calcium and excretion of phosphate.

Low serum calcium levels, by a feedback system, trigger an increase in the production of parathyroid hormone. Magnesium is also important in the release of parathyroid hormone, which acts on bone, kidney, and intestine to increase serum calcium levels. Osteoclasts, in response to parathyroid hormone, release bone salts into the extracellular fluid, thereby raising both calcium and phosphate levels in the plasma. The renal tubular cells, in response to the parathyroid hormone, increase reabsorption of calcium and decrease reabsorption of phosphate from the glomerular filtrate.

Calcitonin, a potent hypocalcemic hormone, has effects opposing those of parathyroid hormone, because it increases renal calcium clearance.

Vitamin D also plays an important role in calcium homeostasis, by increasing the efficiency of intestinal calcium absorption.

Laboratory tests
Serum parathyroid hormone (PTH) assay

Since direct measurement of the parathyroid hormone level by radioimmunoassay has become available and is now practical for clinical use, the indirect measurements of parathyroid function (phosphate clearance and phosphate reabsorption tests) have become obsolete.

The stimulus for PTH secretion is serum calcium; the production of the hormone is stimulated by hypocalcemia and suppressed by hypercalcemia.

Clinical value. When a diagnosis of hyperparathyroidism is strongly suspected in the clinical setting, a serum PTH assay is the single most important test; it must be done in conjunction with serum calcium determinations. In patients with hypercalcemia resulting from hyperparathyroidism, there are elevated calcium and parathyroid hormone levels; in all the other secondary hypercalcemias, the parathyroid hormone level is low.

If a patient has mild, intermittent hypercalcemia, an examiner may have to resort to multiple determinations of parathyroid hormone and calcium levels over several months in order to determine whether the elevated calcium level is accompanied by an elevated parathyroid hormone level or a normal one.

Tests for the localization of parathyroid adenoma or parathyroid hormone secretion

Percutaneous venous catheter sampling of the veins in the neck and thorax can be performed to obtain blood for a parathyroid hormone assay and for localization of an adenoma. However, in diffuse hyperplasia this procedure is of no help.

Selective arteriography, guided by the results of venous catheterization and sampling of parathyroid hormone, can also be used to localize a hypersecreting adenoma.

Phosphate clearance and *phosphate reabsorption tests* provide indirect measurements of parathyroid function. These tests have become obsolete since the advent of the direct measurement of parathyroid hormone level by radioimmunoassay.

Clinical application of laboratory tests
Primary hyperparathyroidism

In primary hyperparathyroidism there is an excessive secretion of parathyroid hormone, usually resulting in hypercalcemia, the most common manifestation of hyperparathyroidism, and hypophosphatemia. Evaluation of parathyroid function and the differential diagnosis in hypercalcemia were discussed in Unit One, in the sections on calcium and phosphate.

Laboratory tests

Skeletal x-ray film. Distinctive radiographic abnormalities of bone, including lesions that are pathognomonic of subperiosteal bone resorption, are found in approximately 20% of patients with primary hyperparathyroidism.

Serum phosphate level. Usually the serum phosphate level is low in hyperparathyroidism. However, it may be normal if there is superimposed renal failure.

Serum chloride level. In hyperparathyroidism the serum chloride concentration is elevated (often 104 mEq/L or greater) and is associated with mild metabolic acidosis.

Chloride/phosphorus ratio. In hyperparathyroidism the chloride/phosphorus ratio is greater than 30; if the hypercalcemia is from other causes, this ratio is less than 30.

Serum magnesium level. Usually, hyperparathyroidism also causes hypomagnesemia, but the serum magnesium level is, of course, influenced by various factors.

Urinary cyclic adenosine monophosphate (cyclic AMP) excretion. Since the secretion of parathyroid hormone is mediated partly by cyclic AMP, increased levels of parathyroid hormone are associated with increased renal synthesis of cyclic AMP, which is indicated by an increased level in the urine. A high level of cyclic AMP in the urine, along with hypercalcemia and hypercalciuria, usually suggests hyperparathyroidism.

Prednisone suppression test. This test requires the administration of 60 to 80 mg of prednisone daily for 2 weeks. In hyperparathyroidism the serum calcium level usually does not decrease, while in other conditions in the differential diagnosis of hypercalcemia there usually is a drop in the serum calcium level.

Hypoparathyroidism

Hypoparathyroidism results from a deficiency of parathyroid hormone production. Pseudohypoparathyroidism results from resistance by the end organs (kidney and bone) to the action of the hormone. In both disorders there is hypocalcemia and hyperphosphatemia; but only in pseudohypoparathyroidism is the blood level of parathyroid hormone elevated.

Differential diagnosis

Serum PTH level. The diagnosis of hypoparathyroidism is usually made because a patient has the neuromuscular symptoms of hypocalcemia, and is then found to be not only hypocalcemic but also hyperphosphatemic with normal renal function. If, in spite of the stimulus of marked hypocalcemia, no parathyroid hormone is found by radioimmunoassay, hypoparathyroidism is the most likely diagnosis. If, however, high concentrations of parathyroid hormone are detected, a diagnosis of pseudohypoparathyroidism is strongly suggested. If this diagnosis is correct, the patient has a normally functioning parathyroid, but there is resistance to the action of the hormone at the target tissues (kidney and bone).

Urinary cyclic AMP excretion. When the concentrations of parathyroid hormone are found to be high, the renal end-organ resistance can be demonstrated by measuring the urinary excretion of cyclic AMP in response to the injection of a standard dose of parathyroid hormone. In normal persons or in persons with idiopathic or postsurgical hypoparathyroidism, there is a tenfold to twentyfold increase in urinary cyclic AMP secretion; in patients with pseudohypoparathyroidism, there is little or no response.

• • •

In all the other secondary hypocalcemias—those resulting from vitamin D deficiency, hypoproteinemia, pancreatitis, acute nutritional deficiencies, or renal failure—the parathyroid hormone level will be increased.

THE ADRENAL GLANDS

Anatomy and physiology

The adrenal glands overlap the upper ends of the kidneys. Each gland (left and right) is composed of two distinct parts, the medullary or inner portion and the cortical or outer portion (Fig. 9-6). The adrenal medulla secretes the catecholamines epinephrine and norepinephrine, and is a part of the sympathetic nervous system. It differs from other ganglia of the sympathetic nervous system because it secretes more epinephrine (adrenaline) than norepinephrine, and it secretes its hormones directly into the blood-

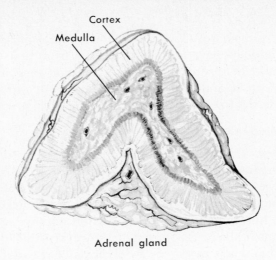

Adrenal gland

Fig. 9-6
The adrenal gland. (From Schottelius, B.A., and Schottelius, D.D.: Textbook of physiology, ed. 17, St. Louis, 1973, The C.V. Mosby Co.)

stream; this classifies it as an endocrine organ. The adrenal cortex secretes the steroid hormones.

The adrenocortical hormones

The steroid hormones of the adrenal cortex and their physiologic effects (Fig. 9-6) are as follows:
1. The glucocorticoids *cortisol* and *corticosterone,* which affect metabolism of proteins, carbohydrates, and lipids
2. The mineralocorticoid *aldosterone,* which predominantly affects sodium and potassium excretion
3. The sex steroids, *androgens* and *estrogens,* which primarily affect secondary sex characteristics

Cortisol, most of which is bound to globulin and albumin, represents 75% to 90% of the plasma corticoids, and its plasma level usually parallels the total corticoid level. Less than 5% of circulating cortisol is free and physiologically active. The free cortisol is filterable by the renal glomerulus, and its level in the plasma regulates adrenocorticotropic hormone (ACTH) release. If cortisol levels are reduced, such as in the adrenogenital syndromes, the secretion of ACTH is increased and the levels of total corticoids and deoxycorticoids increase.

Aldosterone (see also p. 169) is the chief electrolyte-regulating hormone of the adrenal gland and the most potent of the mineralocorticoids. The kidneys require aldosterone for the normal reabsorption of sodium and chloride, which leads to a loss of potassium and hydrogen. Normally, an increase in total body sodium triggers a decrease in the rate of aldosterone secretion, causing the kidneys to lose large quantities of sodium until the total body sodium level returns to normal. If the total body sodium level falls below normal or if serum potassium levels rise, the rate of aldosterone secretion increases so that sodium is retained and potassium lost.

Aldosterone is also important in the maintenance of blood pressure and blood volume. Aldosterone secretion is believed to be regulated primarily by the hormone renin, which is secreted by the kidney cells in hypovolemic or hyponatremic states, and by stimulation of sympathetic outflow to the kidney. The renin-angiotensin-aldosterone system is described on p. 169.

The carbon atoms on the basic steroid nucleus are numbered in sequence from 1 to 17. The steroids derived from this basic nucleus are of two structural types, the C-19 steroids and the C-21 steroids.

The C-19 steroids have predominantly androgenic activity and carry methyl groups at positions C-18 and C-10. If there is also a ketone group at the C-17 position, they are called *17-ketosteroids*.

The C-21 steroids have predominantly glucocorticoid or mineralocorticoid properties. These steroids have 2 carbon side chains (C-20 and C-21) attached at position 17 of the molecule. There are also methyl groups at C-18 and C-19. The C-21 steroids that also possess a hydroxyl group at position 17 of the steroid nucleus are called *17-hydroxycorticosteroids* or *17-hydroxycorticoids*.

Adrenocorticotropic hormone (ACTH)

The role of the anterior pituitary gland in adrenocortical secretion is shown in Fig. 9-7. Adrenocorticotropic hormone is stored in and released from the anterior pituitary gland. The release of stored ACTH is governed by a corticotropin-releasing factor (CRF) in the hypothalamus, which in turn is governed by plasma cortisol levels, stress, and the sleep-wake cycle. The plasma ACTH level roughly follows a diurnal pattern, being highest just prior to waking and lowest just prior to retiring. In certain types of stress (emotional trauma, surgery, pyrogens) the ACTH levels rise. However, the circulating cortisol is the principal regulator of ACTH and CRF release. This is a negative feedback mechanism (Fig. 9-6): a low plasma cortisol level causes an increase in the rate of release of CRF; a high plasma cortisol level causes a decrease in the rate of release of CRF. A low plasma cortisol level increases the responsiveness of the anterior pituitary adrenocorticotropic cells to CRF. Thus a smaller amount of CRF, in the absence of cortisol, will cause an inappropriate increase in the secretion of ACTH.

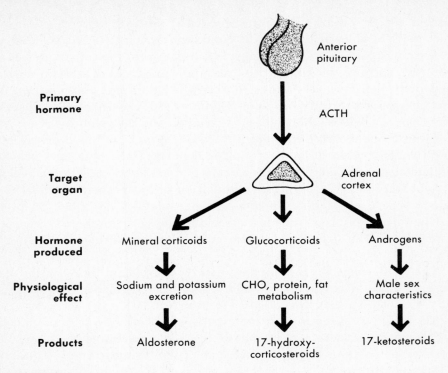

Fig. 9-7
The steroid hormones of the adrenal cortex, their physiological effects and products.

Laboratory tests of adrenal function

In the past most of the tests of adrenal function involved collection of 24-hour urine specimens for determination of hormone secretory rates. These tests have largely been replaced by absolute determinations of individual adrenal hormone levels, which may be done on an outpatient basis. Such determinations are more accurate and less costly to the patient.

Adrenal function tests are divided into two major categories: (1) absolute determinations of individual hormone values in serum and urine and (2) tests that reflect the interdependency between hormones and that evaluate feedback mechanisms.

Absolute determinations of individual adrenal hormone levels

Plasma cortisol level. The plasma cortisol level is measured by radioimmunoassay. Blood samples are obtained in the morning (8 A.M.) and afternoon (4 P.M.). In a healthy person the secretion rate is higher in the early morning hours and lower in the afternoon. This diurnal variation is interrupted if there is any disturbance of the hypothalamopituitary axis or if there is an autonomous lesion in the adrenals producing a high cortisol level.

Clinical value. The clinical value of this test is limited because of the manner in which the hormone is secreted—episodically. Thus a single determination may be misleading. However, a definite reversal in the diurnal variation may help in the diagnosis of an adrenal disorder.

Limitations. Estrogens and oral contraceptives may result in an elevated serum cortisol level in the absence of hypercorticism.

♦ Normal plasma cortisol

A.M.:   5-25 μg/dl
P.M.:   <10 μg/dl

Urinary free cortisol assay. This test measures the level of active urinary free cortisol, by radioimmunoassay; the result correlates well with the level of circulating free cortisol. Only the free, unconjugated cortisol is filtered by the glomeruli. Thus in hypercorticism, when the plasma cortisol concentration exceeds the capacity of the binding sites on cortisol-binding globulins, the plasma free cortisol concentration rises and the free cortisol enters the urine.

Clinical value. This test is important in the diagnosis of hypercorticism, and it is a sensitive test for the various types of adrenocortical hyperfunction.

Disadvantages. Urinary excretion values may not truly reflect the secretion rate, because of improper collection technique, renal disease, or altered metabolism.

♦ Normal value

24-108 μg/24 hr

Aldosterone levels (serum and urine). Aldosterone is the most potent of the mineralocorticoids. Its physiology is discussed on pp. 169 and 238.

Clinical value. Both serum and urinary aldosterone levels are usually measured in cases of hypertension that is thought to be of endocrine origin; in these cases the peripheral plasma renin activity (PRA) may also be determined. (It should be mentioned that the "renin profiling" of hypertensive patients for diagnostic, prognostic, and therapeutic reasons is controversial.)

For the specific diagnosis of hyperaldosteronism (hypersecretion of aldosterone), knowledge of the aldosterone levels is invaluable. The peripheral plasma renin activity is also determined, as a means of identifying the syndromes associated with aldosterone abnormalities. In primary hyperaldosteronism, aldosterone secretion is increased and renin secretion is suppressed. In secondary hyperaldosteronism both the serum aldosterone level and the PRA are elevated.

Limitations. Since the aldosterone level varies widely in accordance with dietary potassium intake and body position (supine or standing), the random determination of the aldosterone level is of no value.

♦ Normal aldosterone levels

Serum: 1-21 ng/dl (morning peripheral vein specimen)
Urine: 2-16 μg/24 hr

Plasma renin activity (PRA). Renin is an enzyme that is secreted by the kidney in response to a fall in glomerular blood pressure, a reduction in the level of sodium at the distal tubule, or sympathetic stimulation. Renin converts angiotensinogen to angiotensin I, which is in turn converted to angiotensin II, a potent vasopressor that also stimulates the adrenal cortex to release aldosterone.

Clinical value. A determination of PRA is performed in conjunction with a measurement of the plasma aldosterone level in the differential diagnosis of primary versus secondary hyperaldosteronism. In addition, a PRA determination is a screening test for essential, renal, or renovascular hypertension.

Limitations. Random PRA measurement is useless because of marked fluctuations in renin activity that result from such variables as time of day and sodium intake.

♦ Normal PRA

Na-depleted (upright; peripheral vein specimen):
       Ages 20-39: 2.9-24 ng/ml/hr
     Ages 40 and up: 2.9-10.8 ng/ml/hr
Na-replete (upright; peripheral vein specimen):
       Ages 20-39: <0.6-4.3 ng/ml/hr
     Ages 40 and up: <0.6-3.0 ng/ml/hr

Plasma adrenocorticotropic hormone (ACTH) level. Adrenocorticotropic hormone, also known as adrenocortical-stimulating hormone, governs the secretion of glucocorticoids by the adrenal glands and the sympathetic response of these glands to stress. The plasma ACTH level is determined by radioimmunoassay.

Clinical value. ACTH levels are useful in differentiating primary adrenal insufficiency from secondary adrenal insufficiency. Both conditions are characterized by low cortisol concentrations, but the ACTH level is high in primary adrenal insufficiency and normal to low in secondary adrenal insufficiency. Extremely high ACTH levels are found in cases of ectopic ACTH-producing tumors and in cases of pituitary adenomas in which there is increased secretion of ACTH.

Limitations. The plasma ACTH level is subject to diurnal variations, and ACTH, like cortisol, is secreted episodically. Thus a plasma level is difficult to evaluate unless it is considered along with other data.

♦ Normal plasma ACTH

<150 pg/ml at 8 A.M.

Urinary excretion of 17-hydroxycorticosteroids and 17-ketosteroids. The urinary levels of these steroids are no longer measured as a screening test to evaluate adrenal function because such a test involves 24-hour urine measurements, which require hospitalization and which may not accurately reflect the secretion rate of a hormone because of improper collection, renal disease, and/or altered metabolism. The most important screening test for hyperadrenalism is the overnight dexamethasone suppression test. However, if a patient is hospitalized for a definitive dexamethasone suppression test, the 24-hour urinary excretion of 17-hydroxycorticoids and 17-ketosteroids is still determined.

♦ Normal 17-hydroxycorticosteroid excretion (24-hr urine)

Male: 5.5-14.5 mg/24 hr
Female: 4.9-12.9 mg/24 hr
Lower in children
After 25 USP units ACTH, given IM: 200%-400% increase

♦ Normal 17-ketosteroid excretion (24-hr urine)

Male: 8-15 mg/24 hr
Female: 6-11.5 mg/24 hr
Children:
12-15 yr: 5-12 mg/24 hr
<12 yr: <5 mg/24 hr
After 25 USP units ACTH, given IM: 50%-100% increase

Tests that reflect interdependency of hormones and evaluate feedback mechanisms

Various tests measure, by means of stimulation and suppression, the integrity of the functions of the hypothalamus and the pituitary and adrenal glands. Stimulation tests can document a hormonal deficiency by measuring the hormonal release after a standardized stimulus. Suppression tests can document hypersecretion of a hormone by demonstrating a decrease in the level of the hormone after standardized suppression.

ACTH stimulation test. This test provides an index of the functional reserve of the adrenal gland to produce cortisol, especially in cases in which cortisol production has been suppressed because of exogenous corticoid administration. In complete adrenal destruction there is no response to ACTH stimulation.

Rapid screening test. Twenty-five units (0.25 mg) of cosyntropin (synthetic ACTH) is injected intramuscularly. The plasma cortisol level is measured prior to the injection and 30 and 60 minutes afterward. If plasma cortisol levels are below normal, the full (intravenous) ACTH stimulation test should be performed.

Normal increment. At least 7 μg/dl above the baseline value.

Disadvantage. Because of the irregular absorption of cosyntropin from the IM injection site, this test can give a false-positive result (that is, indicate adrenal insufficiency).

Twenty-four-hour test. Cosyntropin is given intravenously in 500 to 1000 ml of normal saline, at a rate of 2 units per hour, for 24 hours.

Normal increment. Plasma cortisol levels exceed 40 μg/dl; 17-hydroxy-steroid excretion rates increase by at least 25 mg/24 hr.

Aldosterone stimulation test. Blood volume depletion stimulates renin secretion, which in turn increases aldosterone secretion. Some of the protocols used in this test are sodium restriction, diuretic administration, and upright posture.

In hyperaldosteronism the plasma renin activity and the plasma aldosterone level do not increase with this test.

Aldosterone suppression test (salt-loading test). This test is performed either by intravenous saline infusion or by oral salt loading, either of which expands the extracellular fluid volume and normally results in decreases in circulating plasma renin activity and in aldosterone secretion and/or excretion. Normal persons respond to this test by suppressing renin production and decreasing angiotensin formation, with subsequent suppression of aldosterone secretion; persons with primary hyperaldosteronism resulting from an adenoma do not respond.

Dexamethasone suppression test. This test is based on the fact that the blood level of glucocorticoids determines the amount of ACTH released from the anterior pituitary, which in turn determines the amount of steroid produced by the adrenal gland. Therefore dexamethasone, a potent glucocorticoid, is given to test this feedback mechanism.

Overnight screening test. Because of its simplicity, this is the preferred screening test for Cushing's syndrome. One milligram of dexamethasone is given at midnight. At 8 A.M. the following day the plasma cortisol level is measured. Normally it is less than 5 μg/dl.

Definitive test of adrenal suppressibility. One-half milligram of dexamethasone is administered every 6 hours for 2 days; during this period, and afterward, 24-hour urine specimens are collected. Normally, after the second day, there is a fall in the urinary excretion of 17-hydroxycorticoids to less than 3 mg per day or the plasma cortisol level is less than 5 μg/dl.

Metyrapone test. Metyrapone blocks the action of 11-β-hydroxylase, thus preventing the conversion of 11-deoxycortisol to cortisol and causing more 11-deoxycortisol and less cortisol to be secreted by the adrenals. The diminished cortisol level stimulates the pituitary to produce ACTH so that the adrenals can be stimulated to release 11-deoxycortisol, a biologically inactive precursor of cortisol. This release is reflected in the urine by an increase in the excretion of 17-hydroxycorticoids. Thus, in normal individuals, after the administration of metyrapone (750 mg orally every 4 hours for 24 hours) there is a rise in plasma 11-deoxycortisol levels and an increase in the urinary excretion of 17-hydroxycorticoids, which are the metabolite of 11-deoxycortisol. These two measurements should be made before and after the administration of metyrapone.

Clinical value. This test is used for assessment of the pituitary reserve and secretion of ACTH and for assessment of the adrenal response to ACTH. A poor response usually occurs in both primary and secondary adrenal insufficiency. This test is also used in differentiating among the causes of Cushing's syndrome.

Precautions. This test may occasionally induce an adrenal crisis. Thus the patient should be hospitalized and observed closely for signs of postural hypotension, nausea, vomiting, tachycardia, or diaphoresis.

Limitations. This test is inaccurate if the patient is taking glucocorticoids or drugs that accelerate the metabolism of metyrapone (such as phenytoin).

Normal result. A rise in the urinary excretion of 17-hydroxycorticoids to at least twice basal levels (or a rise of 8 to 10 mg/24 hrs).

Adrenal radiography

Radiographic visualization of the adrenal glands may reveal calcification caused either by tuberculosis associated with Addison's disease or by carcinoma of the adrenal glands.

An intravenous pyelogram and a tomogram may be of value in further delineating the size and shape of the adrenal gland and displacement of other organs resulting from adrenal gland disease.

Adrenal venography and arteriography may be helpful for further radiographic delineation.

Retroperitoneal air insufflation is no longer recommended, since it can be dangerous and there are better ways of delineating and visualizing the adrenal glands.

Adrenal sonography (ultrasound) and total-body CT scanning are being used increasingly often, for better visualization of the adrenal gland and detection of tumors, and are replacing the radiographic tests just mentioned.

Clinical application of adrenal function tests
Hyperfunction of the adrenal cortex

Hyperfunction of the adrenal cortex can be divided into two major categories: excess production of glucocorticoid (for example, Cushing's syndrome) and excess production of mineralocorticoid (for example, primary hyperaldosteronemia). However, these clinical syndromes may have overlapping features.

Cushing's syndrome. Cushing's syndrome may be produced by:
1. Adrenocortical hyperplasia secondary to pituitary ACTH production, which may be due either to pituitary-hypothalamic dysfunction or pituitary ACTH-producing microadenomas or macroadenomas (both conditions are sometimes referred to as "pituitary-dependent Cushing's syndrome.")
2. Adrenal adenoma or carcinoma
3. Ectopic ACTH production

When Cushing's syndrome is clinically suspected, one should proceed as follows to make a definite diagnosis:

An overnight dexamethasone suppression test is the most important screening test. A normal response rules out Cushing's syndrome (cortisol production is suppressed [<3 mg/24 hr] by a small dose of dexamethasone).

If suppression of cortisol production does not occur, one should proceed to the more definitive test, which involves larger doses of dexamethasone (p. 244). In response to a high dose of dexamethasone, a patient with adrenal hyperplasia secondary to pituitary ACTH secretion due to hypothalamic dysfunction will demonstrate a suppression of urine 17-hydroxysteroid levels to less than half the baseline value.

No suppression of urine 17-hydroxysteroid levels occurs in patients with adrenal hyperplasia secondary to a nonendocrine ACTH-producing tumor or in patients with adrenal neoplasia. If suppression does not occur, a determination of plasma ACTH level is done. A normal or low ACTH level suggests adrenal adenoma. A level greater than 400 pg/ml suggests adrenal hyperplasia secondary to an ACTH-producing tumor.

The metyrapone suppression test may be useful in differentiating between adrenal hyperplasia resulting from pituitary ACTH secretion (normal response) and that resulting from adrenal tumors (no response).

If the pathological state is narrowed down to the adrenal glands, three further tests are of help:
1. Retrograde catheterization of adrenal veins and measurement of hormone levels. In bilateral adrenal hyperplasia the cortisol concentration is high in both adrenal veins; in adrenal adenoma there is a significant differential in cortisol concentration.

2. Adrenal scanning with ^{131}I-19-iodocholesterol. In adrenal hyperplasia there is increased bilateral uptake, while in adrenal tumor one side shows increased uptake and not the other.
3. Measurement of the urinary 17-ketosteroid level distinguishes between an adenoma and a carcinoma. This level will be high in adrenal carcinoma and normal or low in adrenal adenoma.

Mineralocorticoid excess syndrome (hyperaldosteronism). This syndrome is usually caused by primary hyperaldosteronism resulting from adenoma (aldosteronemia); it is usually associated with clinical hypertension.

Laboratory tests. The best screening test is the electrolyte panel (pp. 8-18), which would show a low serum potassium level in association with hypochloremic alkalosis and high blood pressure. At this point, before more expensive tests are ordered, the 24-hour urinary excretion of potassium should be measured. If the patient's hypokalemia results from diet or malabsorption, there will be negligible amounts of potassium in the urine. A 24-hour excretion of 30 mEq or more strongly suggests kidney potassium wasting.

Once renal potassium wasting has been established, urinary aldosterone excretion and peripheral plasma renin activity should be measured. The hallmark of primary hyperaldosteronism is elevated 24-hour urinary aldosterone excretion in combination with suppression of plasma renin activity.

In patients with elevated aldosterone excretion, one should also demonstrate suppressed and nonstimulable plasma renin activity, as well as nonsuppressibility of aldosterone production by means of the aldosterone suppression test. In primary hyperaldosteronism there is no response to this test.

Differential diagnosis. The disease state causing primary hyperaldosteronism is usually either an adenoma or bilateral hyperplasia. Therefore once the diagnosis has been made by means of the tests just mentioned, the next step is to measure the aldosterone concentration in blood from an adrenal vein (obtained by catherization). In a case of adrenal adenoma this level is elevated in a specimen obtained from the affected side, while in bilateral hyperplasia there is no difference in the aldosterone concentrations in blood from the two sides. In addition, adrenal scans show an increased uptake of injected ^{131}I-19-iodocholesterol on the side affected with adrenal adenoma, while in bilateral hyperplasia the uptake is increased in both glands.

A diagnosis of Bartter's syndrome is made when hyperaldosteronism is accompanied by hypokalemia, metabolic alkalosis, a marked increase in peripheral plasma renin activity, salt craving, and normal blood pressure.

Hypofunction of the adrenal cortex (adrenal insufficiency)

This disorder is also known as Addison's disease or chronic glucocorticoid deficiency, the signs and symptoms of which are secondary to cortisol deficiency resulting either from an adrenal lesion (primary adrenal insufficiency) or from a defect in ACTH secretion by the anterior pituitary (secondary adrenal insufficiency). Early recognition of Addison's disease may be difficult, but it is important. If the disease is not treated, the prognosis is poor (the disorder can be fatal); however, with early treatment the metabolic anomaly can be corrected.

The cause of the hyperpigmentation that is associated with Addison's disease, and with ectopic ACTH secretion, is uncertain. It has been postulated that the hyperpigmentation is caused by the ACTH rather than by melanocyte-stimulating hormone (MSH), whose existence is in question.

Laboratory tests. Under the stress of being acutely ill, a patient with normal adrenal glands has an elevated plasma cortisol level, while in a patient with adrenal insufficiency, the 8 A.M. plasma cortisol level is low or low normal. A low cortisol level combined with an elevated ACTH level is diagnostic of primary adrenal insufficiency. A low cortisol level in combination with a normal ACTH level reflects secondary hypoadrenalism, which is best evaluated by means of the metyrapone test.

Selective hypoaldosteronism

Selective hypoaldosteronism is a deficiency of aldosterone secretion without an abnormality in cortisol synthesis. It may result from decreased adrenal responsiveness because of chronic lack of stimulation by the renin-angiotensin system. Selective hypoaldosteronism is usually associated with chronic kidney disease that is diabetes related.

The diagnosis is made by demonstrating a lack of response to the aldosterone stimulation test.

Hyperfunction of the adrenal medulla (pheochromocytoma)

A pheochromocytoma is a catecholamine-producing tumor of pheochrome tissue; it is most commonly located in the adrenal medulla. A pheochromocytoma releases abnormally large amounts of catecholamines into the circulation, a small percentage of which is excreted unchanged in the urine. Some of the adrenal medullary hormones appear in the urine as metanephrine, and the major portion of the hormones will be excreted as vanillylmandelic acid (VMA), which is a metabolic by-product of catecholamine degradation.

Laboratory tests. A complete work-up for a patient with a possible pheochromocytoma should include a 24-hour urine collection with determinations of levels of VMA, catecholamines, and metanephrine, any one of which might be elevated in a given case of pheochromocytoma. Pheochromocytoma is characterized by hypertension with marked vasomotor changes and thus enters into the differential diagnosis of hypertensive patients. Computerized tomography (p. 288) localizes the tumor, and has obviated the need for IV pyelography, tomography, venography, and arteriography.

THE PITUITARY GLAND

Anatomy and physiology

The pituitary gland is protected in the bony cavity known as the sella turcica and is covered by the dura mater. The hypothalamus is attached to the pituitary gland by a stalk, and the two act together to control the functions of the target organs. The hypothalamus controls the pituitary by inhibiting and releasing factors. The pituitary, in turn, exerts its effect on various peripheral endocrine organs. The relationships between the pituitary gland, the hypothalamus, and the target organs are shown in Fig. 9-8.

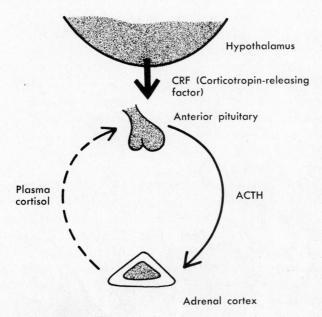

Fig. 9-8
The roles of the hypothalamus and the anterior pituitary gland in adrenocortical secretion.

The six known hormones secreted by the anterior lobe of the pituitary gland are:

1. Growth hormone (GH), which has a general effect on growth
2. Prolactin, which controls the secretion of milk by the mammary glands
3. Thyroid-stimulating hormone (TSH), which stimulates the formation and release of thyroid hormones
4. Adrenocorticotropic hormone (ACTH), which controls the secretion of the adrenal cortex
5. Luteinizing hormone (LH), which initiates ovulation and luteinization in the ovary
6. Follicle-stimulating hormone (FSH), which stimulates estrogen secretion and the growth of the graafian follicle in women and spermatogenesis in men

The releasing factors secreted by the hypothalamus are as follows: corticotropin-releasing factor (CRF), gonadotropin-releasing factor (GRF), thyrotropin-releasing hormone (TRH), and growth hormone–releasing factor (GHRF). In addition, three known inhibiting factors are secreted by the hypothalamus: prolactin-inhibiting factor, melanocyte-inhibiting factor, and a growth hormone–inhibiting factor (somatostatin).

The releasing factors stimulate the synthesis and release of the specific pituitary hormones. These factors reach the pituitary gland by way of the hypothalamic-pituitary venous plexus. The pituitary hormones ACTH, FSH, LH, and TSH are also controlled by a negative feedback loop, in which the concentration of the circulating hormone secreted from the target gland suppresses the elaboration of the corresponding pituitary hormone.

The posterior pituitary hormones are vasopressin (antidiuretic hormone, ADH) and oxytocin; both are manufactured in the hypothalamus and stored in and released from the posterior pituitary gland.

Vasopressin (antidiuretic hormone, ADH) and oxytocin are synthesized in the hypothalamus and reach the posterior pituitary for storage by traveling along the supraopticohypophyseal tract (Fig. 9-9). Vasopressin is stored bound to a protein (neurophysine); both are released into the circulation mainly in response to serum osmolality. Some of the stimulators of ADH release are dehydration, saline infusion, isomolar injection of CHO solutions, decrease in plasma volume or blood pressure, pain, stress, sleep, exercise, and certain drugs (nicotine, morphine, and barbiturates). The following are some of the inhibitors of ADH release: increase in plasma volume, hypoosmolality, exposure to cold, alcohol, and some drugs (phenytoin and glucocorticoids).

ADH stimulates water reabsorption by the distal tubules and collecting ducts. This major physiologic effect determines the final concentration of

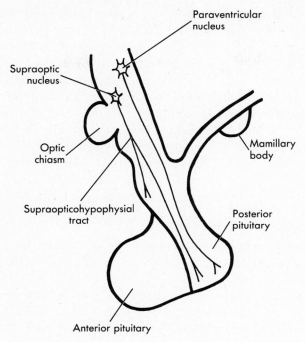

Fig. 9-9
Posterior pituitary gland and the supraopticohypophyseal tract. Vasopressin and oxytocin, synthesized in the hypothalamus, travel along the supraopticohypophyseal tract to be stored in the posterior pituitary.

urine. In the presence of ADH more water is reabsorbed, resulting in concentrated urine; in the absence of ADH less water is reabsorbed, resulting in dilute urine.

Laboratory tests of anterior pituitary function

Most of the tests performed for evaluation of pituitary function have already been described in the sections dealing with the pituitary's target organs, the thyroid and the adrenals. An adenoma of the pituitary gland initially increases secretion by the target organs. For example, there may be increases in the levels of thyroxine and cortisol initially because of stimulation of the thyroid and adrenal glands. Later on, as more pituitary tissue is destroyed, there is diminution of the pituitary secretions and secondary failure of the target organs.

The radioimmunoassay technique for measuring the pituitary hormone levels has significantly simplified the assessment of anterior pituitary function, especially when the hormone level is clearly elevated. However, if the hormone level is low, it is uncertain whether this indicates simply a low normal or if there is in fact pituitary hypofunction. For example, a TSH level of 50 μU/ml clearly indicates hypothyroidism. But a TSH level of 3 μU/ml could be a low normal, or it could be abnormal. Therefore, one measures the hormone level at the target organ. If this level is also found to be low, then there is pituitary hypofunction. For example, if the thyroxine level is low because of primary hypothyroidism, the TSH level will be elevated. However, if the TSH level is also low, primary pituitary failure is indicated. For further documentation, TRH stimulation is done, to which there would be no response in a case of primary pituitary failure. In general, these principles apply to all of the hormones that the pituitary gland regulates.

Measurement of growth hormone level

Growth-hormone excess syndromes. In growth-hormone excess syndromes, the growth hormone levels are elevated; therefore suppression tests are used, the most common being the glucose tolerance test, with simultaneous determination of blood glucose and growth hormone levels. The rationale is that administration of glucose suppresses the growth hormone levels. The demonstration of elevated levels of growth hormone that are unsuppressible is diagnostic of growth-hormone excess syndromes.

Deficiency states or syndromes. Since normal levels of growth hormone may be very low, demonstration of a deficiency state is usually based on stimulatory tests. The two most common tests employed are the insulin tolerance test and the L-dopa test.

Insulin tolerance test. Just as growth hormone secretion is suppressed by glucose administration, it is stimulated by insulin-induced hypoglycemia.

Following the injection of insulin the blood glucose level will fall promptly, reaching its lowest point in about 30 minutes. The mild symptoms of hypoglycemia thus produced will resolve spontaneously in normal individuals. A 50% reduction from the basal value will be enough to increase the growth hormone concentration to 5 ng/ml or more within 45 to 60 minutes of the administration of insulin.

Oral and intravenous glucose should be kept available, since severe hypoglycemia may occur in patients with hypopituitarism and an increased sensitivity to insulin. This test is potentially dangerous; however, it is very specific and reliable and will substantiate the results of other tests.

In addition, the integrity of the pituitary-adrenal axis may be confirmed with this test, since hypoglycemia will also cause a release of ACTH and cortisol.

L-dopa test. L-dopa, 0.5 gm, is given orally, and blood samples for growth hormone determination are obtained every 30 minutes for 2 hours. Normally, the growth hormone concentration rises to greater than 5 ng/ml.

X-ray films of the skull

It is advisable to take an x-ray film of the skull to evaluate the sella turcica, a depression in the sphenoid bone where the pituitary gland rests, for volume and erosion or enlargement. Computerized tomography (p. 288) of the brain has significantly improved this phase of evaluation.

Plasma prolactin level

Measurement of prolactin levels is made by radioimmunoassay. Several prolactin-stimulatory tests have been developed but are not in clinical use.

Clinical value. Certain types of pituitary tumors, in the past thought to be nonfunctional, have been found to be secreting high levels of prolactin (prolactin-secreting microadenomas, or prolactinomas). Most of the chromophobe adenomas fall into this category. In women these tumors are associated with the galactorrhea-amenorrhea syndrome; in men they are associated with secondary hypogonadism with decreased testosterone level.

♦ Normal plasma prolactin

    Men: 1-20 ng/ml
Women: 1-25 ng/ml

Pituitary gonadotropin levels

The two gonadotropins secreted by the anterior pituitary are luteinizing hormone (LH) and follicle-stimulating hormone (FSH).

Gonadotropin-releasing hormone, secreted by the hypothalamus, stimulates secretion of LH and, to a lesser degree, FSH. In women, LH induces ovulation and maintains the corpus luteum, which produces progesterone; in men, LH stimulates testosterone secretion.

In women, follicle-stimulating hormone stimulates the growth of ovarian follicles, in men it stimulates spermatogenesis. After stimulation by FSH, the ovarian follicles secrete estrogen.

Estrogen suppresses the secretion of FSH and, to a lesser degree, LH. Testosterone suppresses the secretion of the LH.

♦ Normal serum estrogens

                Males: 4-14 ng/dl
    Premenopausal females: 4-60 ng/dl
Postmenopausal females: <3-14 ng/dl
            Children: <3 ng/dl

♦ Normal serum testosterone

Total: Male: 300-1200 ng/dl
       Female: 20-80 ng/dl
Free: Adult male: 9-30 ng/dl
      Adult female: 0.3-1.9 ng/dl

Clomiphene stimulation test

Clomiphene is used to test the gonadotropin reserve. Clomiphene competes with estrogen for binding in the target organ. The pituitary gland perceives this situation as a lack of estrogen and responds by secreting FSH and LH. If the gonadotropin reserve is significantly decreased, there is no response.

Clinical application of laboratory tests

Primary hypogonadism

When primary hypogonadism exists in females, the plasma estrogen and estradiol levels are low; in males the testosterone level is low. In addition, in this disorder the FSH and LH levels are high.

Pituitary hypogonadism

When this condition exists in females, both estrogen and estradiol levels are low; in males the testosterone level is low. In addition, this disorder is associated with low levels of FSH and LH.

Hypothalamic hypogonadism

In this condition females have low estrogen and estradiol levels and males have low testosterone levels; the LH and FSH levels are low in both males and females. To distinguish pituitary hypogonadism from hypothalamic hypogonadism, gonadotropin-releasing hormone (GRH) is injected and the serum FSH and LH levels are measured. If these levels fail to rise, pituitary hypogonadism is indicated. However, if there is an increased secretion of FSH and LH, primary hypothalamic hypogonadism is indicated.

The clomiphene stimulation test is used to evaluate the gonadotropin reserve.

Acromegaly-gigantism syndrome

The increased secretion of growth hormone that results from pituitary tumors leads to gigantism before puberty and acromegaly after puberty. The appropriate diagnostic tests are measurement of the growth hormone level, which is not suppressible with the glucose tolerance test, and evaluation of the sella turcica by conventional x-ray techniques and computerized tomography. In addition, since visual impairment may be a result of the presence of a tumor, visual field examinations are performed.

Galactorrhea-amenorrhea syndrome

This syndrome is the result of increased prolactin secretion because of a pituitary microadenoma. In women this secretion leads to amenorrhea and galactorrhea. In men, galactorrhea is usually absent, and there is hypogonadism evidenced by a low testosterone level and depression.

The diagnosis is confirmed by the existence of elevated plasma prolactin levels that fail to respond to stimulation by phenothiazine (Thorazine). Radiologic examination of the sella turcica may be performed, including tomography and computerized tomography, but may fail to demonstrate the presence of the microadenoma.

Laboratory tests of posterior pituitary function
Determination of specific gravity

After overnight fasting a morning determination of specific gravity will give a rough indication of the concentrating ability of the kidney as well as an indication of whether there is an adequate amount of vasopressin.

Vasopressin injection test

In diabetes insipidus a vasopressin (antidiuretic hormone, ADH) deficiency is present. This deficiency is manifested by excessive urine output, which may amount to up to 12 to 15 liters per day. The patient will respond to a vasopressin injection with a decrease in urine output, thus documenting the deficiency and the normal responsiveness of the renal tubules to the hormone.

Water deprivation test

This test is used in suspected cases of diabetes insipidus.

After several hours of controlled water deprivation, the urine should be concentrated. In diabetes insipidus not only will the patient be unable to concentrate the urine, but also, becuase of a continued loss of water, the serum osmolality will be relatively higher in spite of the lower urinary specific gravity or osmolality. Since the kidney tubules function normally in diabetes insipidus, an injection of vasopressin will correct the abnormal concentrating ability of the kidneys and bring the osmolality of both urine and serum back to normal.

Clinical application of laboratory tests
Inappropriate ADH secretion syndrome

Serum osmolality and urine osmolality are measured when inappropriate ADH secretion syndrome is suspected. These tests have already been described on p. 174, in Chapter 7.

Normally, hyperosmolar serum stimulates the osmoreceptors, and the posterior pituitary produces ADH in an attempt to dilute the blood. The individual is also thirsty, a physiologic sign of hyperosmolar blood. Conversely, when there is hypo-osmolarity ADH is not secreted and the individual excretes a diluted urine. In the so-called inappropriate ADH secretion syndrome there is hypo-osmolality of the blood in association with a relative hyperosmolarity of the urine, indicating a malfunction of the normal osmolar response of the osmoreceptors, an excess of exogenous vasopressin, or the production of a vasopressin-like hormone that is not under the regular control of serum osmolarity.

The inappropriate secretion of ADH has been described in many disease entities, such as bronchogenic carcinoma or other types of cancer, congestive heart failure, inflammatory pulmonary lesions, and some metabolic diseases such as porphyria. The syndrome has also been seen in some patients who use diuretics excessively.

The diagnosis should be suspected when there is hyponatremia along with low BUN and uric acid values. The diagnosis can be confirmed by simultaneous measurement of urine and serum osmolality. The serum osmolality will be much lower than the urine osmolality, indicating the inappropriate excretion of a concentrated urine in the presence of a dilute serum.

ADH deficiency

ADH deficiency is manifested by polyuria. The differential diagnosis is among psychogenic polydipsia, hypothalamic diabetes insipidus, and nephrogenic diabetes insipidus.

Laboratory tests include determination of serum and urine osmolality, fluid deprivation tests, and Pitressin administration.

Serum and urine osmolality determinations

Psychogenic polydipsia: both are low
Hypothalamic or nephrogenic diabetes insipidus: serum normal or high; urine low

Fluid restriction test

Psychogenic polydipsia: no change in serum osmolality; urine osmolality usually increases
Hypothalamic diabetes insipidus: serum osmolality increases with no significant increase in urine osmolality
Nephrogenic diabetes: no change

Pitressin administration

Psychogenic polydipsia: sick feeling and no change in serum osmolality; urine osmolality increases
Hypothalamic diabetes insipidus: patient feels better; decrease in serum osmolality; increase in urine osmolality (approaching normal)
Nephrogenic diabetes insipidus: no change

THE HYPOGLYCEMIAS

Hypoglycemia is said to exist when the plasma glucose concentration falls below 55 mg/dl. The blood glucose concentration is dependent on the interaction between glucose production (dietary intake and liver glycogenolysis and glyconeogenesis) and glucose utilization (organs, tissue, and glands). Hypoglycemia may be either reactive or organic. The reactive type develops in response to a high-carbohydrate meal, is transient, and involves inappropriate insulin response. The organic type occurs spontaneously in the fasting state and suggests a defect in hepatic glucose formation or the presence of insulin-producing tumors.

Laboratory tests
Fasting glucose and insulin levels (plasma)

Normally, when glucose concentrations rise, so do insulin levels; and when plasma glucose concentrations fall, insulin release is inhibited. Thus the two levels are measured together, and the insulin level is evaluated in light of the glucose value. The insulin level is measured by radioimmunoassay. In normal persons, when the two levels are measured at 8 A.M. following a 12- to 14-hour overnight fast, the insulin/glucose ratio is always less than 0.3. Patients with insulinoma usually have ratios greater than 0.3, and often greater than 1.0. If the results after an overnight fast are inconclusive, fasting can be prolonged to 72 hours, and the insulin/glucose ratio determined again.

Tolbutamide tolerance test

Tolbutamide (Orinase) is a hypoglycemic agent. In this test it is given intravenously in a dose of 1 gm, after which blood glucose and insulin levels are determined at 0, 5, 10, 20, 30, 60, and 120 minutes. In normal individuals, at 5 to 10 minutes the serum insulin level increases by less than 100 μU/ml, and returns to the baseline value at 40 to 60 minutes. The lowest glucose levels occur at 20 to 30 mintues and return to normal within an hour. Individuals with insulinoma have a greater than normal response to tolbutamide.

Contraindications. Intravenous administration of tolbutamide is contraindicated in hypoglycemic patients. Seizures and death may result.

Precautions. If serious hypoglycemic symptoms develop, an ampule of 50% dextrose in water should be given intravenously.

Limitations. There have been false-positive results.

Clinical application of laboratory tests
Reactive hypoglycemia

This is the most common type of hypoglycemia. It is usually seen in diabetic persons, but it is sometimes seen in prediabetic persons. This type of hypoglycemia is thought to be the result of a lag in insulin release that occurs after the blood glucose level has been high. After a high-carbohydrate meal, the increased blood glucose level normally stimulates the release of insulin. In reactive hypoglycemia there is a slight delay in the release of insulin. Thus the peak of insulin release occurs at a time when the blood glucose level is decreasing, causing the level to drop below normal.

The most frequently employed test is the 5-hour glucose tolerance test (p. 96). In cases of reactive hypoglycemia there is a greater than normal reduction in plasma glucose level 2 to 3 hours after glucose ingestion. Usually the blood glucose level drops below 50 mg/dl and is associated with symptoms

Reactive hypoglycemia may also be diagnosed on the basis of symptoms, a blood glucose level below 50 mg/dl after a high-carbohydrate meal, and resolution of the symptoms after administration of glucose. This method is probably more diagnostic than a 5-hour glucose tolerance test.

Organic hypoglycemia

Hypoglycemia caused by insulin-producing tumors is diagnosed by evaluating the insulin/glucose ratio after a 12- to 14-hour and/or a 72-hour fast, and by the tolbutamide tolerance test.

Iatrogenic hypoglycemia

Both insulin injections and long-acting oral hypoglycemics cause this type of hypoglycemia, the diagnosis of which is made on the basis of a patient's history.

Alcoholic hypoglycemia

This type of hypoglycemia is common in chronic alcoholics who drink for a few days without eating. The diagnosis is made on the basis of a patient's history.

TEN Diagnostic tests
for hematologic disorders

BONE MARROW EXAMINATION

The bone marrow, which produces millions of blood cells daily (hemato-poiesis), is the major site of the formation of blood. In the adult the red bone marrow is found in only a few locations, mainly in membranous bones, such as the vertebrae, the sternum, and the ribs. The most accessible region for bone marrow examination is the sternum, by means of sternal puncture, or the iliac crest. Since the bone marrow is the center of hematopoiesis, the system that actually produces the blood, a bone marrow examination should be performed when a disorder in this production is suspected.

A bone marrow examination is diagnostic in the following diseases.

Leukemias

The examination is helpful especially if there is a differential diagnostic problem with the peripheral smear, such as leukemia versus leukemoid reaction, or in aleukemic leukemia, in which the peripheral smear is not diagnostic of leukemia. In leukemia the bone marrow examination will show the ratio of myeloid cells to erythroid cells to be decidedly increased, with an increase in the number of early immature forms. A decreased leukocyte alkaline phosphatase concentration and the presence of the Philadelphia chromosome are characteristic of chronic myelogenous leukemia but not of leukemoid reaction.

Iron deficiency anemia

In the early stage of iron deficiency anemia a bone marrow examination reveals normoblastic hyperplasia, but the severe iron deficiency that develops later eventually limits erythropoiesis (the formation of red blood cells) to the basal level. The normoblasts are small, with frayed edges. Smears stained for iron reveal storage iron to be absent.

Serum ferritin levels correlate very well with iron bone marrow stores, they can be obtained easily and in a noninvasive manner. Thus, in most cases ferritin level determinations obviate the need for bone marrow examination to obtain iron stains for the diagnosis of iron deficiency anemia.

Megaloblastosis

Although at the present time the levels of vitamin B_{12} and folic acid in the blood are being relied on increasingly for the diagnosis of macrocytic anemia, bone marrow aspiration can reveal megaloblasts in both vitamin B_{12} and folic acid deficiencies. Such a finding would be diagnostic, since the deficiency is responsible for the megaloblastosis.

Multiple myeloma

Bone marrow aspiration can be diagnostic in multiple myeloma if sheaths of plasma cells occupying most of the marrow elements are seen. The plasma cells may vary from less than 1% to over 90% of marrow, depending upon the degree of involvement in the site from which the marrow is aspirated.

Hemolytic anemias

A bone marrow examination is important in determining whether hemolysis is a cause of anemia, although it does not help a physician to differentiate between the various causes of hemolytic anemias.

Hypoplastic or aplastic anemias

The diagnosis of hypoplastic or aplastic anemias can be made only through a bone marrow examination, which would reveal hypocellularity.

Idiopathic thrombocytopenic purpura versus hypoplastic marrow

In bleeding disorders that result from a decrease in the number of platelets, a bone marrow examination is helpful in differentiating between idiopathic thrombocytopenic purpura (normal or increased numbers of megakaryocytes) and hypoplastic marrow (depletion of megakaryocytes). A normal or increased number of megakaryocytes indicates that platelets are being destroyed in the patient's circulation, while the depletion of megakaryocytes indicates a defect in platelet production.

EVALUATION OF BLEEDING DISORDERS

In recent years there has been a complete reevaluation of all concepts of bleeding disorders. New clotting factors have been identified, the use of a uniform nomenclature has been attempted, and the use of routine coagulation studies prior to surgery has made the laboratory evaluation of bleeding disorders practical.

In this section we introduce new concepts and theories of coagulation that have direct relevance to clinical evaluations.

Bleeding disorders usually result from one of the following:

1. A clotting problem, which is exemplified by hemophilia. Such a problem involves bleeding from large vessels or extended bleeding as a result of trauma.
2. A hemostatic plug problem, which usually is the result of a platelet factor abnormality. This problem is characterized by small-vessel bleeding, petechiae, and mucous membrane bleeding.
3. A combination of a plug formation problem and a clotting problem

Hemostasis

Hemostasis (prevention of blood loss) is achieved through the following chain of events: vascular spasm, formation of a platelet plug, blood coagulation, and formation of fibrin threads to strengthen the blood clot.

Vascular spasm and the platelet plug

Immediately after the blood vessel is cut or ruptures, the wall of the vessel contracts locally, permitting platelet plugging and the process of coagulation.

When a vessel wall is injured, factor III (thromboplastin) is released from the damaged cells. The platelets exposed to the recently disrupted endothelial surface of the vessel come into contact with collagen fibers and connective tissue, whereupon they change their characteristics. There follows a very complicated process, greatly oversimplified here.

Platelet aggregation and release reaction

The sequence of platelet plug formation is shown in Fig. 10-1.

Adhesion. Thrombin and collagen both cause platelet aggregation in vivo and in vitro. Thus when the platelets are exposed to the collagen of the in-

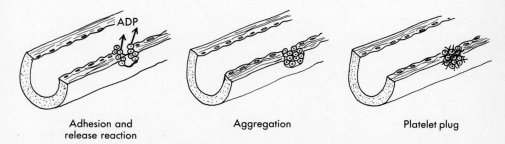

Adhesion and
release reaction

Aggregation

Platelet plug

Fig. 10-1
Sequence of platelet plug formation.

jured vessel wall they begin to adhere to the vessel wall and to clump together.

Release reaction. Adhesion to the vessel wall and exposure to thrombin, which is being generated from the clotting systems, stimulates the platelets to release their intracellular pool of adenosine disphosphate (ADP), adenosine triphosphate (ATP), serotonin, and Ca^{++}.

Aggregation. Platelet aggregation results from the exposure of the platelets to the intracellular pool of ADP and to thrombin. The platelets secrete substances that maintain vasoconstriction, and thus participate in blood coagulation.

Fusion. The vasoconstriction and the platelet aggregation result in the formation of the *platelet plug*, the maintenance of which is achieved through the interaction of platelets, thrombin, and fibrin.

Mechanism of coagulation

Each of the substances involved in coagulation has been assigned a Roman numeral (I to XIII, with VI having been dropped because it was identical to activated factor V).

The activation of the coagulation process involves two sequential pathways, intrinsic and extrinsic, each of which is sometimes described as a "waterfall" or a "cascade" because it involves step-by-step interactions and the dependency of one reaction upon the other. The two pathways are initially independent and then interact to form a common pathway (Fig. 10-2).

The *extrinsic pathway* originates with the injury to the blood vessel, at which time factor III (tissue thromboplastin) is released from the endothelial cells. In the presence of calcium ions (Ca^{++}) and factor VII (a circulating serum prothrombin conversion accelerator), factor III activates factor X, which then joins the intrinsic system to form a common pathway.

The *intrinsic pathway* involves protein-protein interactions and is slower than the extrinsic system. As the name implies, the intrinsic factors are within the blood itself.

Factor XII is the plasma component that is activated by tissue factors, collagen, endotoxin, platelets, endothelial cell membrane, and possibly other activators, including Fletcher factor and Fitzgerald factor. Once activated, factor XII activates factor XI, which in turn, in the presence of Ca^{++}, activates factor IX ("Christmas Factor"), which is synthesized in the liver in a vitamin K–dependent process.

The site of synthesis of factor VIII (antihemophilic globulin, AHG) and its exact function in the intrinsic clotting pathway are not known.

Prothrombin is converted into thrombin by factor X (Stuart-Prower factor), in the presence of Ca^{++} and factor V. Factor X may be activated by the products of either the intrinsic pathway or the extrinsic pathway, and thus begins the *common pathway* of coagulation (see Fig. 10-2).

Factor V, a glycoprotein, acts as a catalyst in the activation of factor X. It thus participates in prothrombin activation.

Thrombin acts as an enzyme to convert fibrinogen into fibrin threads to form a soluble plug, the first visible sign of coagulation. Finally, the clot structure is strengthened by factor XIII, the fibrin-stabilizing factor.

Coagulation tests

Laboratory evaluation of coagulation, combined with a complete history and physical, with emphasis on family history, can greatly facilitate the definitive diagnosis of coagulation disorders.

If there is no family history of bleeding problems, presurgery screening tests include platelet count, bleeding time, partial thromboplastin time, and

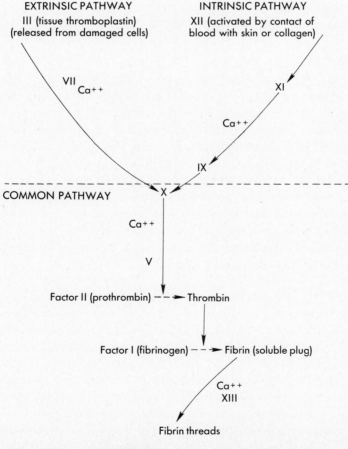

Fig. 10-2
Mechanism of coagulation.

prothrombin time. Bleeding time is the screening test for platelet function in the presence of a normal platelet count; partial thromboplastin time and prothrombin time are the screening tests for intrinsic, extrinsic, and common pathway abnormalities. If an abnormality is found, or if there is a family history of a bleeding problem, then more specific tests are required, such as specific factor assays and tests for qualitative platelet abnormalities.

Platelet count

The platelet count is a screening test for disorders involving platelet factors; it is valuable in the diagnosis of thrombocytopenia. A platelet count involves the determination of the number of platelets per cubic millimeter of blood. The test is indicated when a peripheral smear reveals a lower than normal number of platelets.

> ◆ **Normal platelet count**
> 150,000-350,000/cu mm

Bleeding time

A test of bleeding time provides an indication of the adequacy of platelet function. A small stab wound is made in the earlobe or forearm, and the time required for bleeding to stop is then recorded.

Clinical value. The bleeding time is normal in disorders of coagulation but is abnormal in severe thrombocytopenia, defects of platelet function, or von Willebrand's disease, or when blood fibrinogen is totally absent.

Limitations. The normal range may vary if the puncture is not standard size. Prolonged bleeding may result from heavy alcohol consumption or from the presence of any of the following drugs: aspirin, dextran, streptokinase-streptodornase, mithramycin, and pantothenyl alcohol.

Precautions. If bleeding continues beyond 15 minutes, pressure should be applied and a physician should be notified.

Platelet aggregation test

If the bleeding time is found to be abnormal, the platelet aggregation test, another screening test for platelet dysfunction, is performed. Light transmission through platelet-rich plasma is recorded continuously, and aggregating agents (ADP, epinephrine, connective tissue, and ristocetin, an antibiotic that causes spontaneous aggregation of normal platelets) are added to the glass cuvette of an aggregometer. When the platelets clump, more light passes through the plasma, and is recorded on a strip chart.

Precautions. Specimens left for more than 3 hours at room temperature may lose their aggregating characteristics. Aspirin inhibits the secondary waves of aggregation brought about by ADP and epinephrine, but not the primary wave. Therefore, the patient must not be using aspirin or other non-steroidal anti-inflammatory agents prior to the test.

Normal values. In most laboratories the results are reported in descriptive terms, and are dependent on the concentrations of the aggregating agents.

The addition of ADP (1 µg/ml) to the curette of an aggregometer produces two waves of aggregation. The first is the direct result of the ADP added to the specimen; the second is the result of ADP released from the storage pool in the platelet. Lower concentrations of ADP result in no release reaction; only a primary wave is seen. With larger doses only a single, broad wave is seen.

The addition of epinephrine produces two waves of aggregation in 50%-80% of healthy persons.

The addition of collagen does not produce a primary wave; the effect of collagen is limited to inducing the release of ADP from the storage pool within the platelets.

Partial thromboplastin time (PTT)

Partial thromboplastin time is the time required for recalcified citrated plasma to clot. Abnormal results usually indicate deficiencies of the coagulation factors in the intrinsic and common pathways, and an impairment of clotting factor function to below 15%-20% of normal.

Limitations. PTT is insensitive to platelet function and to deficiencies in factors VII and XIII (extrinsic factor deficiencies).

♦ Normal PT

30-45 sec

Activated partial thromboplastin time (APTT)

The APTT is a modification of PTT. Artificial reagents are used to activate the intrinsic system more rapidly.

♦ Normal APT

16-25 sec

Prothrombin time (PT)

A test of prothrombin time is used to identify defects of the vitamin K–dependent coagulation factors in the extrinsic and common pathways (factors VII, X, and II); the test measures the time taken for recalcified citrated plasma to clot in the presence of tissue thromboplastin. The effect of coumarin anticoagulants on the PT is significant, and heparin may prolong the PT slightly.

♦ Normal PT

11-16 sec or 100% (each laboratory sets its own normal)

Manipulation of prothrombin time and partial thromboplastin time

Over 95% of the inherited coagulopathies are caused by factor deficiencies in the intrinsic system. There are specific in vitro assays for each coagulation factor. In the absence of these assays, however, the partial thromboplastin time and the prothrombin time can be used to identify the absent factor.

For example, substitution experiments using barium sulfate-adsorbed plasma and aged, citrated serum with the tests of prothrombin time and the partial thromboplastin time may pinpoint the deficient coagulation factor. Serum that is aged and citrated is depleted of thrombin and devoid of factors I, II, V, and VIII; adsorbed plasma (barium sulfate–adsorbed oxalated plasma) is devoid of factors II, VII, IX, and X.

Manipulation of prothrombin time. When aged, citrated serum is added to the patient's serum the prothrombin time becomes normal in factor VII and X deficiencies, but remains abnormal in factor I, II, and V deficiencies.

Table 10-1

Use of prothrombin time (PT) to identify deficient factor*

Deficient factor	PT	PT + serum	PT + adsorbed plasma
VII	Abnormal	Normal	Abnormal
X	Abnormal	Normal	Abnormal
V	Abnormal	Abnormal	Normal
II	Abnormal	Abnormal	Abnormal
I	Abnormal	Abnormal	Normal

From Blatt, P.M., Zeitler, K.D., and Roberts, H.R.: Hemophilia and other hereditary defects of coagulation. In Conn, H.F., and Conn, R.B., Jr., editors: Current diagnosis, Philadelphia, 1980, W.B. Saunders Co.
*Normal PT is 12 to 14 seconds. Abnormal is greater than 14 seconds.

Table 10-2

Use of the partial thromboplastin time (PTT) to identify deficient clotting factor*

Deficient factor	PTT	PTT + serum†	PTT + adsorbed‡ plasma
XII	Abnormal	Normal	Normal
XI	Abnormal	Normal	Normal
VIII	Abnormal	Abnormal	Normal
IX	Abnormal	Normal	Abnormal

From Blatt, P.M., Zeitler, K.D., and Roberts, H.R.: Hemophilia and other hereditary defects of coagulation. In Conn, H.F., and Conn, R.B., Jr., editors: Current diagnosis, Philadelphia, 1980, W.B. Saunders Co.
*Normal PTT is 45 to 65 seconds; abnormal is over 65 seconds.
†Serum should be aged to deplete thrombin and should be citrated (1 part 3.2 per cent citrate to 5 parts serum). Serum contains factors VII, IX, and X and is devoid of I, ii, V, and VIII.
‡BaSO$_4$-adsorbed oxalated plasma or Al (OH)$_3$-adsorbed citrated plasma removes factors II, VII, IX, and X.

A factor deficiency can be further pinpointed with the addition of absorbed plasma to the patient's serum, in which case the prothrombin time becomes normal in deficiencies of Factors I and V. By the same token, if the prothrombin time does not normalize, the deficiency cannot be in factors I or V, but must be in factors II, VII, IX, or X. In either case a specific assay would be required for an accurate diagnosis, but the field would have been narrowed (see Table 10-1).

Manipulation of partial thromboplastin time. If the partial thromboplastin time becomes normal with the addition of aged, citrated serum to the patient's serum, the deficiency is in factor IX, XI, or XII; it remains abnormal only in factor VIII deficiency.

With the addition of adsorbed plasma to the patient's serum the partial thromboplastin time normalizes in factors VIII, XI, or XII deficiency; if it remains abnormal, the deficiency can only be in factor IX (see Table 10-2).

Thrombin time (TT)

Thrombin time is the time required for plasma to clot after the addition of thrombin. Two strengths of thrombin are used.

Clinical value. The thrombin time is abnormal in fibrinogen deficiencies and in disseminated intravascular coagulation (because of the presence of DIC-circulating anticoagulants).

♦ Normal TT

With the stronger thrombin solution: 9-11 sec (a prolongation of 3 sec over this time is considered abnormal)

With the weaker thrombin solution: 25-35 sec (a prolongation of 5 sec over this time is considered abnormal)

Clinical application of coagulation tests
Platelet-related disorders

The thrombocytopenias. Thrombocytopenia is the most common bleeding disorder involving platelets. It may be the result of decreased production or increased destruction of platelets, or it may result from redistribution of platelets, with splenic pooling. *Bone marrow aspiration* is the most useful diagnostic test for thrombocytopenic disorders. Bone marrow depletion of megakaryocytes implies a defect in platelet production; the presence of normal or increased numbers of megakaryocytes implies a platelet-destructive mechanism within the patient's circulation.

Thrombocytopenias are usually caused by one of the following:

1. *Defects in platelet production*, resulting from chemotherapy, radiotherapy, or malignant invasion of the bone marrow, or as part of the clinical picture of generalized aplastic anemia, acquired or congenital. Such a defect is diagnosed because of a reduced number of megakaryocytes in the bone marrow.

2. *Excessive destruction of platelets* in the patient's circulation, usually because of an autoantibody (idiopathic thrombocytopenic purpura, systemic lupus erythematosus) or drug sensitization. This situation is diagnosed because of normal or increased numbers of megakaryocytes in the bone marrow.
3. *Abnormal platelet distribution* because of hypersplenism, in which large numbers of platelets become trapped in the enlarged spleen, causing an increased number of megakaryocytes in the bone marrow. The platelets, however, have a nearly normal life span.

Disorders caused by defective platelets. The qualitative platelet disorders may be either congenital or acquired, but they all are characterized by a *prolonged bleeding time*, a *normal platelet count*, and *normal results of clotting tests*. The mechanism responsible for and the degree of a platelet defect can be identified through the measurement of *platelet adhesion, platelet aggregation,* and *platelet factor III availability*.

Bernard-Soulier syndrome. This is an inherited disease, somewhat dominant, that is characterized by the failure of platelets to aggregate with ristocetin in the presence of normal plasma. Platelets aggregate normally with ADP, epinephrine, collagen, and thrombin.

Storage pool disease. This disorder may result from (1) a congenital deficiency of the intracellular platelet pool of ADP and serotonin or (2) a defective release mechanism, in which case although there is enough ADP and serotonin to accomplish the secondary wave of aggregation, they are not released.

Laboratory tests. In both types of storage pool disease, the *bleeding time* is abnormal. *Aggregation* with ristocetin is normal, but with epinephrine or ADP the secondary wave of aggregation is absent. Differentiation between the two subgroups requires special tests that are not readily available.

Thrombasthenia (Glanzmann's disease). Glanzmann's disease is a rare congenital disorder in which there is a defect of primary platelet aggregation; the platelets do not aggregate with any concentration of ADP, epinephrine, connective tissue, or thrombin.

Drug-induced defects. Aspirin and the other nonsteroidal anti-inflammatory agents inhibit the platelet release reaction, an effect that lasts the life span of the platelet (48 to 72 hours after ingestion). There is a prolonged bleeding time, the secondary waves of aggregation with ADP and epinephrine are inhibited, and primary aggregation is inhibited with connective tissue.

Other coagulation abnormalities

The hemophilias. Hemophilia is a congenital bleeding disorder. It may be divided into hemophilia A (classic hemophilia) and hemophilia B (Christmas disease) by laboratory tests, but the two are clinically indistinguishable. (Another hereditary coagulopathy, separable from hemophilia A, is von Willebrand's disease.)

Hemophilia A (classical hemophilia). This is a deficiency in factor VIII *clotting activity;* in this disorder there are, however, normal amounts of circulating factor VIII. This disease is usually found in males and carried by females. Sons of affected males will be normal; daughters will be carriers. Thus the disease appears to skip a generation. Its severity depends upon the level of factor VIII clotting activity.

Laboratory tests. In the routine screening test the partial thromboplastin or activated partial thromboplastin time will be prolonged; prothrombin time, bleeding time, and thrombin time are all normal.

The definitive diagnosis is made by specific assay. If a specific assay is not available, a diagnosis can be made by means of the partial thromboplastin time. If the PTT is corrected with barium sulfate–adsorbed plasma but not with aged serum, the deficiency is in factor VIII.

Differential diagnosis. Mild hemophilia A is distinguished from von Willebrand's disease by laboratory tests measuring factor VIII clotting activity (decreased in hemophilia A) and the factor VIII antigen level (normal or high in hemophilia A), which is obtained by immunoelectrophoresis. The bleeding time and the ristocetin-induced platelet aggregation are normal in hemophilia A and abnormal in von Willebrand's disease.

Hemophilia B (Christmas disease). This is a factor IX deficiency; it is characterized by a prolonged partial thromboplastin time. Hemophilia B is distinguished from hemophilia A by a specific factor IX assay. If such an assay is not available, hemophilia B may be diagnosed as follows: if the partial thromboplastin time normalizes with the addition of aged serum but not with the addition of barium sulfate–adsorbed plasma, the deficiency is in factor IX.

Von Willebrand's disease. This inherited bleeding disorder appears to result from a deficiency of the factor VIII molecule, which under certain circumstances is required for the aggregation of platelets.

Laboratory tests. The diagnosis is based on family history, prolonged bleeding time, and decreased factor VIII activity. Platelet aggregation in the presence of ristocetin is decreased.

Differential diagnosis. Factor VIII (the von Willebrand factor) possesses an activity related to platelet function, in addition to its coagulant and antigenic activities. In von Willebrand's disease the platelet function of factor VIII is abnormal, and so is bleeding time; in hemophilia A the coagulation sequence of factor VIII is abnormal, and thus bleeding time is normal. The level of the factor VIII–related antigen is usually decreased in von Willebrand's disease but normal or increased in hemophilia A.

Table 10-3

Coagulation factors

Factor	Synonyms	Deficiency state	Inheritance pattern	Abnormal tests
I	Fibrinogen	Afibrinogenemia	Autosomal recessive	BT, PT, PTT, TCT
		Dysfibrinogenemia	Autosomal dominant	PT, PTT, TCT
II	Prothrombin	Hypoprothrombinemia	Autosomal recessive	PT, PTT
		Dysprothrombinemia	? Autosomal recessive	PT, PTT
III	Tissue thromboplastin	None		
IV	Calcium	None		
V	Accelerator globulin (proaccelerin)	Factor V deficiency‡	Autosomal recessive	PT, PTT, BT (prolonged in ⅓)
VII	Proconvertin	Factor VII deficiency†	Autosomal recessive	PT
VIII	Antihemophilic factor	Classic hemophilia† (hemophilia A)	X-linked recessive	PTT
		von Willebrand's disease	Autosomal dominant	BT, PTT
IX	Plasma thromboplastin component	Hemophilia B† (Christmas disease)	X-linked recessive	PTT
X	Stuart factor	Factor X deficiency†	Autosomal recessive	PT, PTT
XI	Plasma thromboplastin antecedent	Factor XI deficiency†	Autosomal recessive	PTT
XII*	Hageman factor	Factor XII deficiency†	Autosomal recessive	PTT
Fletcher*	—	Fletcher factor deficiency	Autosomal recessive	PTT
Fitzgerald*	—	Fitzgerald factor deficiency	Autosomal recessive	PTT
Passavoy	—	Passavoy factor deficiency	Autosomal recessive	PTT
XIII	Fibrin stabilizing factor	Factor XIII deficiency†	Autosomal recessive	Clot solubility increased in 5 M urea

From Blatt, P.M., Zietler, K.D., and Roberts, H.R.: Hemophilia and other hereditary defects of coagulation. In Conn, H.F., and Conn, R.B., Jr., editors: Current diagnosis, Philadelphia, 1980, W.B. Saunders Co.
Key: BT = bleeding time; PT = prothrombin time; PTT = partial thromboplastin time; TCT = thrombin clotting time.
*No clinical symptoms.
†Genetic heterogeneity identified with some patients showing "true" deficiency of factor synthesis while other patients have abnormal molecules incapable of supporting procoagulant activity yet present in antigenically normal quantity.
‡Genetic heterogeneity suggested by variable levels of factor V activity.

Pitfalls. Pregnancy and the use of birth control pills can normalize many of the test results that are usually abnormal in von Willebrand's disease.

One or more of the laboratory tests may have normal results when most of the laboratory tests and the clinical picture support the presence of the disease.

The test results can vary from day to day or month to month in one patient.

Factor XIII deficiency. Factor XIII transforms the initial fibrin clot into the strengthened, cross-linked fibrin clot. Thus the absence of factor XIII allows delayed bleeding. This is a rare disorder, but it is easily diagnosed.

Laboratory tests. The prothrombin, partial thromboplastin, and thrombin times are all normal; the deficiency is detected by a simple screening test, which is based on the solubility of the clot in 5M urea. Normal clots are stable for days; in the absence of factor XIII, however, a clot dissolves within approximately an hour, and often within minutes.

• • •

The abnormal laboratory test results that characterize other defects of coagulation factors are listed in Table 10-3.

Disseminated intravascular coagulation (DIC). DIC is an acquired bleeding and thrombotic disorder that is usually secondary to serious systemic disease; it is characterized by intravascular formation of fibrin thrombi, along with reductions in the levels of clotting factors, platelets, and fibrinogen, resulting in the activation of the fibrinolytic system. The fibrinolytic process produces potent circulating anticoagulants. The levels of factors I, II, V, and VIII, and platelets, are frequently decreased.

Etiologies are varied and many; they include obstetric conditions such as abruptio placenta, septic abortion, and amniotic fluid embolus; extensive trauma or surgery, particularly prostatic surgery; certain disseminated malignancies; infections that lead to endotoxic shock; prolonged hypotension and shock; and acidosis from any cause.

Laboratory tests. Prothrombin time and partial thromboplastin time are increased; the platelet count and the fibrinogen level are decreased. Definitive tests are an assay for fibrinogen degradation products, which will have a positive titer, and thrombin time, which will be increased. The peripheral blood smear will show fragmented red cells.

EVALUATION OF HEMOLYTIC DISORDERS

Hemolysis

The term "hemolysis" refers to the premature destruction of red blood cells, resulting in the release of hemoglobin into the surrounding medium. In the *hemolytic anemias* this process is a prominent feature. Recognition of its presence and determination of its degree are based upon the identification of compensatory red blood cell production (erythropoiesis) and increased red blood cell destruction.

Red blood cells are usually destroyed in the reticuloendothelial system; afterward the hemoglobin is degraded, converted to bilirubin, and conjugated by the liver. The resulting bilirubin glucuronide is excreted via the biliary system, and is measured in the blood as the direct-reacting fraction. The unconjugated bilirubin is measured as the indirect-reacting fraction. If the rate of bilirubin formation exceeds the liver's capacity to conjugate and excrete, there will be an increase in the amount of "indirect" bilirubin in the serum. The unconjugated bilirubin is not found in the urine, because it is not water soluble and thus is not cleared by the kidney.

Routine screening tests for hemolysis
Tests for compensatory red blood cell production

The blood film provides a rough index of the degree of reticulocytosis, but a reticulocyte count is more specific; and it also measures the number of red cells recently delivered to the blood from the marrow, per 100 erythrocytes. If compensatory red blood cell production is occurring, examination of the bone marrow reveals erythroid hyperplasia and early megaloblastic changes resulting from folic acid deficiency.

♦ Normal reticulocyte count

0.5-1.5%

Examination of the peripheral blood film may also be a way of spotting anisocytosis, macrocytosis, and poikilocytosis. In addition, the following may be suggested from careful examination of the blood film:
1. Marked spherocytosis suggests a diagnosis of hereditary spherocytosis. Mild spherocytosis suggests hemoglobin C disease. Mild spherocytosis combined with a positive reaction to Coombs' test suggests autoimmune hemolysis.
2. Hemolysis, with a significant amount of elliptocytosis, suggests hereditary elliptocytosis.
3. The presence of schistocytes in significant numbers or of helmet cells suggests microangiopathic hemolytic anemia (for example, anemia associated with an aortic valve prosthesis).
4. The presence of heinz bodies during a hemolytic crisis strongly suggests hemolysis due to red cell enzyme deficiency.

Tests for increased red blood cell destruction

Destruction of red cells is reflected by an increase in the level of indirect-reacting bilirubinemia and a reduction in the level of haptoglobins. If the hemolysis is intramuscular and severe, one sees *hemoglobinuria* (see p. 46), which indicates that the amount of plasma hemoglobin exceeds the amount of haptoglobin available to bind it; *hemosiderinuria,* which indicates chronic hemoglobinuria (iron from the plasma hemoglobin is filtered by the kidneys to produce this condition); and increased amounts of plasma *lactic dehydrogenase (LDH)* (see p. 21).

Serum haptoglobin level. Haptoglobins are produced by the liver to act as transport proteins for hemoglobin. The haptoglobin level declines either because there is too much free hemoglobin to bind (as in intravascular hemolysis) or because of a production failure (liver failure). Levels are increased by infection, inflammation, and malignancy.

♦ **Normal serum haptoglobin**

40-180 mg/dl

Plasma hemoglobin level. A qualitative assessment of plasma hemoglobin level usually suffices as a means to detect acute intravascular hemolysis.

Limitations. The test is reliable only when the plasma level exceeds 50 mg/dl, the threshold for visual estimation. However, a free hemoglobin level below 30 mg/dl is not clinically important.

♦ **Normal plasma hemoglobin**

<100 mg/dl

Additional tests for hemolysis

Hemolysis usually can be documented with the screening tests just mentioned, unless in addition to hemolysis there is bone marrow depression as a result of infection or drugs, in which case there would not be reticulocytosis. If hemolysis is low grade and the serum bilirubin level is borderline, other tests may be used to document the hemolysis and to suggest diagnostic possibilities.

Osmotic fragility

This is a measurement of the ability of a cell to hold extra water. A normal red blood cell is biconcave; in a hypotonic medium, it will fill with water until the osmotic pressure is the same inside and outside of the cell. At a certain critical volume (about 1.8 times the resting volume), a normal cell becomes a perfect sphere and further entry of water produces lysis. A cell that is already spherical can admit less water before it lyses.

Clinical value. This test can be used to document the presence of hemolysis. A low value for osmotic fragility strongly suggests hereditary spherocytosis.

Autohemolysis

This test is used to document the presence of hemolytic disease, and it is helpful in the diagnosis of atypical hereditary spherocytic anemia.

Hemolysis gradually occurs when red cells are incubated in their own serum. In hereditary spherocytosis the addition of glucose to a specimen will significantly diminish the degree of hemolysis, while in congenital nonspecific hemolytic anemias only partial reduction of hemolysis may occur with administration of glucose.

♦ Normal values

<3.5% at the end of 48 hr without added glucose
<0.6% at the end of 48 hr with added glucose

Erythrocyte survival measurements

Erythrocyte survival measurements involve the labeling of erythrocytes with radioisotopes. This test may be indicated when every other effort to establish the presence of hemolysis has failed.

Limitations. The procedure is expensive and inconvenient, requiring repeated blood sampling for several weeks.

Direct Coombs' test

A direct Coombs' test is used to detect immunoglobulin (IgG) and/or complement coating the erythrocytes of patients with warm-antibody autoimmune hemolytic anemia. Coombs' reagent is an antiglobulin that reacts in vitro with IgG and/or complement on the erythrocytes to cause agglutination (a positive result of a direct Coombs' test). Additional antisera react specifically with either the IgG or the complement.

Clinical value. A direct Coombs' test is most useful in the differentiation of acquired immunologic hemolytic anemias from secondary hemolytic anemias that result from diseases such as lymphoma. If globulin is detected on the red cells, an immune mechanism is thought to be the cause of the hemolysis.

Limitations. For any of the following reasons, a direct Coombs' test may have a positive result in a patient who does not have autoimmune hemolytic anemia:

1. The patient is receiving cephalosporin drugs, resulting in nonspecific absorption of globulins by red cells.
2. The patient has reticulocytosis, which may occasionally result in a weakly positive reaction because of the binding of transferrin (a globulin) to the reticulocyte membranes.
3. The patient had a transfusion that resulted in minor blood group incompatibility of the transfused red cells.

Indirect Coombs' test

In this test, the patient's serum and the red cells of a compatible donor are mixed and incubated. The result is positive if, after the addition of Coombs' reagent, agglutination occurs, indicating that the patient has antibodies to the donor red cells.

Clinical value. The result of this test is positive in many cases of warm-antibody hemolytic anemia. If the indirect Coombs' test has a positive result and the direct test has a negative result, the patient does not have an autoimmune hemolytic anemia but has been sensitized to a red cell antigen through transfusion or pregnancy. The indirect Coombs' test is also used to detect IgG antibodies (anti-Rh_0[D]); to demonstrate other antigen-antibody reactions, involving white cells, platelets, and tissue cells; and to demonstrate the presence of hypogammaglobulinemia or agammaglobulinemia.

Erythrocyte enzyme assays

At least 14 forms of hemolytic anemia are associated with a deficiency of erythrocyte enzymes. Although quantitative assays are necessary for the identification of most of these anemias, simple screening tests are available for the more common ones: glucose-6-phosphate dehydrogenase deficiency (favism, G-6-PD), pyruvate kinase (PK) deficiency, triosephosphate isomerase (TPI) deficiency, NADH diaphorase deficiency, and glutathione reductase deficiency.

Hemoglobin electrophoresis

Electrophoresis is useful for detecting hemoglobins A, S, C, E, and D. Like protein (protein electrophoresis is described on p. 278), hemoglobin will migrate in solution in response to an electrical current. However, this migration is relative. Therefore, known reference hemoglobins are important to the test. In normal adult red blood cells, hemoglobins A_1, A_2, and F are present, the latter two only in trace amounts.

The most common abnormal hemoglobins are hemoglobin S, which causes sickle cell disease if homozygous and sickle cell trait if heterozygous, and hemoglobin C, which may cause mild hemolytic anemia.

Measurement of the hemoglobin A_2 level is important in the diagnosis of the thalassemias and is commonly ordered in conjunction with tests for the level of hemoglobin F, since both may be increased in thalassemia.

Laboratory tests in the differential diagnosis of the hemolytic anemias

Once a diagnosis of hemolytic anemia has been made, a differential diagnosis should be done to determine the cause of the anemia, and the appropriate test for documentation should be performed.

A hemolytic disorder may be caused by a defect in the red blood cells, which may be either congenital or acquired, or by an extraneous factor, such as transfusion incompatibility or a chemical agent, or by mechanical trauma resulting from valve replacement, particularly insertion of an aortic valve prosthesis. The following are the more commonly encountered hemolytic anemias, along with the laboratory tests most helpful in differential diagnosis.

Hemolytic anemias caused by defective erythrocytes

Congenital
1. Membrane defects. Besides hereditary spherocytosis, there is hereditary elliptocytosis and stomatocytosis. (All are characterized by a negative result of Coombs' test, an increase in osmotic fragility, and autohemolysis.)
2. Hereditary deficiencies in the Embden-Meyerhof pathway (anaerobic glycolysis), such as occur in pyruvate kinase deficiency (low levels of erythrocyte pyruvate kinase [PK] shown by specific assays of the red blood cell glycolytic enzymes)
3. Abnormalities of the phosphoglucokinase oxidative pathway, such as glucose-6-phosphate dehydrogenase (G-6-PD) deficiency. More than 100 varieties have been described. Hemolysis is precipitated sometimes by the ingestion of various drugs or by the ingestion of fava beans. These abnormalities are detected with erythrocyte enzyme assays.
4. Qualitative abnormalities in globin peptides—for example, hemoglobinopathies such as hemoglobin C disease and sickle cell disease (both detected with hemoglobin electrophoresis)
5. Quantitative abnormality in globin peptide synthesis—for example, thalassemias (hemoglobin electrophoresis shows an increase in the level of hemoglobin F in thalassemia major; a decrease in hemoglobin A_1 and a relative increase in hemoglobin A_2 in thalassemia minor)

Acquired
1. Vitamin B_{12} deficiency (as shown by serum B_{12} levels, Schilling test)
2. Paroxysmal nocturnal hemoglobinuria (shown by plasma hemoglobin determination, sucrose hemolysis test, or acid hemolysis test)
3. Acquired hemolytic anemia mediated by an immune mechanism
   a. Hemolytic transfusion reaction
   b. Hemolytic diseases of the newborn
   c. Erythroblastosis fetalis (Coombs' test positive)
   d. Idiopathic acquired hemolytic anemias (Coombs' test positive)
   e. Hemolysis associated with certain mycoplasmal infections, such as that caused by *Mycoplasma pneumoniae* (indicated by elevated levels of cold agglutinins)

   f. Acquired hemolytic anemia resulting from drugs

   g. Infection with an autoimmune component

Extracorporeal factors causing hemolytic anemias

1. Chemical agents and drugs such as phenylhydrazine, benzene, and lead (peripheral smear for lead)
2. Infection
3. Liver disease
4. Splenomegaly of any cause
5. Mechanical injury such as that caused by aortic valve prosthesis
6. Certain poisons
7. Thermal injury
8. Osmotic injury

Secondary hemolytic anemias (Coombs' negative)

This group of anemias is associated with sarcoidosis (shown by node biopsy and Kveim test), liver disease (shown by liver function tests), Hodgkin's disease (node biopsy), disseminated lupus erythematosus (antinuclear antibodies), renal cortical necrosis (renal sediment and renal function tests), and thrombotic thrombocytopenic purpura (bone marrow examination and peripheral smear).

EVALUATION OF THE GAMMOPATHIES

Normal human serum contains proteins that can be separated into different types by serum protein electrophoresis. These types are albumin, alpha I globulin, alpha II globulin, beta globulin, and gamma globulin.

The gamma globulins may be further divided into the following immunoglobulins: immunoglobulin G (IgG), immunoglobulin A (IgA), immunoglobulin M (IgM), immunoglobulin D (IgD), and immunoglobulin E (IgE).

All of the immunoglobulins contain combinations of light and heavy polypeptide chains, which are classified according to molecular weight. The normal immunoglobulins in the body are involved in the antigen-antibody reactions that protect the human organism from infective agents and thus are of paramount importance in immunologic or allergic reactions.

The gammopathies are a group of disorders in which neoplastic cells produce an excess of a single immunoglobulin. The abnormal proteins produced by the cell tumors are called paraproteins or M components (M stands for myeloma or macroglobulinemia) and belong immunologically to one of the immunoglobulin groups described above.

The two major gammopathies are multiple myeloma and Waldenstrom's macroglobulinemia.

Tests for the gammopathies
Protein electrophoresis

The serum proteins, part of which are immunoglobulins in solution, will migrate and separate into distinct layers in response to an electrical current passed through a solution. This is because each immunoglobulin has its own specific electrical charge, rate at which it moves, size, and shape.

The solution to be charged is placed on paper or cellulose acetate strips. After the proteins separate, they are stained. The normal pattern will be diffuse, since no single protein is in excess, and the immunoglobulins will diffuse in the gamma band. However, if a single protein does dominate, there will be a peak or a spike at the gamma band, or less frequently at the beta band, of electrophoresis. This peak is often called the M component. Serum protein electrophoresis will give a quantitative numerical value for the amount of protein in each electrophoretic band. Sometimes the results are expressed as percentages of the total proteins.

Immunoelectrophoresis

The purpose of immunoelectrophoresis is to classify immunoglobulins found in the serum. Usually this test is performed after simple serum protein electrophoresis shows a spike in the gamma band, thus identifying the type of the excess immunoglobulin. The immunoglobulins are designated immunoglobulin G (IgG), immunoglobulin M (IgM), immunoglobulin A (IgA), immunoglobulin D (IgD), and immunoglobulin E (IgE).

Immunodiffusion

After serum electrophoresis identifies a spike (M component) and immunoelectrophoresis identifies the type of immunoglobulin in the M component, immunodiffusion quantitates the amount of abnormal immunoglobulin. This test uses an antiserum to produce a reaction between antibody and antigen in a supporting medium.

Nonspecific tests

1. Sedimentation rate: markedly elevated
2. Blood smear: rouleau formation
3. Hyperuricemia, reflecting abnormal cell turnover
4. Alkaline phosphatase level: increased

Clinical application of tests

In *multiple myeloma* bone marrow study reveals the presence of plasma cells in sheaths or isolated islands. Serum or urine protein electrophoresis reveals a homogeneous spike in the gamma range, the alpha I range, or the alpha II range. Immunoelectrophoresis usually yields abnormal quantities of immunoglobulin G. However, some multiple myelomas have been reported to be associated with abnormal production of immunoglobulin A, immunoglobulin D, or immunoglobulin E.

In the *macroglobulinemias* serum protein electrophoresis yields mainly immunoglobulin M. Bone marrow study reveals infiltration with lymphocytes rather than plasma cells.

In *benign monoclonal gammopathy*, so called because the tumor is thought to stem from a clone of cells, there will usually be a spike on serum protein electrophoresis even though the patient is asymptomatic. This situation may represent a latent form of multiple myeloma, which may develop into an active form, or it may represent an extensive immunologic response to some unknown antigen and have a perfectly benign course.

Also classified as gammopathies are heavy chain disease, alpha heavy chain disease, gamma chain disease, and light chain disease. However, it is beyond the scope of this book to discuss these entities, since they are extremely rare.

ELEVEN Diagnostic tests
for neurologic disorders

ANATOMY AND PHYSIOLOGY OF THE BRAIN

The brain consists of three major parts: the cerebrum, the cerebellum, and the brain stem. The cerebrum is the largest division and is divided into two hemispheres, each of which has four lobes—frontal, temporal, parietal, and occipital. The *cerebrum* is the highest integrative center of the nervous system; it is responsible for sensation, perception, memory, consciousness, judgment, and will. The *cerebellum*, located just below the posterior portion of the cerebrum, functions in the control of skeletal muscles. The *brain stem* is composed of the midbrain, the pons, and the medulla oblongata, which connects the brain with the spinal cord and controls breathing, heart rate, and blood pressure. (See Fig. 11-1.)

The three meninges or membranes that envelop the brain and spinal cord are the *dura mater,* the *arachnoid mater,* and the *pia mater* (Fig. 11-2). Their names imply their qualities: the dura is the strong, tough outer layer; the arachnoid is a delicate layer between the dura mater and the pia mater; and the pia adheres to the brain surface like a delicate skin. The pia, which could also be compared to a delicate, transparent layer of cellophane, contains numerous capillaries and arterioles. It is the pia and arachnoid membranes that become inflamed and thickened as a result of infection or hemorrhage and that account for the headache and neck stiffness occurring in those conditions.

A potential space, called the *subdural space,* lies between the dura mater and the arachnoid mater. Between the arachnoid mater and the pia mater lies an actual space, called the *subarachnoid space,* which is filled with cerebrospinal fluid (CSF).

Cerebrospinal fluid is produced by filtration from blood circulating through the richly vascular tissue of the choroid plexuses, which are secretory modifications of the pia mater that project into the ventricles of the

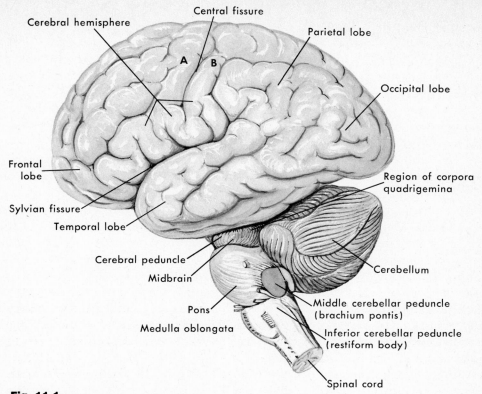

Fig. 11-1

The brain. (From Schottelius, B.A., and Schottelius, D.D.: Textbook of physiology, ed. 17, St. Louis, 1973, The C.V. Mosby Co.)

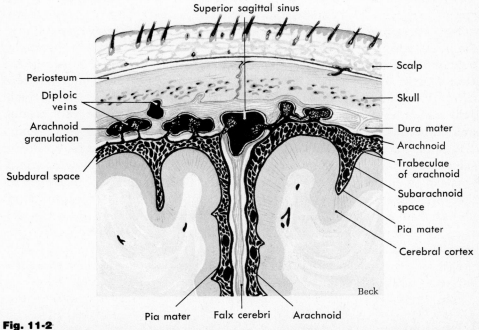

Fig. 11-2

The meninges of the brain as seen in coronal section through the skull. (From Anthony, C.P., and Kolthoff, N.J.: Textbook of anatomy and physiology, ed. 9, St. Louis, 1975, The C.V. Mosby Co.)

brain. The continuously formed, fresh cerebrospinal fluid must drain out of the ventricles through the apertures in the fourth ventricle, in the brain stem. It must freely circulate through the subarachnoid spaces and over all the surfaces of the brain and spinal cord. It is then mostly reabsorbed into the venous system by specially modified arachnoid tissue, called arachnoid granulations (see Fig. 11-2).

The skull can expand in response to increasing intracranial pressure resulting from hydrocephalus or tumor, until skull sutures ossify at age 12 or 13. After that age, increasing pressure inside the then rigid skull pushes the brain downward and backward into the foramen magnum. This foramen is the largest opening in the skull; it surrounds the lower brain stem and its junction with the spinal cord. Increasing intracranial pressure resulting from trauma, hemorrhage, tumor, infection, or hypoxia can force the cone-shaped brain stem ever lower into the bony foramen magnum until the brain stem and the adjacent cerebellar tonsils become tightly wedged or impacted in the foramen magnum. This situation is invariably accompanied by rapid clinical deterioration, as evidenced by decreased responsiveness to stimuli, coma, dilated and/or nonreactive pupils, and Cheyne-Stokes respiration, apnea, or other abnormal respiratory patterns.

Another special area of brain vulnerability is the midbrain. Here the cerebral peduncles, which connect each hemisphere with the brain stem, must pass through a small, semicircular, sharp-edged opening, the incisura in the tentorium, a strong dural structure on each side of the brain stem that forms the roof of the posterior fossa. Any substantial increase in the volume of one cerebral hemisphere, whether from head injury, hemorrhage, tumor, abscess, or large infarction, can wedge the inferior and medial portion of the temporal lobe (the uncus) down into this semicircular opening in the tentorium. This forces the mid-brain laterally into the opposite knifelike dural edge of the tentorium and usually results in multiple hemorrhages in the midbrain and compression of either the ipsilateral or the contralateral third nerves as they sweep around the lateral margins of the midbrain en route to the orbits.

Despite the remarkable versatility of the brain, it reacts to most clinical insults by either localized or generalized swelling. Thus the following conditions can all cause serious problems in clinical management of increased intracranial pressure: traumatic head injury; hypertensive or idiopathic intracerebral hemorrhage; subarachnoid hemorrhage caused by ruptured aneurysms; large infarcts resulting from thrombosis or cerebral embolus; hypoxia resulting from cardiac arrest, drowning, or neonatal asphyxia; bacterial meningitis or viral encephalitis; brain abscess; electrolyte depletion; and poisoning with lead or mercury.

Continuous monitoring of intracranial pressure

The most critical practical considerations in regard to brain anatomy and physiology are the fact that the size of the skull is fixed, allowing no room for expansion of an injured and swollen brain, and the fact that brain swelling is the end result of most metabolic insults. Continuous monitoring of intracranial pressure is therefore becoming widely used in large intensive care units; a manometer is placed in a skull burr hole by a neurosurgeon. Continuous monitoring is of considerable advantage in assessing the need for:

1. Medical decompression by means of dexamethasone (Decadron), mannitol, or urea
2. Controlled hyperventilation to lower Pco_2
3. Intravenous administration of barbiturates to further lower intracranial pressure in certain head injuries
4. Surgical decompression of the brain by ventricular drainage, by evacuation of intracerebral blood clots or necrotic brain tissue, or by ventricular shunts. Surgical decompression is used when medical decompression is inadequate or not the method of choice.

LABORATORY TESTS

Cerebrospinal fluid examination

A lumbar spinal tap is a relatively harmless procedure; it can be quickly and easily done on cooperative patients by physicians with some experience. Cisternal puncture, however, is very hazardous unless done by experienced physicians; patients must be cooperative or sedated. Fortunately, a cisternal tap is only rarely necessary—for example, in the treatment of fungal meningitis, when it is indicated for installation of a small amount of amphotericin into the cisternal cerebrospinal fluid.

Clinical value

A spinal tap is essential in the diagnosis and management of herpes simplex encephalitis, bacterial or fungal meningitis, or meningeal leukemia or carcinoma. When cerebral hemorrhage is suspected, clear evidence of hemorrhage on a CT scan of the brain usually eliminates the need for a spinal tap. However, a normal CT scan does not eliminate the possibility of a small subarachnoid hemorrhage, and a spinal tap would still be necessary if clinical suspicion were not dispelled by the normal CT scan.

Patient positioning

The patient is usually placed in the lateral decubitus position, with his back even with the edge of the mattress and the knees folded up against the chest to the extent consistent with comfort. Drapes obscure landmarks and are best avoided. If the patient is obese or apprehensive or has scoliosis, the procedure is best accomplished with the patient sitting across the bed with legs extended and trunk flexed forward to the extent consistent with comfort.

The Queckenstedt maneuver

The Queckenstedt maneuver involves temporary compression of both jugular veins to see if the cerebrospinal fluid level promptly rises in a manometer and then promptly falls with jugular release. This maneuver is dangerous when intracranial pressure is elevated; it *should not be done* under the following circumstances:

1. When opening pressure on the spinal tap is elevated
2. When the diagnosis is uncertain
3. When an intracranial mass, hemorrhage, or edema is suspected

This maneuver is only justified when compression of the spinal cord as a result of tumor, blood clot, or acute vertebral fracture is suspected.

Normal opening pressure is 180 mm of water in relaxed patients who are in the lateral decubitus position. The cerebrospinal fluid level is at or below the level of the foramen magnum in patients who are in the sitting position.

Clinical significance of gross appearance of cerebrospinal fluid

Grossly clear cerebrospinal fluid sample. Routine cerebrospinal fluid tests on grossly clear specimens include red cell and white cell counts, determination of glucose and protein levels, and the venereal disease research laboratories (VDRL) test.

Blood in the cerebrospinal fluid sample. The presence of blood could result from recent intracranial or intraspinal bleeding, or it could result from the needle striking a small vein or capillary as it penetrates the arachnoid membrane to enter the lumbar subarachnoid space, a fairly common occurrence that causes diagnostic confusion. The most reliable method of distinguishing this mere "bloody tap" from preexisting and critically important recent intracranial or intraspinal hemorrhage is to take the tubes of cerebrospinal fluid *immediately* to the laboratory and have one tube centrifuged *at once*. If the blood in the cerebrospinal fluid has been freshly released as a result of needle puncture of the arachnoid membrane, the spun supernatant cerebrospinal fluid will be crystal clear because red cells will not yet have hemolyzed and caused staining of the supernatant fluid.

Intracranial or intraspinal hemorrhage that has occurred an hour or more prior to the tap usually has resulted in enough hemolysis of red cells so that supernatant cerebrospinal fluid is slightly pink or straw colored, or yields a positive *Hematest* result. This centrifuge test is much more reliable than determining the percent of crenated red cells in the cerebrospinal fluid or the degree of clearing of blood in serial tubes of cerebrospinal fluid.

IMPORTANT: Since red cells in tubes of cerebrospinal fluid can hemolyze in 20 to 30 minutes while sitting at nursing stations or in laboratory receiving areas, all cerebrospinal fluid specimens should be sent to the laboratory *stat* and processed immediately upon arrival. This promptness is also crucial to accurate red cell and white cell counts, to accurate glucose level determinations, and to valid cerebrospinal fluid cytologic or cell button examinations.

Cloudy cerebrospinal fluid sample. Cloudy fluid requires a *stat* gram stain and usually acid-fast stains as well as cultures for aerobic, anaerobic, and acid-fast bacteria. It is a good policy for hospital laboratories to telephone all results of gram and acid-fast stains and all abnormal cell counts and low glucose values to the physician promptly so that he or she may initiate additional bacterial or other studies while the remaining cerebrospinal fluid specimen is still fresh.

The findings of 100 or fewer lymphocytes, a normal or modestly increased protein level, a negative gram stain, and a normal glucose level are characteristic of viral meningoencephalitis. The same spinal fluid, except for the substitution of a low glucose level, suggests tuberculous or fungal meningitis, meningeal leukemia, meningeal carcinoma, or incompletely treated bacterial meningitis.

Acute bacterial meningitis usually produces cloudy or turbid cerebrospinal fluid containing many hundreds or thousands of white cells per cubic millimeter, predominantly polymorphonuclear cells. Protein levels in such cases often are greater than 250 mg/dl and can reach 800 to 1000 mg/dl.

Tuberculous (TB) meningitis usually produces several hundred white cells, predominantly mononuclear cells, along with low glucose levels and high protein levels (more than 200 mg/dl). The low cerebrospinal fluid chloride level long reported to be associated with TB meningitis is thought by some to be correlated with systemic chloride depletion as a result of repeated vomiting rather than with any intrinsic disturbance of chloride metabolism in the spinal fluid. An acid-fast stain is sometimes diagnostic; acid-fast cultures are often not positive for 4 to 6 weeks.

The differential diagnosis of TB meningitis often includes fungal meningitis, in which case india ink preparations and cerebrospinal fluid tests for cryptococcal antigen and for antibodies to *Coccidioides immitis* are helpful.

Glucose in the cerebrospinal fluid sample. Normally the glucose level in the cerebrospinal fluid is two-thirds the blood glucose level, or about 45 to 70 mg/dl in the fasting adult. Because of the filtration of glucose into the cerebrospinal fluid from blood, the glucose level of the cerebrospinal fluid bears a direct relationship to the current blood level. Therefore, the lower limit of the normal cerebrospinal fluid glucose concentration for a particular patient can be reliably determined only by means of a simultaneous blood glucose determination. Thus, whenever a central nervous system infection is suspected, a blood glucose determination should also be performed at the time of spinal puncture.

Cytologic examination of cerebrospinal fluid

In cases of suspected neoplasm—particularly meningeal leukemia or lymphoma, meningeal carcinoma, or medulloblastoma, but also other neo-plasms—cytologic examination of cerebrospinal fluid may be of diagnostic help.

The laboratory should be alerted beforehand so that it can expedite the handling of the specimen upon receipt. Expeditious processing is important to the validity of the results of cytologic cerebrospinal fluid examinations.

Venereal Disease Research Laboratories (VDRL) test

The VDRL test on cerebrospinal fluid should be performed in cases of suspected CNS syphilis, particularly when there is no history of syphilis and there is a question as to whether a positive result of a blood serologic test is a false positive. VDRL or other similar serologic tests are now routine on all cerebrospinal fluid specimens sent to hospital laboratories.

X-ray films of the skull and spine

Skull films can give clues to the existence of chronic increased intracranial pressure. If such pressure exists, these films may show erosion of the dorsum sellae and the clinoid processes in adults and suture separation in children. In addition, skull films are better than routine CT scans in the diagnosis of pituitary tumors. In older patients, who are likely to have physiologic calcification in the pineal gland, the presence of a tumor in a hemisphere or a subdural hematoma may be suspected when there is lateral displacement of the normally midline pineal gland, as best seen in the Towne projection.

Films of the lumbosacral spine are invaluable in the evaluation of low back pain, especially when the pain radiates down the back of one or both legs, a situation that suggests the presence of degenerated discs at lower lumbar levels. In such cases, x-ray findings of narrowed intervertebral disc spaces in lateral views and of calcified spurs in intervertebral foramina in oblique views are quite common. Occasionally, x-ray film may reveal the collapse of vertebral bodies as a result of osteoporosis, trauma, or metastases. The evaluation of patients with unexplained bladder or bowel incontinence, accompanied by leg weakness or numbness, with or without back or leg pain, usually includes dorsal and lumbar spinal x-ray films, and often cervical films as well.

Myelography is done when a physician suspects that the nerve roots or spinal cord are being compressed by degenerated discs or tumors, or as a result of fracture dislocations of the spine. Most patients are kept fasting and are sedated before the procedure. An iodinated contrast agent is injected into the lumbar subarachnoid space, and anterior-posterior (AP), lateral, and oblique films of the area of interest are made. A disc protrusion or a tumor causes a filling defect in the column of contrast material, as shown in Fig. 11-3.

Both oil-based (Pantopaque) and water-soluble (Amipaque) dyes are in common use. Pantopaque contrast medium is usually used when a pathologic condition is suspected in the cervical or upper dorsal spine, since a fluoroscopist can more readily prevent this material from going up into the cerebral subarachnoid spaces. Such patients are ordinarily kept flat in bed for 4 hours or more after the procedure; however, 10% to 15% of patients still develop a "postspinal" headache and must be kept flat for an additional 12 to 24 hours.

When Amipaque contrast material has been used, the patient should be kept semirecumbent, with the head elevated at 20 to 30 degrees, for the next 8 hours, in order to minimize the diffusion of the water-soluble dye into

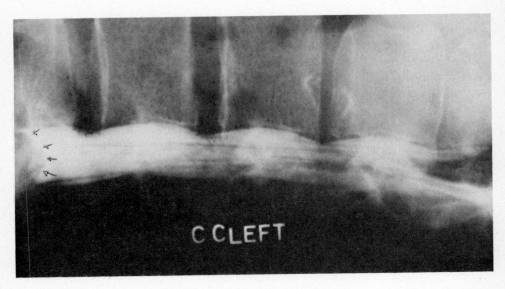

Fig. 11-3
Myelogram. Lateral view of lumbar area. Arrows outline a filling defect in dye column that, during surgery, proved to be a neurofibroma attached to the right SI nerve root. For 3 years this 21-year-old man had complained of low back pain radiating down the back of the right leg. (Courtesy Valley Presbyterian Hospital Radiology Department, Van Nuys, Calif.)

cerebral subarachnoid spaces. Since high concentrations of Amipaque in cerebral subarachnoid fluid can cause confusion and even seizures, the patients should be observed frequently by the nursing staff for 8 to 12 hours after the myelogram has been obtained.

Isotope brain scanning

This test requires that the patient be either cooperative or sedated, so that the head can be immobilized under the gamma camera.

Clinical value

This test, which is essentially risk free, often shows cerebral perfusion defects immediately after the onset of cerebral thrombosis or embolism and fully 2 or 3 days before infarcts can be seen in CT scans. In addition, isotope scans are quite accurate in identifying chronic subdural hematomas, including the 5% or 10% of subdural hematomas that are not seen on CT scans because the x-ray density of the encapsulated mix of blood breakdown products and spinal fluid is equal to the x-ray density of the underlying brain.

Computerized tomography (CT scanning)

An x-ray generator tube and a series of xenon gas–filled detector tubes rotate axially or coronally around the patient's head.

Clinical value

Subtle differences in resistance to the passage of the x-ray beam between normal brain tissue and tumor tissue or fluid-filled ventricles are recorded in the CT computer. These differences are later retrieved to construct photographic slices of the brain that nicely outline the cerebral sulci and gyri, ventricles, and subarachnoid cisterns, as well as pathologic conditions such as tumors, hemorrhages, hematomas, hydrocephalus, or atrophy. Fig. 11-4 is a CT brain scan showing a large hemorrhage into the left basal ganglia. Fig. 11-5 shows a circular mass in the upper left parietal-occipital area; the mass is surrounded by a dense rim. Surgery revealed the mass to be an abscess, which was evacuated.

Certain tumors are "enhanced," or seen better, on a CT scan when Hypaque or a similar iodinated dye is given intravenously just before or during scanning.

Pitfalls

Occasionally renal shutdown may result from large amounts of dye injected into elderly, dehydrated, and/or diabetic patients. An occasional patient will not be a candidate for Hypaque enhancement because of iodine allergy. The only other drawback to CT scans is their cost, which runs from $300 to $500.

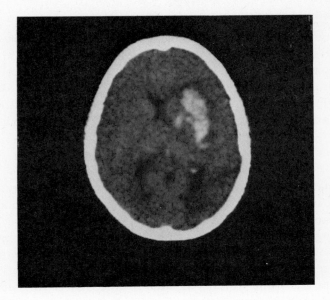

Fig. 11-4
CT scan of brain, showing large hemorrhage into the left basal ganglia. This 40-year-old man developed sudden loss of speech and weakness of the right limbs, followed by seizures. (Courtesy Valley Presbyterian Hospital Radiology Department, Van Nuys, Calif.)

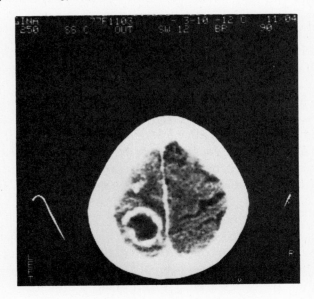

Fig. 11-5
CT scan of brain, showing circular mass in the upper left parietal-occipital area, surrounded by a dense rim. During surgery the mass proved to be an abscess and was evacuated. This 77-year-old patient was well until 3 days before admission to the hospital, when the onset of right-sided seizures and a minimal right-sided limb weakness occurred. (Courtesy Valley Presbyterian Hospital Radiology Department, Van Nuys, Calif.)

Electroencephalography

An electroencephalogram (EEG) provides the most complete information when the patient is cooperative, but it can also provide valuable information on an uncooperative patient who can be sedated. The two cerebral hemispheres normally produce electrical rhythms that are quite symmetric in older children and adults. Thus focal slowing or disorganization of background alpha activity, or the appearance of focal spike or sharp waves, usually correlates with the presence of underlying brain lesions.

Clinical value

Spikes that recur with characteristic location and/or rhythmicity are clues to petit mal epilepsy, Jakob-Creutzfeld disease, herpes encephalitis, or, in some instances, recent temporal lobe infarction.

The finding of generalized slow activity in an EEG of a patient with coma of unknown origin is more suggestive of hypoxia or other metabolic disorders than of a focal structural brain lesion.

Although a CT brain scan usually takes precedence over an EEG in the evaluation of head injuries that have produced stupor or coma, EEGs are abnormal in over 80% of cases of brain tumors and subdural hematomas. Electroencephalography thus remains a very useful and economical screening test for these diseases.

Indications

An EEG is indicated in almost all patients with unexplained episodes of confusion or unconsciousness, and in all patients presenting with first seizures.

Electroencephalography has assumed an important role in establishing brain death. Normally, one or two "flat" (isoelectric) EEGs assist a clinician in determining when brain death has occurred.

IMPORTANT: A "flat" EEG does not support the diagnosis of brain death if the patient's temperature is below 94° at the time of the recording, or if hypnotics or sedatives are present in the patient's serum.

Patient preparation

The patient should be asked to void before going to the EEG laboratory, in order to avoid this necessity once the 21 scalp and ECG electrodes are in place. Other than this no special preparation is required. Patients who are taking anticonvulsive drugs need not have them withheld.

Sleep electroencephalography

Some patients with seizures, particularly those who have temporal lobe seizures or seizures only during sleep, may not have EEG abnormalities when they are awake. Such abnormalities may be revealed by EEGs taken during either natural or sedative-induced sleep. In infants and small children, natural sleep is preferable and safer; the test can best be performed at the child's usual nap time or after feeding.

Evoked brain potentials

These tests use four or more EEG amplifier channels linked to a stimulus signal generator and a computer. The extremely small stimulus-linked cerebral potentials resulting from repetitive visual, auditory, or peripheral sensory nerve stimuli can be stored and amplified by the computer. A smooth, flat baseline is achieved as a background for the desired evoked potentials, because the computer averages out unwanted background resulting from random EEG and artifactitious waves.

Clinical value

These new methods of evaluating nerve conduction through the central nervous system are coming into increasing use in adults with suspected tumors of the brain stem or of the eighth nerve, or with suspected multiple sclerosis. In infants who have sustained a large variety of serious perinatal insults, auditory brain stem evoked potentials can provide evidence of abnormal conduction through the brain stem structures and of hearing impairment.

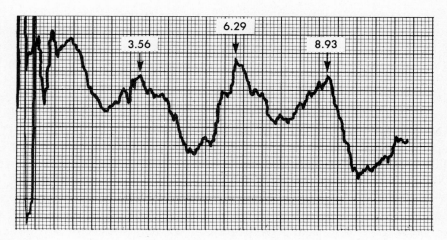

Fig. 11-6
Brain stem auditory evoked responses to click stimuli in an infant born without a right ear canal and external earlobe. Responses prove the presence of an underlying functioning right cochlea and auditory nerve. Stimulus intensity was 80 db HL, with white noise masking on the normal left side. (Courtesy Valley Presbyterian Hospital Neurology Department, Van Nuys, Calif.)

In a patient known to have normal hearing prior to suspected brain death, the absence of brain stem auditory evoked potentials constitutes additional or confirmatory evidence of brain death when EEGs are equivocal because of an unusual artifact, or when they are suboptimal for other technical reasons.

Fig. 11-6 shows brain stem auditory evoked responses to click stimuli of 80 db HL in an infant born without a right ear canal and external earlobe. The responses prove the presence of the underlying right cochlea and auditory nerve.

Echoencephalography

In echoencephalography a sound transducer-receiver placed against the scalp beams sound waves of very high frequency through the brain. Whenever the sound waves pass through an interface between brain tissue and a substance of different sound transmission properties, such as cerebrospinal fluid in the ventricles or blood from an intracerebral hemorrhage, echoes are reflected back to the receiver, thus outlining the structures encountered by the sound waves.

Advantages

This test can be done on agitated patients, and it is inexpensive. However, it has been superseded by the widespread availability of CT scans.

Clinical value

Echoencephalography remains very useful in neonatal intensive care units, where two-dimensional echoencephalograms are valuable in the bedside screening of infants for intracerebral hemorrhage.

Electromyography

An electromyogram (EMG) facilitates an analysis of voluntary and spontaneous muscle action potentials in selected muscles of one or more limbs or limb girdles and in paraspinal muscles. These potentials are examined (1) on needle insertion, (2) with complete muscle relaxation, (3) with minimal voluntary muscle contraction, and (4) with maximal contraction.

Clinical value

An EMG is most useful in cases of suspected cervical or lumbar disc disease, polymyositis, muscular dystrophy, motor neuron disease, myasthenia gravis, and a myasthenia-like disease (Eaton-Lambert syndrome), which occurs with certain cancers.

Nerve conduction velocities

The velocity of electrical impulse conduction along motor or sensory nerves is frequently measured in conjunction with an electromyographic examination.

Clinical value

Velocities are generally low in persons with poorly controlled diabetes, in long-term renal dialysis patients, and in patients who have polyneuritis resulting from any of a variety of other causes. Focal slowing of median nerve velocity across the wrist or of ulnar velocity across the elbow is good evidence of entrapment neuropathy at those locations.

Angiography

Angiography is performed by cannulation of a femoral artery, through which a catheter is advanced to the aortic arch or into the orifices of carotid or vertebral arteries for injection of an iodinated contrast medium. Arch injections do not permit evaluation of intracerebral arteries but often suffice when there is a strong suspicion of atherosclerotic stenosis of the internal carotid artery in the neck.

Clinical value

Although CT brain scanning has lessened the need for angiograms in many cases of brain tumor, intracerebral hemorrhage, and subdural hematoma, they are still of utmost importance in the identification and localization of ruptured aneurysms or of arteriovenous malformations and in providing a surgeon with accurate preoperative information about the blood supply of certain tumors.

Risks

If cerebral angiography is performed by an experienced physician, the risk of stroke, allergic reaction to the dye, bleeding after catheter withdrawal, or other complication is in the 0.5% to 1% range.

Patient preparation

A patient ordinarily should take nothing by mouth for at least 3 hours prior to angiography, and dentures should be removed before he leaves his hospital room. A baseline neurologic assessment—including state of alertness, fluency of speech, and estimates of the symmetry of limb strength or tone and the symmetry of pedal pulses—should be made before premedication is given.

After the procedure the patient should be kept flat and should be instructed to avoid flexing the thigh that was cannulated for at least several hours, to reduce the risk of late bleeding at the site of femoral artery puncture. Patient complaints of groin pain or coldness of the leg, or a nurse's observation of inguinal swelling or pallor or coldness of the leg, or loss of a pedal pulse distal to the arterial puncture site, should be reported to the physician *promptly.*

Digital-subtraction angiography

This new procedure provides arterial imaging of good quality by means of an x-ray image intensifier linked to a computer, which enables small differences in x-ray absorption between an artery and surrounding tissues to be converted to digital information and stored.

A "mask" exposure of the area of interest is made a few seconds before the injection of an intravenous iodinated contrast medium. Four or more exposures are then made while the contrast medium is circulating through the arteries. The computer then subtracts the pre-injection "mask" image from the postinjection images, thus removing all undesired tissue images (such as bone) and leaving arterial images of high contrast and high quality.

As in conventional angiography, patients should take nothing by mouth for at least 3 hours prior to testing, and elderly or diabetic patients should be instructed to increase fluid intake for 24 hours afterward. Outpatients are routinely discharged from the x-ray department immediately after the test.

Pneumoencephalography

A lumbar spinal tap is performed so that air can be injected into the lumbar subarachnoid space. The patient must be in the sitting position so that the air rises to the head and outlines the cerebral cisterns and the ventricles. X-ray film is then exposed in a variety of views and head positions.

Clinical value

Conventional pneumoencephalograms have almost become obsolete in the last few years because of the improved quality of the CT brain scan. Still, small injections of air, perhaps 5 or 10 ml, or small amounts of a water-soluble contrast medium are occasionally introduced into the lumbar subarachnoid space to provide better contrast in CT scanning for suspected posterior fossa tumors.

Noninvasive cerebrovascular flow tests

These tests are increasingly available and useful in the identification of patients who may be at risk of stroke because of embolic or thrombotic lesions in the internal carotid system. While a patient who has a history of internal-carotid-system transient ischemic attacks ordinarily proceeds directly to angiography if he is otherwise a surgical candidate, many histories are less clear and the physical examination may not reveal carotid bruits. A patient who has had *no* cerebral symptoms but who needs heart surgery, a hip prosthesis, or other major surgery may have a carotid bruit on physical examination. Hearing this bruit should trigger the physician to order noninvasive cerebral flow tests *before* the operation. A seriously obstructed carotid artery should ideally be identified and rendered patent *before* the contemplated major surgery is performed.

A commonly available battery of these tests consists of the following:
1. Oculoplethysmography, which involves evaluation of retinal artery pressures and/or pulse waves (see also p. 126)
2. Doppler evaluation of arterial pulses in periorbital arteries connecting the internal and external carotid arterial systems
3. Phonoangiographic recording of bruits over the cervical portion of the carotid arteries

Larger hospital laboratories often offer two additional tests: Doppler evaluation of flow velocity at the carotid bifurcation and ultrasound imaging of the carotid bifurcation.

The availability of digital-subtraction angiography will probably reduce the utilization of some of these noninvasive cerebral flow tests, but will undoubtedly not replace them.

CLINICAL APPLICATION OF LABORATORY TESTS

Cerebral thrombosis

Usually there is an onset over a period of minutes to a few hours of a neurologic deficit such as limb weakness or numbness or speech impairment, which slowly improves or even resolves over the next few days, weeks, or months.

When history, physical findings, and hospital course are all well documented and consistent with the clinical impression of cerebral thrombosis, extensive laboratory evaluations are usually not required.

Patients who fell at the onset of their neurologic symptoms, or who were found on the floor, and/or have scalp contusions or other evidence of recent injury should have *skull films*.

Patients who develop headaches, vomiting, seizures, neck stiffness, decreasing alertness, or decreasing speech or limb function after hospital admission should have *CT brain scans* to rule out intracranial hemorrhage, hematoma, or brain swelling secondary to infarction. A *spinal tap* is usually not required in an ordinary case of cerebral thrombosis, but it is of value in ruling out hemorrhage when a patient's condition deteriorates in the hospital and CT scans are not available. *Electroencephalograms* are not routine when the history and physical are fairly characteristic of cerebral infarction, unless there is a clinical suspicion of seizure activity.

Stroke in progress

An occasional patient who shows progressive or stepwise deterioration after admission to the hospital will have a normal CT scan but will have an isotope perfusion scan that shows a focal perfusion defect. Many such patients have progressive strokes; if these patients are normotensive, they may be candidates for intravenous heparin treatment, after clear spinal fluid has first been demonstrated.

Cerebral embolus

Because there is not time for development of a collateral source of blood flow in a case of cerebral embolus, unlike the situation in an instance of a slowly enlarging atheroma in a cerebral thrombosis case, the onset of embolic stroke is often more dramatic and rapid than the onset of cerebral thrombosis and the neurologic deficits can peak in a few minutes.

The following are common predisposing conditions: recent myocardial infarction, with formation of a mural thrombus; atrial fibrillation; ulcerated plaque in the aortic arch or in the common or internal carotid artery; fibrin or platelet emboli resulting from prosthetic heart valves; mitral stenosis, with enlarged left atrium; mitral valve prolapse syndrome; and subacute bacterial endocarditis.

If cholesterol crystals or fibrin emboli are seen on *funduscopic examination,* or if an *echocardiogram* and other cardiac evaluations suggest a source for an embolus, the risk posed by the possibility that additional cerebral emboli will occur is usually greater than the risks involved in anticoagulation therapy (in normotensive patients). There is, however, a controversy over whether to begin anticoagulation therapy immediately or to wait a few days or a week.

The indications for *EEG, spinal tap,* and *CT or isotope scans* are similar to those described for cerebral thrombosis patients. In some patients no cardiac source for a suspected embolus is present, and careful funduscopic examination may show small quantities of cholesterol or fibrin debris lodged in retinal artery branch points. In such a case, if the residual neurologic deficit is not severe and the patient is otherwise a surgical candidate, *arch angiograms* should be done to look for ulcerated atheromatous plaques in the common and internal carotid arteries.

Intracerebral hemorrhage

Long-standing and poorly controlled hypertension is the most significant risk factor for an intracerebral hemorrhage. Such hemorrhages usually occur deep in the hemispheres—in the basal ganglia and the internal capsule—but they also occur in the pons and the cerebellum. The onset is often announced by a sudden headache in a previously well patient, usually followed quickly by nausea, vomiting, and disturbed speech (if the hemorrhage is in the dominant hemisphere or the brain stem), and by hemiparesis.

A *spinal tap* can be hazardous in such a patient if intracranial pressure is elevated; it is not ordinarily necessary for diagnosis when CT scans can be quickly obtained. Emergency surgical drainage of hemorrhages is often done when they occur in cerebellar hemispheres or in nondominant cerebral hemispheres and the patient is still thought to have a chance to recover.

Subarachnoid hemorrhage

A subarachnoid hemorrhage is most commonly the result of the rupture of an aneurysm on the circle of Willis, which is located at the base of the brain. A subarachnoid hemorrhage typically causes sudden headache, followed within 1 or 2 hours by neck stiffness and pain caused by blood free in the basal cisterns diffusing down into the cervical subarachnoid space. A leaking aneurysm of the anterior communicating artery usually causes no physical findings except for neck stiffness; a leaking aneurysm of the posterior communicating artery frequently causes diplopia and third-nerve weakness; a leaking aneurysm of the middle cerebral artery often causes varying degrees of contralateral hemiparesis and may cause dysphasic speech if it is in the dominant hemisphere.

Since small amounts of subarachnoid bleeding can be missed on a *CT scan*, a *spinal fluid examination* is still necessary in cases in which a CT scan is normal but clinical suspicion of a subarachnoid hemorrhage remains strong.

Transient ischemic attacks (TIA)

Transient ischemic attacks are caused by brief but critical periods of blood flow reduction distal to an atherosclerotic narrowing of an internal carotid, vertebral, or basilar artery, or by small emboli that lodge temporarily at cerebral artery branch points and then break up and move on into small, more distal arteries. Such attacks last from 1 or 2 minutes to several hours, with the average being 15 minutes. Carotid system TIAs most often produce transient monocular blindness ("amaurosis fugax") or transient hemiparesis and hemisensory loss with or without dysphasic speech. Vertebral basilar transient attacks are suggested by the presence of one or more of the following transient symptoms: diplopia, numbness of the lips and tongue, slurred speech, drop attacks, ataxia, or hemiparetic episodes that alternate from one side of the body to the other.

One third to one half of all patients who have cerebral thrombosis have a warning TIA hours, days, or weeks before the completed stroke, and 10%-

15% of all untreated patients who have a TIA develop a completed stroke within 1 year. Most of these strokes occur in the first 5 or 6 months after the TIA.

When the history is typical and reliable, a patient is usually referred for *arch angiography* or *selective cerebral angiograms*. When a history of TIA is doubtful or less reliable, *noninvasive cerebral flow studies* can be most helpful in identifying internal carotid flow restriction.

Patients who are found to have significant atheromatous stenosis at the internal carotid artery origin or ulcerated plaques at that location are ordinarily advised to have a carotid endarterectomy. This procedure has been shown to reduce the incidence of subsequent TIAs and of strokes, and it has had a combined operative mortality and morbidity of less than 3% in many hospitals. In cases in which internal carotid stenosis is not severe and no ulcerated plaques are present, anticoagulants or antiplatelet drugs may reduce the incidence of further TIAs and of strokes.

Acute head injury

Skull films should be obtained after any acute head injury that leads to a period of unconsciousness or that is followed by vomiting or confusion. A nondepressed skull fracture is not in itself of much clinical significance, but it could indicate that a blow has been strong enough to cause injury to the brain or meningeal arteries. Fractures through the base of the skull into the ear or sinuses should be suspected when trauma is followed by clear or serous drainage from an ear or the nose. Such patients often are given broad-spectrum antibiotics to reduce the risk of intracranial infection.

Anterior-posterior and lateral cervical spinal films should be made, along with skull films, in any case of acute head injury in which the patient does not move all limbs well, is confused, or has depressed consciousness.

An *emergency CT brain scan* is invaluable in the case of a head-injured patient who has a depressed state of consciousness or whose neurologic status deteriorates (as reported by relatives, if the patient has been at home, or by hospital personnel). Such deterioration in a previously awake and talking patient suggests acute epidural or subdural hematoma. Such findings on a CT scan or, if a CT scanner is not available, on an angiogram ordinarily call for prompt neurosurgical intervention.

An electroencephalogram is usually not very helpful in evaluating acute head injuries, but it can be of prognostic help in subacute and recovery stages.

A *spinal tap* is usually unnecessary and can be hazardous. It is performed only if a head injury is suspected of being complicated by intracranial infection.

Intracranial pressure monitoring by means of an epidural, subdural, or intraventricular manometer placed through a skull burr hole is being used in large hospitals. The procedure is being used in certain cases of severe head injury in which high intracranial pressure is life threatening.

Spinal cord injury or tumor

Plain spine films are indicated whenever spinal injuries or spinal cord tumors are suspected.

Myelography, performed promptly, is in order when clinical suspicion is increased because of the history and the physical findings of progressive limb weakness and numbness, with or without back pain or impaired bladder control. This procedure should generally not be delayed for performance of a spinal tap, a Queckenstedt test, or EMG. Myelographic findings of partial or complete spinal canal block resulting from fracture-dislocation or from a tumor usually call for prompt neurosurgical and/or orthopedic consultation. Some cases of cord compression resulting from metastatic cancer may be treated with dexamethasone (Decadron) and irradiation as an alternative to surgery.

Myopathic disorders

The most common cause of generalized muscle weakness in hospital patients is hypokalemia; serum potassium levels should therefore be checked in such patients. High doses of steroids, alcoholism, myxedema, and occult carcinoma are examples of other causes of generalized myopathy, which often appears first in the hip girdle muscles. Such patients must use their arms to push themselves up out of low chairs. Muscular dystrophies typically are characterized by very slowly progressive and painless weakness of the limbs and limb girdles without any sensory impairment. Careful inquiry into a patient's family history will usually reveal that other family members are also affected. Duchenne dystrophy is unique in that the weakened leg muscles of affected young boys usually appear larger than normal and both the boys and their asymptomatic carrier mothers have elevated serum levels of creatine phosphokinase.

Special histochemical stains and electron microscopic studies of muscle biopsy specimens are the most useful laboratory examinations in muscle disease; they have resulted in the classification of many subtypes of muscular dystrophy in recent years. The identification of a carnitine enzyme deficiency in some forms of limb-girdle dystrophy has enabled affected patients to be treated with carnitine supplements.

Seizure disorders

In seizure disorders the work-up varies according to individual circumstances, but a few general principles can be stated.

Focal seizures have a higher correlation with structural brain lesions, such as tumors, hemorrhages, abscesses, than do generalized seizures.

Seizures in pediatric patients are less likely to be caused by structural brain lesions than are seizures in adults.

Seizures that first appear in patients who are hospitalized for other conditions are often of metabolic origin. Among the occasional inciting causes are the following: hyponatremia; excessive use of, or withdrawal from the use of, alcohol or hypnotic or tranquilizing drugs prior to admission; high serum levels of aminophylline or lidocaine; and cerebral hypoxia.

Laboratory tests usually include electroencephalography, skull x-ray films, and, in adults, a CT scan as well. An EEG is abnormal in about 75% of patients with seizures. Sleep EEGs may be useful in patients who have normal routine EEGs but who have primarily nocturnal seizures or temporal lobe seizures.

When seizures are suspected to be of metabolic origin, the following tests are usually done: serum electrolytes levels, calcium levels, magnesium levels, blood glucose levels, and, in selected patients, arterial blood gas determinations and serum lidocaine and aminophylline levels.

If a patient has a history of seizures and has been prescribed anticonvulsants, determinations of serum anticonvulsant drug levels are helpful in assessing the patient's compliance with the physician's instructions. Such determinations also help a physician to adjust an anticonvulsant drug regimen.

Headaches

Since headaches can have dozens of causes, the extent of laboratory investigation depends heavily on the history and the physical examination. In general, headaches that are constant or progressive in intensity or frequency, awaken patients from sleep, or are accompanied by stiff neck, anorexia, nausea, or vomiting require fairly extensive laboratory investigation. Headaches that are episodic, with interim periods of good health, begin during the day in fairly regular relation to job or other stresses, remit during vacations, and are relieved by simple analgesics are usually less extensively investigated. The most common headaches seen in outpatient practice are migraine and tension headaches.

Migraine headaches are typically periodic temporal-frontal-orbital headaches that occur in persons who are otherwise well; these headaches often are accompanied by photophobia or bright scotomas in the visual fields and by nausea or vomiting. They often are severe enough to prevent a person from continuing his current activity. Migraine headaches are frequently alleviated by ergotamine-containing medications and by sleep. A family history of migraines is common.

Tension headaches are usually occipital, cervical, or generalized. They begin during the day, they are often associated with environmental stresses, and they do not awaken a person at night. Such a headache often remits on holidays or during vacations, and it frequently clears as a result of simple analgesics, reassurance, and rearrangement of daily schedules to minimize frustrations and stresses.

A rare cause of headaches in persons over 55 years of age is temporal arteritis. Any patient over that age presenting with headaches should have a *Westergren sedimentation rate test* done, which is an excellent screening tool. It is important to identify this disease because, although rare, it carries with it a significant risk of blindness if undiagnosed and untreated. Treatment consists of the administration of steroids.

A frequent cause of headaches that regularly begin on *awakening* in the morning is undiagnosed or inadequately controlled hypertension. Blood pressure control usually results in prompt headache relief.

If the history and the physical examination lead a clinician to order laboratory investigation of the cause of a patient's headaches, one generally starts with *skull films, sinus films,* and an *electroencephalogram*. If the suspicion of an intracranial mass persists, the clinician goes on to a *CT brain scan,* if it is available, or to an *isotope brain scan*. Most patients who have unremitting headaches accompanied by unexplained fever or persistent neck stiffness and who have negative brain scans should also have *cerebrospinal fluid examinations* to rule out minimal subarachnoid hemorrhage or central nervous system infections.

Coma

The causes of coma are legion. A clinician's first task is to determine whether a patient's coma is of primary (central nervous system) origin or of metabolic origin. This determination is complex and beyond the purposes of this book. However, a few generalizations can be made. Localized abnormalities, as shown by neurologic examination or an electroencephalogram, suggest a central nervous system cause; generalized or symmetrical abnormalities usually correlate with metabolic causes.

Laboratory tests for metabolic causes of coma might include most or all of the following: *serum hypnotic screening panel, blood alcohol level, electrolyte levels, and levels of calcium, phosphorus, magnesium, BUN, creatinine, triiodothyronine, thyroxine, blood glucose, arterial blood gases, SGOT, SGPT, alkaline phosphatase,* and *serum ammonia*.

Suspected central nervous system causes of coma ideally would be investigated by *EEG* and by *CT* or *isotope brain scans* before a physician proceeds to *cerebrospinal fluid examination*. However, when a comatose patient has an unexplained fever, and petechiae, or there is other reason to suspect acute meningitis, time is of critical importance; in most such instances the physician should do a spinal fluid examination promptly, without waiting for an EEG or scans.

TWELVE Diagnostic tests for collagen vascular diseases

The systemic rheumatic diseases include rheumatoid arthritis, systemic lupus erythematosus, rheumatic fever, and progressive systemic sclerosis, to name a few. These disorders are also known as connective tissue diseases and were formerly called collagen diseases.

The following laboratory procedures are the ones most commonly used in the diagnosis and management of rheumatic diseases.

LABORATORY TESTS FOR RHEUMATIC DISEASES

Radiologic studies of joints

Although x-ray film can be of help in the early diagnosis of certain entities, such as sacroiliac involvement in ankylosing spondylitis, seldom can one make a specific diagnosis through radiologic studies.

Usually, in diseases associated with joint involvement one sees erosion of the joint margins, narrowing of joint spaces, and diffuse osteoporosis of the involved joints. A bamboo appearance of spinal joints is characteristic of ankylosing spondylitis, and in certain infectious conditions there will be bony erosion and lytic lesions.

In addition to the initial radiologic evaluation of rheumatic diseases, x-ray films are usually taken to follow the course of the disease.

Synovial analysis

Synovial fluid is contained within articulations having a joint cavity. This viscous dialysate of blood plasma, along with hyaluronate from the synovial membrane, provides the perfect frictionless film for the bony surfaces. It also nourishes the cartilaginous structures of the joints.

An examination of synovial fluid will provide information regarding the underlying synovial tissue reaction to a specific irritant causing inflammation.

Routine synovial fluid analysis includes determination of clarity, color, and viscosity; evaluation of mucin clot formation; white cell count; and polarized light microscopy. In special situations levels of synovial fluid complement, protein, and glucose can be measured; rheumatoid factors and the lupus erythematosus cell phenomenon can be looked for. When there is a suspicion of septic arthritis, it is essential that a gram stain of the synovial fluid and the appropriate cultures be performed.

Normal synovial fluid is straw-colored and transparent; it has normal viscosity, good mucin clot formation, a WBC count of less than 200/cu mm, and a neutrophil count of less than 25/cu mm. The glucose content is the same as that of blood.

In disease states the clarity is lost; the fluid may become cloudy, milky, grayish, or red, depending on the underlying disorder. Viscosity will be poor in fluid from chronically inflamed joints.

Polarized light microscopy aids in the differential diagnosis between gout and pseudogout, since it enables a clinician to distinguish between urate and pyrophosphate crystals. In gout one sees negative birefringence under polarized light, while in pseudogout weakly birefringent crystals are seen.

Patient preparation and care for arthrocentesis

The patient should be fasting for 6 to 12 hours; otherwise glucose and lipid evaluations are invalid. The knee joint is most frequently used, although synovial fluid from any articulation may be aspirated. The area from which fluid is to be aspirated is prepared as for surgery, and rigid aseptic technique is observed to avoid the only complication of this procedure, infection in the joint.

Titers of rheumatoid (RA) factors

Rheumatoid factors are antiglobulin antibodies, which react to immunoglobulins of the IgG class. The principal fractions measured are the IgM rheumatoid factors, although they also exist in the other two major immunoglobulin classes (IgG and IgA), in which case the disease would be milder.

High titers of rheumatoid factors are usually associated with active disease. Low titers are sometimes found in other nonspecific connective tissue diseases, as well as in an estimated 16% to 20% of the elderly population.

Complement analysis

The complement system is a group of nine serum proteins that react with each other to mediate the immunologic response that follows the interaction between antigen and antibody. These serum proteins are normally inactive in the blood serum. When activated they function as enzymes.

Activation occurs when IgG or IgM antibodies are altered following union with their respective antigens. The activated components are designated C1 to C9.

There is also an alternative pathway called the properdin system, which is activated in a wide variety of defense mechanisms.

The C3 component of the complement correlates very well with the total hemolytic complement. It is diminished in lupus, and is usually associated with kidney involvement.

C4 component is significantly diminished in lupus nephritis.

The importance of the other components of the complement system, as well as of the alternative pathway, is under intense research.

Lupus erythematosus (LE) cell test

This test involves visualization of the LE cell phenomenon, which consists of an autoantibody (LE factor) complexing with leukocyte nucleoprotein as the antigen. The characteristic LE cell is thus produced in vitro only. A substantial level of LE factor must be in the blood before a positive LE test is produced.

Test for antinuclear antibodies (ANA)

The antinuclear antibodies are immunoglobulins, usually of the IgM class, but they may be IgG or IgA. They react with the nuclear component of leukocytes and are detected by the immunofluorescent method. They include antibodies against RNA, DNA, ribosomes, and lysosomes as well as other cytoplasmic constituents.

Four nuclear fluorescence patterns are characteristic of this test:
1. Diffuse or homogeneous. This is the most common pattern; it is produced when the antinuclear antibody binds to nucleoprotein. The diffuse pattern is characteristic of systemic lupus erythematosus (SLE), but is seen in other disorders as well.
2. "Shaggy" or peripheral pattern. This pattern is produced by antibodies to DNA; it is seen almost exclusively in SLE, especially when there is associated lupus nephritis.
3. Speckled pattern. This pattern is produced by an antibody against a nuclear glycoprotein.
4. Nucleolar pattern. This pattern is rare.

Test for anti-DNA antibodies

Antibodies to DNA (deoxyribonucleic acid) are important in evaluating lupus nephritis. A negative anti-DNA test result usually is associated with the absence of acute nephritis.

Test for anti-ENA antibodies

The antibodies to extractable nuclear antigens (ENA) form a speckled pattern with the fluorescent antinuclear antibody test and usually occur in SLE. However, they are also commonly present in the so-called mixed connective tissue diseases.

HLA-B27 antigen test

HLA-B27 is a tissue transplantation antigen found in human cell C6 chromosomes. It is a genetically determined marker that remains unchanged throughout a person's life. It has become important in the diagnosis of rheumatic diseases, particularly in the differential diagnosis of seronegative rheumatic variants.

In 90% of patients with either ankylosing spondylitis or Reiter's syndrome the findings of this test will be positive. Therefore, the test is very useful in distinguishing ankylosing spondylitis from other arthritic conditions, and Reiter's syndrome from gonococcal arthritis.

In some cases of juvenile rheumatoid arthritis, the presence of the HLA-B27 antigen indicates the possibility of ankylosing spondylitis.

In patients with psoriatic arthritis or inflammatory bowel disease associated with arthritis, the HLA-B27 test will help to predict the development of ankylosing spondylitis.

Antistreptolysin O (ASO) titer

The ASO titer is elevated in approximately 80% of streptococcal pharyngitis patients who develop rheumatic fever or glomerular nephritis. It is elevated in 60% of patients with uncomplicated streptococcal disease—except in streptococcal pyoderma, in which only 25% of patients have an elevated ASO titer, even though acute glomerular nephritis may also be present.

Other streptococcal antibody tests

Other streptococcal antibodies include antihyaluronidase (AH), anti-deoxyribonucleotidase B (anti-DNase B), antistreptokinase (ASK), and anti-streptozyme (ASTZ). Tests for these antibodies are most advisable when there is a low or borderline ASO titer. The ASTZ test in particular is a very sensitive indicator of recent streptococcal infection.

Tests performed for muscle disease

The tests performed to determine the presence of muscle disease include measurement of the levels of the enzymes released when there is muscle destruction. These enzymes (CPK, LDH, GOT) have been discussed in previous chapters. In addition, the aldolase level is elevated in certain muscular dystrophies and in polymyositis.

LABORATORY TESTS NOT DIRECTLY RELATED TO RHEUMATIC DISEASES

The following is a brief listing of some immunologic tests performed by specialized rheumatology diagnostic laboratories; however, these tests have no bearing on strictly rheumatic diseases.

1. *Antimitochondrial antibodies*—found in 95% of patients with biliary cirrhosis and also in some patients with chronic active hepatitis
2. *Antimyocardial antibodies*—found in 80% to 90% of patients with Dressler's (postmyocardial infarction or postcardiac surgery) syndrome
3. *Anti–parietal cell antibodies*—found in 84% of pernicious anemia cases
4. *Antireticulin antibodies*—found in 60% of children with untreated gluten-sensitive enteropathy and 30% of adults with gluten-sensitive enteropathy; also in 25% of patients with dermatitis herpetiformis
5. *Anti–skeletal muscle antibody*—found in patients with myasthenia gravis
6. *Anti–smooth muscle antibodies*—found in patients with chronic active hepatitis
7. *Antithyroglobulin antibodies*—found in patients with thyroiditis and Hashimoto's disease, in 30% of patients with Graves' disease, and in 25% of patients with papillary carcinoma of the thyroid (antithyroid microsomal antibodies are also found in the same conditions)

CLINICAL APPLICATION OF LABORATORY TESTS

Rheumatoid arthritis

Rheumatoid arthritis is a chronic systemic disease of unknown origin. The primary manifestation is inflammation of the peripheral joints.

In the pathogenesis of rheumatoid arthritis the rheumatoid factors (antiglobulin antibodies) combine with antigens (usually IgG) in the synovial fluid to form immune complexes. Polymorphonuclear leukocytes are thus attracted to the joint space, causing destruction of joint structures.

The *RA factor* is found in significant titer in 75% of patients with rheumatoid arthritis, and in 95% of patients when the disease is associated with subcutaneous nodules. At the beginning of the disease the titers may not be elevated. It will take approximately 6 months for a significant elevation of titer, with a high titer indicating more severe disease. It should be remembered that a positive RA factor test result is not diagnostic of rheumatoid arthritis; such a result should be correlated with the total clinical picture.

Antinuclear antibodies are present in 20% to 60% of cases; and the *LE cell test* has a positive result in 10% to 20%. The *serum complement* level is normal or sometimes slightly diminished in vasculitis associated with rheumatoid arthritis.

The *synovial fluid* will have diminished viscosity, with poor mucin clot formation. The leukocyte count will be approximately 15,000/cu mm, with 75% being neutrophils. Glucose levels will be low; the result of the test for RA factor will be positive, and complement levels will be diminished, indicating complement binding.

In addition to these specific findings, patients with rheumatoid arthritis also have nonspecific laboratory findings, such as anemia, leukocytosis, and elevated erythrocyte sedimentation rate.

Systemic lupus erythematosus (SLE)

Systemic lupus erythematosus is a disease of unknown origin, occurring most frequently in women of childbearing age. It is a disorder of connective tissue, with many and varied immunologic abnormalities.

A positive result of the *LE cell test* is no longer considered the hallmark of SLE, since LE cells are found in other diseases as well. This test is not helpful in determining a prognosis. The test for *antinuclear antibodies* is much more specific, since the titer correlates well with the activity of the disease.

The *anti-DNA antibody test* is highly specific for SLE, since this antibody is not found in any other collagen vascular disease. A positive test result usually indicates associated immune injury to the kidneys.

Serum complement levels, specifically those of C3 and C4, are significantly diminished in lupus nephritis. This finding actually heralds the exacerbation of renal involvement 1 or 2 months ahead of time.

The *rheumatoid factor* is found in approximately 20% of patients with SLE.

Synovial fluid examination reveals decreased viscosity, a white cell count of around 5,000/cu mm, LE cells, and diminished complement levels.

X-ray films of the joints are neither characteristic nor of much diagnostic importance.

Nonspecific laboratory findings are leukopenia and elevated erythrocyte sedimentation rate.

Rheumatic fever

Rheumatic fever is an inflammatory disease related to previous infection with group A β-hemolytic streptococci; the disease is manifested by acute migratory polyarthritis. The arthritis, as such, is a self-limiting condition. However, it becomes of clinical importance because of its association with the nonsuppurative complications of streptococcal infection—for example, carditis and glomerular nephritis.

A *throat culture* is performed for isolation of the β-hemolytic streptococcus.

The *ASO titer* will be 250 or more Todd units. The levels of the other streptococcal antibodies, such as antihyaluronidase, antideoxyribonucleotidase B, antistreptokinase, and antistreptozyme, can also be measured. Virtually all patients with rheumatic fever have antistreptozyme titers greater than 200 units per milliliter.

Electrocardiographic findings are important; the disease is characterized by a prolonged P-R interval.

The production of *C reactive protein* is a nonspecific acute phase reaction.

X-ray studies are unnecessary.

Progressive systemic sclerosis (scleroderma)

Progressive systemic sclerosis is characterized by alterations in connective tissue, leading to fibrosis involving the skin (scleroderma) and internal organs; the disorder is accompanied by immunologic abnormalities. The diagnosis, however, is strictly clinical.

Immunologic abnormalities include an elevated immunoglobulin G (IgG) level, the presence of the RA factor in 20% of cases, and the presence of antinuclear antibodies in 40% to 80%. A low titer of extractable nuclear antibodies in a "speckled." pattern suggests mixed connective tissue disease.

Mixed connective tissue diseases

Affected patients have clinically overlapping features of scleroderma, SLE, and polyarthritis.

The sera of these patients contain high titers of antibodies to nuclear ribonucleoprotein. Thus on fluorescent antibody testing a speckled pattern is produced.

Polymyositis and dermatomyositis

Polymyositis and dermatomyositis are the most common primary myopathies in adults. The term "polymyositis" is used if the disease is restricted clinically to the striated muscles. "Dermatomyositis" is used if the skin is involved.

The diagnosis, as in progressive systemic sclerosis, is mainly clinical.

Laboratory tests employed include serum enzyme (CPK, aldolase, GOT, and GPT) determinations, electromyography (see p. 292), and muscle biopsy.

Ankylosing spondylitis

Ankylosing spondylitis is a chronic inflammatory disease involving spinal articulations, especially the sacroiliac joints. In the past ankylosing spondylitis was classified as a variant of rheumatoid arthritis. However, with the advent of the recently perfected HLA-B27 antigen test, it is recognized as a distinct entity.

Radiologic studies show early sacroiliac joint involvement and typical pathology of the axial skeleton and the symphysis pubis. The spine has a bamboo appearance in later stages.

In ankylosing spondylitis the *RA factor* is absent; the *HLA-B27 antigen* is present in 90% of cases.

Reiter's syndrome

The triad of arthritis, urethritis, and conjunctivitis characterizes Reiter's syndrome. The arthritis of Reiter's syndrome has some similarities to ankylosing spondylitis, particularly because of the involvement of the sacroiliac joint.

X-ray films show some soft tissue swelling of the joints along with the sacroiliitis. In long-standing cases there is some bony erosion.

The RA factor is absent; the HLA-B27 antigen is present.

Differential diagnosis

Because of the urethritis, a differential diagnosis must sometimes be made between gonococcal arthritis and Reiter's syndrome. In gonococcal arthritis the HLA-B27 antigen is absent, and usually a positive culture is obtained. However, if there is doubt, the treatment for gonococcal arthritis is indicated. This treatment will not affect Reiter's arthritis.

Psoriatic arthritis

Psoriatic arthritis is one of the so-called seronegative arthritic diseases—in other words, it is RA factor negative. This disease is associated with hyperuricemia and has characteristic *x-ray features*. There is some destruction of isolated joints, osteolysis, and some ankylosing. The level of *HLA-B27 antigen* is elevated in 40% of cases. This level is also elevated in 70% of cases of inflammatory bowel diseases associated with arthritis. This finding may indicate a possible association with ankylosing spondylitis.

Gouty arthritis

Gouty arthritis is an acute clinical manifestation of gout, usually appearing abruptly, with the initial attack involving the great toe in 50% to 70% of cases.

Radiologically, it is impossible to differentiate gouty arthritis from pseudogout. Although in gouty arthritis there is usually an elevation of the uric acid level, in the final analysis the diagnosis is made by aspiration of synovial fluid. In gouty arthritis there will be negative birefringence of crystals under polarized light. In pseudogout the crystals are those of calcium pyrophosphate, which show weakly positive birefringence under polarized light.

Septic arthritis

Septic arthritis is usually monoarticular; the disorder is considered a medical emergency.

X-ray films may show soft tissue swelling, bony erosion, and lytic lesions.

Joint aspiration is imperative; it usually demonstrates an initially cloudy and later purulent synovial fluid. The leukocyte count is between 50,000 and 100,000/cu mm, with 90% or more being neutrophils. The glucose concentration will be decreased. A gram stain and culture should be performed on the synovial fluid right away to establish the definitive diagnosis and treatment.

Degenerative arthritis or osteoarthritis

Degenerative arthritis is found in 85% of persons over the age of 70; it usually is not associated with systemic abnormalities. The results of *serologic tests,* including those for rheumatoid factor, antinuclear antibodies, and sedimentation rate, are usually normal. *Radiologic changes* are quite characteristic. *Synovial fluid* has decreased viscosity, good mucin clotting ability, and a white cell count of less than 200/cu mm. The glucose level is normal.

THIRTEEN Diagnostic tests for infectious diseases

GRAM STAIN

A gram stain permits the classification of bacteria into four basic groups: gram-positive or -negative rods and gram-positive or -negative cocci. After staining with gentian violet and Gram's iodine, the morphology can be visualized. A blue stain is designated gram-positive, and a red stain is gram-negative. Such a classification has important clinical implications. For example, identification of a gram-positive chain of cocci immediately narrows down the differential diagnosis of an infectious process, thus guiding therapy 24 to 48 hours before the specific cultural identification and sensitivity testing have been completed. The types of groups in which the bacteria arrange themselves can also be seen on a gram stain. This is another guide to therapy. For example, the finding of gram-positive diplococci suggests *Pneumococcus*, while the presence of gram-positive organisms in clumps suggests *Staphylococcus*. Of course, eventually the culture and sensitivity tests should be performed for definitive diagnosis and adequate treatment, since even after positive gram stain identification it may be very important to have culture identification and sensitivity testing of all isolates.

ACID-FAST BACILLI (AFB) STAIN

The acid-fast, or Ziehl-Neelsen, stain is used mainly in the diagnosis of tuberculosis, tuberculous infections, and leprosy. The causative organisms of these diseases will appear red against a blue background when stained by this method. Since it usually takes 2 to 3 weeks to culture the tubercle bacilli, results of the AFB stain can indicate the need for the immediate initiation of therapy. It is diagnostically most helpful if seen in sputum or the cerebrospinal fluid; the AFB stain is used for follow-up evaluation as well.

BACTERIAL CULTURE AND SENSITIVITY TESTING

Usually, identification of bacteria and determination of their sensitivity to specific antimicrobial drugs are done after the initial gram stain analysis. Most frequently the identification of a specific organism must be accompanied by a sensitivity study. An exception to this generalization is the finding of β-hemolytic streptococci in a throat culture, since the sensitivity of these organisms to antibacterial drugs is well known. However, because of the changing patterns of resistance of other bacteria to antibacterial agents, sensitivity studies are essential.

There are three methods of sensitivity testing: Kirby-Bauer disk, agar diffusion, and tube dilution. Up until recently the Kirby-Bauer disk method was most commonly used clinically, with organisms being described as "sensitive," "intermediate," or "resistant" to tested antibiotics. This method is being replaced by the tube-dilution method, which, up until now, was time-consuming and cumbersome. However, there are now available commercially prepared microfilter plates that allow the laboratory to report sensitivities in terms of concentration of antibiotic effective against an organism.

Blood culture

In fevers of unknown origin, when bacterial infection is suspected, it is usually advisable to take three cultures, aerobically and anaerobically, at 30-minute intervals. This method helps to increase the yield of an organism, and it confirms a diagnosis when the same organism is obtained in separate blood cultures.

In bacterial endocarditis it is usually easy to identify the organism in culture because of the constant shedding of the bacteria into the bloodstream. In other types of infection, the yield is greatest if cultures are obtained just prior to an expected chill and a subsequent rise in temperature. However, since this event is difficult to predict, the next best period is during the chill, when the temperature is rising.

Sputum culture

Sputum should be collected after deep cough and production of thick, purulent sputum. It is important that the specimen be truly sputum and not saliva. When accurate bacteriologic diagnosis and sensitivity testing are of paramount importance, transtracheal aspiration of sputum is done.

Urine culture

Since most urinary tract infections are caused by gram-negative bacilli, identification and sensitivity testing are of primary importance.

The clean-catch, midstream technique is considered in clinical practice to be an adequate means of obtaining an uncontaminated urine specimen. To obtain such a specimen, the urethral meatus is cleansed with an antiseptic solution and the initial third of the urine is discarded. The second third of the urine is then collected for culture and sensitivity studies. The quality of the specimen thus obtained correlates well with that of a specimen obtained with a catheter, since the normal bacterial flora of the distal urethra and urethral meatus is eliminated from the culture. With this method there is no need to catheterize patients simply for the purpose of obtaining uncontaminated urine. In patients who already have a catheter in place, the specimen is obtained through the catheter. When the catheter is removed, urine from the distal end of the catheter should be cultured.

IMMUNOLOGIC METHODS OF DIAGNOSIS

The immunologic or serologic methods of diagnosis give information about past or present infection by (1) demonstrating the presence of antibodies against a particular organism and (2) detecting components of causative organisms. In addition, an antibody titer can be followed from the acute phase to the convalescent phase of a disease by observing at least a fourfold elevation of titer and then a gradual decrease. Thus in the majority of cases a diagnosis will be retrospective and of more epidemiologic use than immediate clinical value.

Immunologic methods are employed for detecting the presence of antibodies against specific organisms. The choice of tests depends on ease and practicality and has no bearing on the type of infection, organism, or pathogenesis.

The most frequently used serologic tests are discussed below.

Precipitin tests

Precipitates will form when soluble antigens are combined with antiserum containing specific antibodies. These tests are used mainly in the identification of bacterial exotoxins and the antibodies of certain fungi.

Neutralization tests

An antigen is said to be neutralized when it loses the ability to produce an injurious effect. An antigen-antibody combination causes such an effect. Neutralization tests are usually used in viral identification. An incubated known virus and a test serum are inoculated into a tissue culture, and the effects are noted. Animals may also be used for such a test. The test serum is given, and the animal is then challenged with the toxin or microorganism. If the antibody is present in the test serum, the animal will be protected against infection.

Agglutination tests

Antibodies are capable of clumping antigen molecules and bacteria together. This process is called *agglutination*. Agglutination reactions can be performed on a slide or in a test tube by mixing the patient's serum with the specific antigen. The presence of agglutination or clumping is then observed.

These tests are used, for example, in the diagnosis of *Brucella* and *Salmonella* infection. The heterophil agglutination tests are used to diagnose infectious mononucleosis.

Complement fixation tests

A complement fixation test involves a more tedious procedure. Complement is a substance found in normal serum that produces lysis of red blood cells when it is combined with antigen-antibody complexes. The patient's serum is first incubated with the antigen to be tested and a specific amount of complement. If an antigen-antibody reaction takes place, the complement will "fix" to the antigen-antibody complexes. Erythrocytes coated with antibodies are then added to the combination, and lysis occurs if there is any free complement left in the serum. The failure of lysis to occur implies that all of the complement was used up in the first phase of the test, indicating the presence of the particular antibody for which the test was performed. An example of a complement fixation test is the VDRL test.

Fluorescent antibody methods

In such a test antibody attachment to an antigen is identified under a fluorescent microscope through the use of a fluorescent dye. The clinical material is fixed on a microscope slide and overlaid with a specific preparation of antibodies conjugated to dye. An antigen-antibody reaction is noted if fluorescent microorganisms are seen. The FTA-ABS test for the diagnosis of syphilis is an example of a fluorescent antibody method.

An indirect immunofluorescence test uses antibodies to human immunoglobulins, which may be prepared in animals and then conjugated with fluorescein.

Skin tests

A skin test is an intradermal test for delayed hypersensitivity caused by certain infections, such as TB. The sensitization occurs in the T-lymphocytes.

The antigen is injected intradermally several inches below the elbow, on the volar surface of the forearm. An induration of 10 mm or more appearing 48 to 72 hours after injection is diagnostic of delayed sensitivity. In tuberculin testing false negative results (from 5% to 20%) can be caused by depletion of T-lymphocytes because of overwhelming infection, pleural effusions, or an anergic state such as Hodgkin's disease or sarcoidosis.

CLINICAL APPLICATION OF LABORATORY TESTS

Bacterial pneumonias

Chest x-ray film is nearly always essential in the diagnosis of bacterial pneumonias. In addition to substantiating the existence of an inflammatory infectious condition, the consolidation pattern may indicate the cause. For example, a lobar distribution usually indicates that the cause is a pneumococcus organism, while a bronchial distribution will suggest other gram-positive organisms. *Klebsiella* and staphylococci also have some unique radiologic characteristics.

A *gram stain* of the sputum may be suggestive enough to indicate therapy before a culture is available. Occasionally, transtracheal aspiration of sputum will be necessary, especially in anaerobic infections.

Blood cultures are useful both in substantiating the sputum culture result and in indicating bacteremia, thus raising the possibility of distant metastatic infection and the need for modification of therapy.

Arterial blood gas determinations are helpful in documenting the degree of hypoxemia.

A *pleural tap* may yield the offending organism if there is associated pleural fluid.

Bronchoscopy is performed to exclude obstruction in the tracheobronchial tree when the pneumonia is recurrent or slowly resolving.

An untreated or inadequately treated bacterial pneumonia may resolve into a lung abscess. All of the diagnostic tests helpful in pneumonia are employed in the diagnosis of lung abscess. Occasionally, surgical evacuation is needed for specific bacteriologic diagnosis.

Mycoplasmal pneumonia

Mycoplasmal pneumonia has also been called Eaton's agent pneumonia and PPLO (pleuropneumonia-like organisms) pneumonia. Specific diagnosis is important because *Mycoplasma pneumoniae* does not respond to penicillin. Effective drugs are tetracycline and erythromycin.

Chest x-ray film and the clinical picture aid in the diagnosis. *Cold agglutinins* are present in up to 90% of severe cases. This test is also helpful in predicting the possibility of hemolysis associated with the pneumonia.

Serologic tests are available for retrospective diagnosis.

Viral pneumonias

There are at least twelve groups of viruses and 150 different serotypes that can cause pneumonias. In general, viral infections are a common cause of upper respiratory infections that last 2 to 3 days and that are usually of no clinical consequence. Since there is no specific treatment for viral infections, no specific diagnosis is necessary, except for epidemiologic purposes.

Secondary bacterial infection may occur in some patients (particularly in smokers), usually in the form of bronchitis. In such a case there will be purulent sputum and normal chest x-ray film. The infecting organism is usually *Pneumococcus* or *Hemophilus influenzae*.

Specific serologic diagnosis of viral upper respiratory infections and pneumonias is available for epidemiologic surveys; preventive vaccination is available for specified populations.

Rare types of pneumonia
Tularemia

Tularemia (rabbit fever, deer fly fever, Ohara's disease) is transmitted to humans from animals by direct contact or through an insect host. The causative organism is *Pasteurella (Francisella) tularensis*, a gram-negative bacillus.

The *agglutination test* for this disease uses a suspension of the bacterium *Francisella tularensis*. In patients with tularemia, titers of 1:80 are reached during the second week of infection; titers rise to 1:640 and above in 2 to 3 months and then fall. Since cross-reactions with *Brucella* and *Proteus* OX-19 can occur, both should be tested to make the diagnosis of tularemia.

Cultures from mucocutaneous lesions and sputum should be obtained for definitive diagnosis.

Psittacosis or ornithosis

Psittacosis, also known as ornithosis, is transmitted from birds to humans by inhalation; it results in a pneumonitis and involvement of the reticuloendothelial system.

Chest x-ray film shows patchy pneumonitis resembling *Mycoplasma* infection.

The diagnosis is made by isolation of the *Chlamydia psittaci* organism from the sputum and by serologic testing (mainly complement fixation of antibodies) in the acute and convalescent stages.

Legionnaires' disease

Legionnaires' disease is a specific bacterial infection that is so named because it caused an outbreak of pneumonia at a convention of American Legionnaires at a Philadelphia hotel in 1976. The acute disease is a patchy pulmonary infiltrate and consolidation, which may result in respiratory failure.

After painstaking investigation, a gram-negative bacillus was isolated and documented as the cause. This organism can be isolated directly in vitro on special media. However, this method is difficult. Clinically, the *indirect fluorescent antibody test* of the patient's serum is the most practical method of diagnosis.

Serologic testing has shown that other outbreaks of this disease have occurred and that subclinical infection is not uncommon but that it is detectable only by serologic testing.

Viral and bacterial infections of the central nervous system
Meningitis and brain abscesses

In cases of meningitis or brain abscesses it is extremely important to make an etiologic diagnosis. Common bacterial infections, in order of frequency, are those caused by *Meningococcus* organisms, *Hemophilus influenzae* (especially in children), and *Pneumococcus* organisms, and tuberculosis. Less common causative agents are *Escherichia coli*, *Streptococcus* organisms, and *Staphylococcus* organisms. *Listeria monocytogenes* may be found in immunosuppressed and terminally ill patients.

The most important test is the *spinal tap*, discussed on p. 283. The cerebrospinal fluid is analyzed for protein, glucose, and lactate concentrations, and a cell count is determined. A gram stain and an acid-fast stain may be diagnostic of the specific bacterial or tuberculous nature of the infection, and an india ink stain may be diagnostic of a cryptococcal infection (a fungus). Culture and sensitivity tests are always performed.

Blood cultures may be important, especially if the CSF contains no bacteria.

Skull x-ray films may show osteomyelitis and mastoiditis. These results may help in determining where to obtain cultures, and in establishing a specific diagnosis and a possible etiologic agent.

Chest x-ray film is necessary, since bacterial meningitis may be secondary to underlying pneumonitis.

Bacterial meningitis

In florid bacterial meningitis the spinal fluid is purulent, with significant increases in the number of white blood cells (mainly neutrophils) and in the protein level and a marked decrease in the glucose level. The CSF lactate level is increased.

Tuberculous meningitis

In tuberculous meningitis the WBC count in the CSF is less prominent and consists mainly of monocytes and lymphocytes.

In the differential diagnosis between tuberculous meningitis and viral meningitis, the glucose level becomes important: it is decreased in tuberculous meningitis and normal in viral or aseptic meningitis.

Viral meningitis

In the CSF the protein level is usually elevated, the WBC count is slightly elevated (mainly with lymphocytes), and the glucose level is usually normal. The CSF lactate levels are not elevated.

Brain abscess

The CSF pressure is definitely elevated, and the WBC count is between 50 and 300/μl, mainly lymphocytes. If the abscess communicates with the ventricular system, the WBC count will increase in the CSF, with an increase in the number of polymorphonuclear leukocytes, and the infecting organism can be cultured. If there is no such communication, the findings will indicate a space-occupying lesion of the brain (p. 283).

Urinary tract infections

Since urinary tract infections are very common in females, the usual practice is to assume that such an infection is a lower urinary tract infection accompanied by cystitis, with no predisposing factors. It is acceptable practice to base treatment on this assumption, without elaborate laboratory work-ups. However, in repeated urinary tract infections in either females or males, urinalysis should be performed, with a gram stain and a culture. The necessary tests for possible predisposing factors, such as urinary tract obstruction, should be performed.

In asymptomatic bacteriuria a colony count of 100,000/ml or more of gram-negative rods is considered diagnostic of infection. A colony count of only 10,000/ml of enterococci is accepted as diagnostic.

In genitourinary tuberculosis, the most common finding is asymptomatic pyuria and hematuria. In the elderly such a combination should alert the clinician to order the proper cultures to rule out tuberculous involvement of the urinary tract.

Pharyngitis and tonsillitis

The differential diagnosis in acute tonsillitis and pharyngitis is between bacterial infection, mainly with β-hemolytic streptococci, and viral infection. Unless one is already committed to the use of penicillin, it is essential to identify the organism by throat culture because of the complications of β-hemolytic streptococcal infection. There is no need for sensitivity testing once the culture identifies the organism. If the result of the culture is negative, a viral infection is usually indicated.

ASO titers will help in diagnosing β-hemolytic streptococcal infection; however, it takes longer for such a titer to be elevated than for the culture results to be obtained.

Diphtheria

Diphtheria is an infection of the mucous membranes of the pharynx, with toxin production causing widespread inflammation, trauma, and destruction. If the disease is suspected, antitoxin should be administered immediately, even before any specific diagnosis is attempted. However, antibiotics should be withheld until cultures have been taken. A *gram stain* will show gram-positive rods.

Testing for *toxigenicity* is done either by animal inoculation or by in vitro testing, the purpose being to demonstrate that the suspected bacteria are capable of producing toxin.

Testing for *immunity* is accomplished through the *Schick test*. Diphtheria toxin is given intradermally. A positive reaction indicates that the patient does not have circulating antibodies.

Pertussis

Pertussis, or whooping cough, is an acute infection of the mucous membranes of the respiratory tract.

The organism responsible for this condition *(Bordetella pertussis)* is isolated from the upper respiratory tract; it can be cultured only on special media.

Serologic tests are not practical, since the antibodies are in low titer and appear only after 2 weeks.

The *blood count* reveals a leukocytosis—from 15,000 to 40,000 cells/cu mm, with 90% being lymphocytes.

Salmonella infection (typhoidal form)

Salmonella typhi causes typhoid fever. The organisms are ingested, they enter the bloodstream, and they are sequestered in the liver, spleen, and bone marrow. They then multiply within the reticuloendothelial system, being discharged into the intestine from the bile. Three percent of patients will become carriers, with subclinical infections of the gallbladder and the biliary tract.

Blood cultures will have positive results in 70% to 90% of patients during the first week. By the third week only 30% to 40% of patients will have positive results.

The results of *bone marrow cultures* may be positive in partially treated patients when blood culture results are negative.

The results of *throat cultures* will be positive in 10% to 15% the first week, increasing to 75% by the third week.

Serologic tests show an increase in agglutinins against the typhoid bacillus antigens after the first week of illness, rising to a peak by the fifth or sixth week. Such a rise is highly supportive of the presence of infection with the typhoid bacillus, but is not specific, since other organisms will also produce such a rise.

The *blood count* reveals leukopenia during the acute, febrile phase. A sudden appearance of leukocytosis suggests a complication, such as rupture of the bowel.

Salmonella gastroenteritis

Salmonella gastroenteritis usually causes severe nausea, vomiting, and diarrhea. The organism can be isolated from suspected food and from the feces of the patient.

Blood cultures are usually negative.

Shigellosis

The *Shigella* organism will cause acute enterocolitis, with fever, abdominal pain, and diarrhea.

A *stool culture* will confirm the diagnosis.

The *WBC count* will range from 5,000 to 15,000/cu mm. Usually there will be electrolyte abnormalities, depending on the severity of the nausea, vomiting, and diarrhea.

Venereal diseases
Syphilis

Syphilis is a systemic infection caused by *Treponema pallidum*. It is usually transmitted sexually, with the initial manifestation being a chancre.

Microscopic dark field examination is essential in evaluating the moist lesions of primary syphilis. This test must be repeated at least once daily for 3 days before the result can be declared to be negative.

In the secondary stage, when the lesions are nonpruritic, it is more difficult to obtain the organism from the lesion. However, the diagnosis can be made without the microscopic dark field examination if the lesions are characteristic and the results of the serologic tests are positive.

Serologic diagnosis depends on two types of antibodies being produced, the nonspecific reaginic antibody and the specific antitreponemal antibody.

The presence of reaginic antibodies is detected by (1) flocculation tests, the most common being the Venereal Disease Research Laboratories (VDRL) test; (2) complement fixation tests (Kolmer method); and (3) an agglutination test (Rapid Plasma Reagent [RPR] test). All of these tests are nonspecific, with false positives occurring in a significant number of cases.

The presence of antitreponemal antibodies (a specific test) is detected by immunofluorescence technique—the fluorescent treponemal antibody absorption test (FTA-ABS), in which false-positive reactions occur only about 1% of the time.

At present, most institutions and clinics use the VDRL test as a screening test. If the result is positive, the FTA-ABS absorption test is performed. If both results are positive, then the chances of a false positive become extremely remote.

The treponema immobilization test (TPI) will be diagnostically conclusive, but it is tedious to perform and is not routinely used.

Gonococcal infections

In gonorrhea the organism *Neisseria gonorrhoeae*, transmitted by sexual contact, penetrates the mucous membrane of the urogenital tract. In the male, there is a purulent urethritis; in the female, Bartholin's and Skene's glands and the uterine cervical glands are usually infected.

A *gram stain* of the urethral or endocervical discharge will reveal intracellular gram-negative diplococci, which are characteristic and nearly diagnostic.

A *culture* is necessary if one cannot find intracellular gram-negative diplococci by gram stain and the diplococci are extracellular. The culture medium in such a case should have 3% to 10% carbon dioxide, to promote growth. In homosexual patients, cultures must be taken from the throat and the anal canal.

Serologic tests (complement fixation or immunofluorescent techniques) are advisable for systemic infections or in patients with gonococcal arthritis when it is difficult to isolate the organism.

Chancroid

Chancroid is a venereal disease caused by *Hemophilus ducreyi*, which penetrates mucous membranes or broken skin. The disease is manifested as a painful ulcer on the genitals.

Diagnosis is made by exclusion of other genital lesions with which it can be confused, such as herpes progenitalis, syphilis, and lymphogranuloma venereum. When all of these have been eliminated, a response to sulfa drugs is diagnostic.

Culture of *Hemophilus ducreyi* is extremely difficult and impractical.

Granuloma inguinale

Granuloma inguinale is an ulcerative disease caused by *Donovania granulomatis;* it affects the skin and mucous membranes of the external genitalia.

A *punch biopsy* of the lesion is fixed and stained. The finding of Donovan bodies, which are coccobacilli, is diagnostic.

Lymphogranuloma venereum

The organism causing lymphogranuloma venereum is usually transmitted by sexual contact. The first manifestation is a genital lesion, with regional lymph nodes being involved weeks to months later.

A *complement fixation* test with rising titers is evidence of active infection, while a negative result rules out lymphogranuloma.

Herpes progenitalis

Viral isolation techniques are used to diagnose this condition, caused by herpesvirus Type II. If these are not available, cytologic tests and a Pap smear will show multinucleated cells and intranuclear inclusion bodies.

Tuberculosis

Tuberculosis is caused by *Mycobacterium tuberculosis*, which usually infects the lungs but may also involve the kidneys, meninges, spine, and lymph nodes.

An *acid-fast stain* from sputum and gastric washings is sufficient for a tentative diagnosis and initiation of therapy. However, a *culture* of the organism is the only absolute proof of existing infection. For this, multiple sputum specimens and gastric washings are needed for a sufficient positive yield.

An acid-fast stain of spinal fluid, if the result is positive, is fairly diagnostic; it indicates the need for immediate initiation of therapy.

Radiologic methods give valuable information and provide a tentative diagnosis, but never a definitive one. X-ray films are also useful in follow-up and treatment.

The *tuberculin skin test* (purified protein derivative, PPD) does not differentiate between present active infection and dormant and subclinical infections, nor does a negative result rule out active tuberculosis, since anergic states such as Hodgkin's disease, sarcoidosis, massive infection, and pleural effusion will cause false-negative results.

When the result of a routine *urine culture* is negative in the presence of hematuria with pyuria, one should suspect tuberculous infection of the kidney and perform a culture of the urine for the tubercle bacilli.

A *biopsy* of the liver, bone marrow, or lymph nodes may be diagnostic of miliary tuberculosis.

A pleural biopsy may be very helpful in the presence of pleural effusion, which is usually an exudate. Bacteriologic study and fluid analysis should also be performed.

The needle pleural biopsy usually reveals the typical granuloma of tuberculosis, with giant cells showing caseation necrosis. Such findings are sufficiently diagnostic to initiate therapy.

In order to increase the yield, multiple biopsy specimens should be taken at one sitting.

Rickettsial diseases

The rickettsias are intracellular parasites maintained by a cycle involving an insect vector and an animal reservoir, with man being an incidental victim. The organism typically invades the endothelial cells of small blood vessels, with perivascular infiltration and thrombosis. Diagnosis is important because the treatment is specific.

Serologic tests are used in the diagnosis because isolation of the organism is difficult, impractical, and hazardous.

The *Weil-Felix test*, which employs *Proteus* OX-19 and OX-2, gives positive results in patients with Rocky Mountain spotted fever or murine typhus and negative results in patients with rickettsialpox or Q fever.

A *complement fixation test* employing group-specific rickettsial antigens will clinically differentiate among the most common infections. A rise in titer in a week or two, with a fall in titer later, is diagnostic of the specific rickettsia.

Actinomycosis

In the past actinomycosis, a chronic granulomatous infection, has been classified under diseases caused by fungi. However, the causative organism is *Actinomyces israelii*, a gram-positive rod or filament that is normally present in the mouth. Actinomycosis is most common on the face and neck, manifesting a week or more after tooth extraction or mandibular fracture as a painful indurated lesion over the jaw. From there, or from foci in the lung or intestines, actinomycosis may spread to the liver, kidneys, spleen, brain, genitalia, and subcutaneous tissues.

Diagnosis is made by detecting the organism in pus from abscesses, by gram stain, by anaerobic culture, or by biopsy.

A *gram stain* is used when clumps of the organism have formed. Such clumps, which are called "sulfur granules," are crushed and stained.

An *anaerobic culture* is utilized when the sulfur granules are not present, and *biopsies* are employed when the culture is negative.

Nocardiosis

Nocardiosis is caused by an aerobic actinomycete found in the soil, which is either inhaled or introduced into the subcutaneous tissue by trauma. Lung abscesses may result, and they may spread to the brain.

Diagnosis is made by isolation of the gram-positive organism from sputum or abscesses.

Mycoses (diseases caused by fungi)
Cryptococcosis

Cryptococcosis is a pulmonary infection caused by *Cryptococcus neoformans,* an encapsulated yeast. The most virulent strain of this organism is found in pigeon droppings, the dust of which may be inhaled. The organism has an affinity for the central nervous system, with lesions developing in the meninges at the base of the brain. This is one of the causes of aseptic meningitis.

Diagnosis is made by isolating the organism from the cerebrospinal fluid on Sabouraud's agar, and by gram stain and microscopic examination of the spinal fluid.

Blastomycosis

The organism *Blastomyces dermatitidis,* which causes blastomycosis, gains entrance to the body through the lungs to cause systemic infection.

Diagnosis is made by culturing the organism from sputum, pus, or biopsied material on Sabouraud's agar. The value of a skin test is limited. A complement fixation test may also be employed.

Coccidioidomycosis (San Joaquin Valley or desert fever)

The infection coccidioidomycosis is caused by inhalation of the organism *Coccidioides immitis.* After inhalation the organism may be killed or arrested, causing an acute respiratory disease; or in some cases the organism will proliferate and the disease will become chronic.

Diagnosis is made by isolating the organism on Sabouraud's agar. Serologic methods include tests for complement-fixing antibodies and precipitin tests.

Histoplasmosis

In histoplasmosis the organism *Histoplasma capsulatum,* after being inhaled from the soil, causes a pulmonary infection very similar to tuberculosis.

Diagnosis is made by isolating the organism on Sabouraud's agar and by pulmonary radiologic findings. Serologic and skin tests have limited usefulness.

Candidiasis (moniliasis)

Candidiasis is a mild mucocutaneous infection caused by *Candida albicans.* When the mucous membranes are involved, the disease is known as thrush. The disease may enter the bloodstream when it is a complication of other, severe, debilitating diseases.

The fungus can be isolated from a scraping of white patches in the mouth.

In deep, disseminated candidiasis biopsy material from tissues involved will reveal the presence of the organism. In *Candida* endocarditis the organism is isolated from blood cultures. Candidiasis is a common form of vaginal infection.

Mucormycosis (Zygomycosis)

Mucorales organisms, found in soil, manure, and starchy foodstuffs, may become pathogenic for humans in cases of severe underlying disease, particularly diabetic acidosis. The organisms enter through the nasal turbinates or the paranasal sinus and may eventually spread to the brain or cause pulmonary infection.

Diagnosis is made by demonstration of the presence of the organisms in biopsied infected tissue.

Viral infections

Most of the viral infections seen clinically, particularly those of the upper respiratory tract, are not specifically diagnosed, because of their benign nature and short duration. By the time a causative organism could be isolated or serologic test produce diagnostic results, the infection would have subsided. However, for retrospective diagnosis and for epidemiologic purposes, isolation and tissue culture techniques for specific viruses, as well as multiple serologic tests, are available.

Another reason for not attempting specific virologic diagnoses is the fact that there is no specific antiviral therapy.

When pericarditis or myocarditis is diagnosed and a viral etiology is suspected, it is helpful clinically to make as specific a diagnosis as possible. This diagnosis is based on serologic testing of sera taken during the acute and convalescent phases. The results of this test could not be used therapeutically, even if specific therapy for viral infections were available. The main reason for specific diagnoses in such cases is for prognostication and to rule out other possible causes of pericarditis and myocarditis. The acute and convalescent sera are usually sent to a reference laboratory with all of the clinical information. In a case of suspected myocarditis or pericarditis, the laboratory is asked to do serologic testing for all possible viruses that could cause these specific conditions: Coxsackie A and B, poliomyelitis, influenza, adenovirus, ECHO, rubeola, and rubella. If the acute and convalescent sera shows a fourfold rise in titer of any of the above viruses in a suspected case of myocarditis or pericarditis, a definitive diagnosis is established.

Herpes simplex hominis

Herpes simplex hominis, which is caused by herpesviruses, usually involves mucocutaneous lesions, which may disseminate in an immunosuppressed patient. Type I herpesvirus causes naso-oropharyngeal lesions. Type II herpesvirus causes genitourinary tract lesions and is considered a venereal disease in transmission. This type is associated with carcinoma of the cervix.

A smear from the base of a vesicle shows multinucleated giant cells and eosinophilic inclusion bodies.

Immunofluorescent staining can demonstrate the presence of viral antigens in the cells.

Cat-scratch disease

Cat-scratch disease is a suppurative, regional lymphadenitis; cats act as a vector for the disease.

Diagnosis is made by a skin test, which, if the result is positive, shows a delayed tuberculin type of reaction.

Mumps

Mumps results in parotitis, epididymitis, orchitis, and pancreatitis, and it is one of the causes of aseptic meningitis.

The diagnosis usually is serologic (complement fixation test). Between the acute and convalescent phases the serum will show a fourfold increase in titer.

Varicella (chickenpox)

The diagnosis of varicella is usually clinical. However, laboratory findings will verify the clinical impression.

A smear from the base of a vesicle demonstrates varicella giant cells with intranuclear bodies.

Serologic tests, mainly immunofluorescent staining, will confirm the diagnosis.

Cytomegalovirus infection

Cytomegalovirus causes a disease very similar to infectious mononucleosis. It usually occurs in patients who receive large amounts of fresh blood. In the past, patients undergoing open heart surgery would receive large amounts of such blood. The syndrome following open heart surgery was called postperfusion syndrome. Eventually it was found to be caused by cytomegalovirus.

The diagnosis is made by examining a stained sediment of urine, saliva, or gastric washings, which will demonstrate the cytoplasmic inclusion bodies.

Isolation of the virus is possible; serologic tests include complement fixation and neutralization tests.

Variola (smallpox)

The smallpox virus, which gains entrance through the respiratory tract, causes vesicular and pustular eruption, accompanied by fever.

Diagnosis is made by smears taken from the bases of the lesions. When stained, the typical viral particles are visible. Fluorescent antibody tests, both direct and indirect, may also be used.

Isolation of the virus is possible; serologic tests, mainly complement fixation, hemagglutination, and neutralization tests, show rising titers.

Influenza

Influenza is a generalized, acute, febrile disease sometimes associated with upper respiratory infections. Diagnosis is made mainly clinically in a given epidemiologic setting. However, isolated cases can be definitively diagnosed by isolating the virus from chick embryos inoculated with sputum or throat washings. Fluorescent antibody staining of nasal epithelial cells will provide a diagnosis in the first days of the disease. Serologic tests require a fourfold increase in antibody titer between the acute and the convalescent sera.

Infectious mononucleosis

The causative virus for infectious mononucleosis has recently been isolated; it has been called the Epstein-Barr (EB) virus. It causes sore throat and lymphadenopathy. The disease may be very mild, or it may be severe, with hepatomegaly, hepatitis, and sometimes meningitis.

The diagnosis is made because of marked lymphocytosis, with Downey cells (atypical lymphocytes).

High titers of heterophil antibodies are present in the serum of 80% to 90% of affected persons. These agglutinins against sheep red blood cells are normally found in low titers in the blood of most people. Since the titer is elevated in a variety of infections, the heterophil antibody test is nonspecific.

Recently, a rapid method of detecting heterophil agglutinins has been developed; it requires a drop of the patient's blood and a reagent. Known as the Mono-Spot test, it is used mainly for screening purposes.

Diagnostic titers of antibodies to the EB virus range from 1:80 to 1:160. These titers are demonstrated by immunofluorescence techniques.

When there is liver involvement and hepatitis, the results of liver function tests are usually abnormal, including elevated SGOT, SGPT, bilirubin, and alkaline phosphatase levels.

Parasitic diseases
Malaria

Malaria is transmitted by the female *Anopheles* mosquito, the causative organism being protozoa of the genus *Plasmodium*. Malaria has a chronic, relapsing course, with fever, chills, splenomegaly, and anemia.

A blood smear, treated with Wright's, Giemsa's, or Field's stain and taken a few hours after an episode of chills, will usually demonstrate the presence of the parasite. There are four species of the *Plasmodium* protozoa, the identification of which requires experience.

Serologic tests, such as the indirect fluorescent antibody test and hemagglutination tests, are available but not widely used.

Pneumocystis carinii

The parasite *pneumocystis carinii* causes pneumonia in debilitated or immunosuppressed persons.

Chest x-ray film is usually diagnostic, showing diffuse, typical pulmonary and alveolar infiltration.

Definitive diagnosis is achieved by needle biopsy of the lung.

Toxoplasmosis

The protozoan *Toxoplasma gondii* enters the body as a result of the ingestion of poorly cooked, infected meat. The organism causes lymphadenopathy and myalgia, and can cause central nervous system disease. Transplacental infection causes congenital toxoplasmosis, manifested in the infant by rash, fever, chorioretinitis, and encephalitis.

Diagnosis is made by the indirect fluorescent antibody test. Titers of 1:256 or higher indicate recent infection, and titers of 1:1024 or higher indicate active disease.

A complement fixation test will have a positive result in active disease.

Trichinosis

The organism *Trichinella spiralis* gains entry to the body as a result of the ingestion of undercooked meat, particularly pork.

The most characteristic laboratory finding is a marked eosinophilia.

Serologic tests include complement fixation tests, the precipitin test and the fluorescent antibody test. The results of these tests will become positive about the third week of the disease. The tests are most helpful in the diagnosis if initially negative results are followed by significant changes in titer.

Definitive diagnosis is done by muscle biopsy. The most frequently involved muscles are those of the extremities; the throat, and the diaphragm.

Amebiasis

The causative organism of amebiasis is *Entamoeba histolytica,* a protozoon that causes intestinal disease with diarrhea and colitis, as well as hepatic abscess.

Diagnosis is made by identification of the organism in stools and tissues.

Indirect hemagglutination is usually helpful in diagnosing hepatic abscess. In areas where the disease is endemic, a negative serologic test result is important in ruling out the disease.

Trypanosomiasis (sleeping sickness)

Trypanosomiasis is caused by *Trypanosoma brucei,* a protozoon that is transmitted by the tsetse fly. In trypanosomiasis the patient has lymphadenopathy followed by encephalitis.

The diagnosis is made by finding the trypanosomes in blood or the aspirate from lymph glands or cerebrospinal fluid.

The main serologic tests used are the complement fixation test and the indirect fluorescent antibody test.

Giardiasis

Giardiasis, which causes "traveler's diarrhea," is the result of infestation of the duodenum and jejunum by *Giardia lamblia,* a protozoon. Occasionally malabsorption will result.

Diagnosis is made by finding the trophozoid stage of the organism in duodenal washings.

Trichomonas vaginalis infection

Trichomonas vaginalis, a protozoon, causes vaginal infection with discharge.

Diagnosis is established by examination of the vaginal discharge or seminal fluid by a wet stain or with a Giemsa-stained preparation.

FOURTEEN Diagnostic tests
for sleep disorders

SLEEP PHYSIOLOGY

Sleep is a complex, active process. Its primary function remains unknown, although it occurs in most vertebrates and all mammals. The control of sleep and wakefulness resides in the central nervous system (CNS). As understood today, the CNS has three principal operating states:

1. Waking or arousal
2. Synchronized (S) sleep, also called non–rapid-eye-movement (NREM) sleep, which comprises stages 2, 3, and 4 of the sleep cycle
3. Desynchronized, dream (D), or rapid-eye-movement (REM) sleep

Sleep physiology is studied in the laboratory through examination of electroencephalograms (EEG), electro-oculograms (EOG), and electromyograms (EMG). These recordings indicate the presence or absence of sleep and the type of sleep.

Sleep and wakefulness are characterized by a circadian rhythmicity; that is, the two states alternate in a regular, periodic way during every 24-hour span of time. During the sleep phase, REM sleep occurs in a cyclic fashion, alternating with periods of NREM sleep. Each REM-NREM cycle lasts 70 to 120 minutes. NREM sleep normally begins as a person falls asleep and becomes decreasingly conscious of the external environment. Although this initial process of falling asleep seems to be a slow and gradual event, the moment of disengagement from the outside world is precise and sudden. The sleep state that follows the onset of NREM sleep is characterized by progressively decreasing brain activity; this state has been arbitrarily divided into four stages, with stage 1 being light sleep and stage 4 being deepest sleep. Stage 4 sleep is considered to represent the lowest level of physiologic, neurologic, and psychologic activity. During stage 4 sleep it is most difficult for a person to be aroused. Stage 4 sleep may be the most restorative phase of sleep, while REM sleep is considered essential for health.

REM sleep is characterized by an intensely active brain within a paralyzed body. There is profound motor inhibition, paralyzing all reflex and voluntary movement. Simultaneously, there is increased EEG activity, indicating CNS "arousal" because of increased metabolic activity of the brain—a situation that is similar to that in the waking state. External manifestations of this active state include penile erection, phasic eye movements, and changes in the heart rate and the respiratory rate. Dream recall is enhanced; persons awakened from REM sleep have an exceptional ability to recall the details of dreams. Fig. 14-1 distinguishes REM sleep from NREM sleep, on

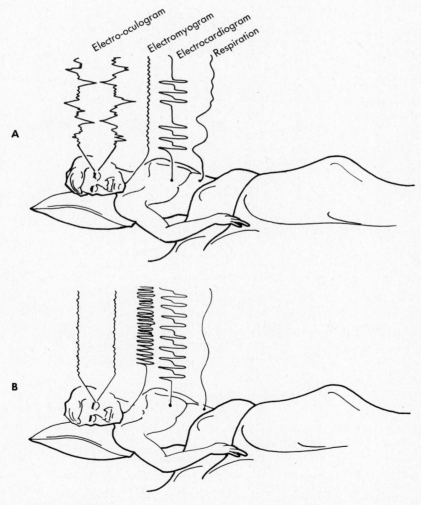

Fig. 14-1
Polysomnographic records during REM **(A)** and NREM **(B)** sleep.

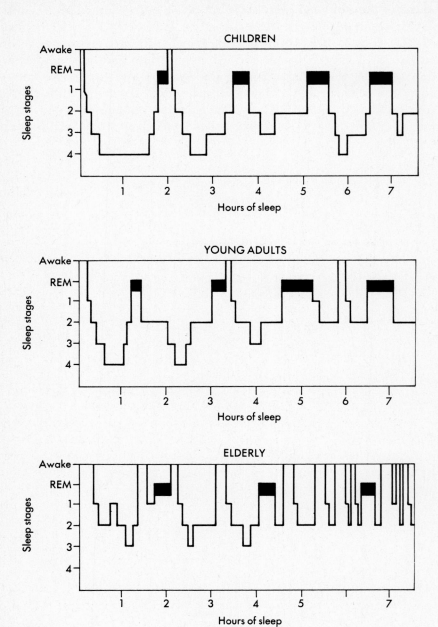

Fig. 14-2
An idealized night's sleep in children, normal young adults, and the elderly.

the basis of polysomnographic differences. The functions of REM sleep are not known, but this phase of normal sleep is considered essential for health.

A single night of normal sleep consists of four to six cycles, each of which includes both NREM sleep and REM sleep, as shown in Fig. 14-2.

Sleep duration and patterns in normal individuals vary extensively. Most normal adults sleep 7 to 8 hours, although normal sleep can be as short as 4 hours and as long as 10 to 12 hours. The duration and quality of normal sleep change with age. Infants sleep up to 18 hours a day, and they spend more time in stage 4 sleep and in REM sleep than children or adults do. With increasing age, stage 4 sleep diminishes, sleep latency (the time required to fall asleep) increases, and sleep disturbances become more frequent. The clinical significance of altered sleep patterns in the aged is not understood (Fig. 14-2).

The biochemistry of normal sleep is under intense study but remains poorly understood. Several neurotransmitters are involved, including serotonin, norepinephrine, and dopamine. The production of various hormones is related to the sleep cycle. Growth hormone is released during stage 4 sleep. Plasma levels of cortisol peak within 1 hour of waking. The circadian rhythm of sleep is closely related to the secretion of neurotransmitters and hormones, but the mechanisms have not yet been classified.

The scientific study of sleep and sleep disorders is a relatively new development in clinical medicine. During the past decade, various sleep-related medical disorders have been described and treatment methods have been proposed. The medical history and the patient's presentation and complaints remain the most important diagnostic clues. Once a significant sleep disorder is suspected, specialized diagnostic studies may be indicated, both for confirmation of the clinical diagnosis and for quantitation of the problem and assessment of the severity of the disorder. Such a study, which generally involves *polysomnography*, is conducted in a specially designed sleep laboratory.

THE SLEEP LABORATORY

Sleep studies are performed in a specially designed "laboratory," which provides an optimal environment for sleep. The room should be quiet, well ventilated, and not excessively warm. Controlled lighting is necessary, but absolute darkness is not required. The room should be equipped with a television camera and a sound monitor to observe the patient and to follow his movements and his noises. Special wiring should lead from the patient's bed to a recording laboratory (to the polysomnograph) to permit continuous recording of various data with minimal interference with the patient's sleep.

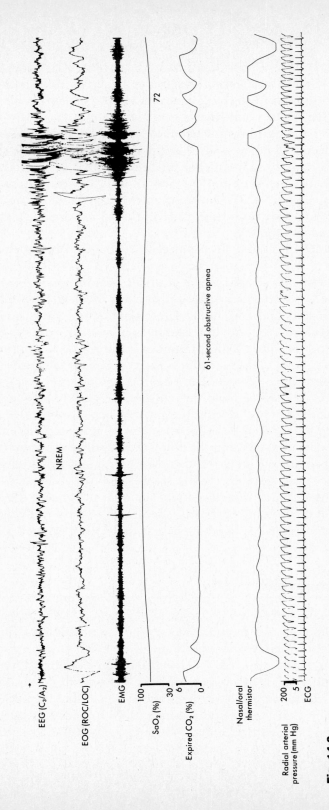

Fig. 14-3

Polygraphic recording during sleep in a patient with obstructive sleep apnea. Obstruction is overcome and respiration is resumed after 61 seconds of apnea. *ECG,* Electrocardiogram. *SaO₂,* Percent oxygen saturation. *EMG,* Electromyogram. *EOG,* Electro-oculogram. *EEG,* Electroencephalogram.

The standard polysomnogram

The polysomnograph is the basic diagnostic tool in the sleep laboratory. It consists of a multichannel (8, 12, or 16) physiologic recorder that continuously performs the following functions:

1. Identifies fluctuations in voltage, by means of electrodes attached to the patient's scalp (electroencephalography). Data from several leads is recorded simultaneously to help determine the presence and stage of sleep.
2. Detects eye movement by noting electrical potentials through electrodes on the face (electro-oculography). Rapid eye movement is one of the features of REM sleep.
3. Monitors submental or digastric muscles (electromyography) to determine periods of muscular paralysis, which characterizes REM sleep
4. Evaluates respiration, by means of one or more of the following:
   a. Thermistors (oral or nasal temperature-sensing probes that monitor air flow)
   b. Strain gauges, either thoracic or abdominal, which sense respiratory muscular activity
   c. Oximetry. Oxygen saturation can be monitored by means of an ear oximeter. Oxygen tension can be estimated by skin electrodes.
   d. Nasal or oral probes that monitor expired carbon dioxide
5. Monitors heart rate variations and rhythm changes

The first three functions are necessary to determine the presence of sleep and monitor its stage.

By means of the respiratory data, diagnosis of apnea and types of apnea may be determined. Fig. 14-3 is a polygraphic recording during sleep in a patient with obstructive sleep apnea.

Special studies

In addition to the functions of the standard polysomnogram, the following can also be monitored:

1. Penile tumescence. Erection of the penis normally occurs during REM sleep. Absence of any penile tumescence during REM sleep would suggest an organic dysfunction (vascular or neural). Penile tumescence is monitored to distinguish psychogenic impotence from organic impotence.
2. Intraesophageal pressure. The monitoring of intraesophageal pressure is one of the best ways of distinguishing central apnea, which is characterized by the cessation of all respiratory efforts, from obstructive apnea, which is characterized by airway occlusion and continuing ventilatory efforts.
3. Intraesophageal pH. The intraesophageal pH is monitored in suspected cases of nocturnal gastrointestinal reflux and esophagitis.

4. Movement of peripheral muscles. In cases where myoclonic jerks of the leg are suspected (nocturnal myoclonus), a peripheral EMG is obtained.
5. Hemodynamics. Early research studies involved *invasive* hemodynamic monitoring of both systemic and pulmonary artery pressures, as well as cardiac output. Invasive methods are now used very infrequently in clinical sleep studies. Noninvasive blood pressure monitoring methods have not been adequately tested in sleep laboratories.

A diagnostic sleep study is tailored to the needs of the individual patient and the problem or disorder being studied. It is both inconvenient and wasteful to record all of the preceding data during all studies.

THE COMMON SLEEP DISORDERS

Narcolepsy

Narcolepsy, a chronic sleep disorder, is characterized by recurrent and uncontrollable attacks of daytime sleepiness. The episodes are sudden and usually brief. The attacks can come at inappropriate times—for example, during coitus or while a person is driving a car—and they can be quite disabling. In addition to the attack of sleepiness, narcolepsy is characterized by *cataplexy*, a flaccid paralysis frequently triggered by strong emotion; *sleep paralysis*, a paralysis that occurs in the transition period between sleep and wakefulness; and *hypnagogic hallucinations*, vivid and terrifying dreams just before or just after sleep.

The laboratory hallmark of narcolepsy is the appearance of the REM phase of sleep at the *onset* of sleep instead of after 70 to 100 minutes of sleep in stages 1 through 4. The cause is not known; a malfunction of the neurochemical process regulating sleep and wakefulness evidently exists, permitting the abrupt intrusion of REM sleep into the waking state. A standard polysomnographic examination that documents the presence of the REM phase at onset of sleep confirms the clinical diagnosis. A complete nocturnal study is advisable to exclude other sleep disorders.

Sleep apneas

Disorders of breathing can occur during sleep. Such a disorder may be related to upper airway obstruction (obstructive sleep apnea) or to a CNS dysfunction (central apnea). With apnea there will be hypoxemia, hypercapnia, respiratory acidosis, systemic and pulmonary hypertension, and arrhythmias. The apnea recurs cyclically, and greatly disturbs the patient's sleep. The most frequent presenting complaint is excessive daytime sleepiness. This can lead to an erroneous diagnosis of narcolepsy. The other manifestations of narcolepsy (cataplexy, sleep paralysis, hypnagogic hallucinations) are not present.

A diagnostic sleep study would clearly distinguish excessive daytime sleepiness caused by sleep apnea syndromes from narcolepsy, since in sleep apnea there is no REM at the onset of sleep. A polysomnographic study will allow a clinician to classify the apnea as central, obstructive, or mixed and to assess the severity of the disorder in terms of the frequency and duration of airway occlusion and the degree of arterial oxygen desaturation. The information obtained during the laboratory polysomnographic study will help in formulating a treatment plan, which may involve CNS or respiratory stimulants, weight reduction, or surgery. Surgical procedures include tonsillectomy and adenoidectomy, palatoplasty, tracheostomy, and insertion of a phrenic nerve–stimulating pacemaker.

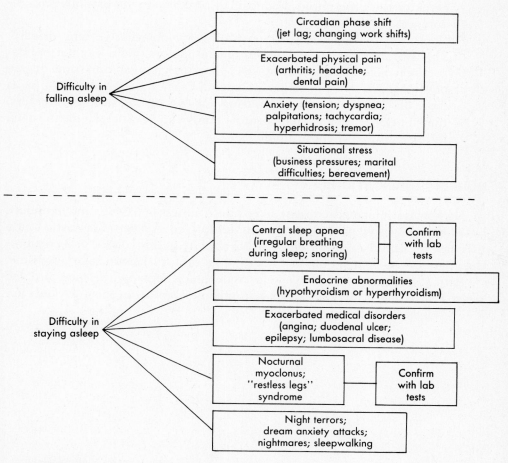

Fig. 14-4
Diagnostic chart for underlying causes of insomnia.

Insomnias

There are many causes of insomnia. Common ones include depression, drug abuse, nocturnal myoclonus, restless leg syndrome, nocturnal seizures, and disturbances of the circadian rhythm (chronic jet lag). Sleep apnea of CNS origin can also be manifested as insomnia. A polysomnogram is helpful in making a diagnosis and in excluding other causes (Fig. 14-4).

EVALUATION OF OTHER MEDICAL CONDITIONS

A sleep diagnostic study can be modified to help evaluate the following problems:

1. Impotence. Penile tumescence (erection) can be measured in terms of both degree and duration during sleep. As discussed earlier, such a test helps in the differential diagnosis of organic versus psychogenic impotence.
2. Nocturnal oxygen desaturation in chronic obstructive lung disease. This situation may be related to several factors, including normal depression of respiration during sleep, posture changes, and some degree of upper airway obstruction. In such a case, a sleep study will focus more on the respiratory monitoring and less on the sleep parameters. Information from a sleep laboratory study can help determine the need for oxygen treatment at night.

NURSING IMPLICATIONS

No special informed consent is required unless invasive, and therefore possibly hazardous, procedures are contemplated. A sleep diagnostic study may last for only 1 night, or on occasion a study will involve 2 or 3 consecutive nights. A patient should arrive at the laboratory 1 hour before bedtime.

Patient preparation involves electrode placement on the face and the scalp. Ear oximetry may be somewhat uncomfortable, but most patients are able to sleep even on the first night.

FIFTEEN Diagnostic tests
in nutritional disorders

An adequate nutritional state is important to protein synthesis, resistance to infection, and wound healing. Protein and calorie requirements are increased by surgery, stress, sepsis, trauma, or hypermetabolic disease processes, and dramatically increased by burns. Thus attendance to the caloric needs of a patient is often a critical factor in his prognosis.

Tests for nutritional assessment are employed for the following purposes:
1. Pretreatment evaluation of a nutritionally deficient patient
2. Evaluation of the progress of a patient while he is being treated
3. Differentiation between nutritional deficiencies—for example, kwashiorkor (protein-calorie malnourishment) versus marasmus (generalized malnourishment)
4. Diagnosis of individual nutritional dificiencies, such as iron deficiency or folic acid deficiency
5. Evaluation of subclinical nutritional deficiency, as yet an ill-defined area in clinical medicine

The quickest and easiest way to determine the presence or absence of malnutrition is to evaluate the body height/weight index and the anthropometric measurements (body measurements). The anthropometric measurements include the *triceps skinfold* and the *arm muscle circumference*, which is calculated from the *mid–upper arm circumference* and the triceps skinfold. Visceral protein status is determined from the serum albumin and/or transferrin levels; it is a guide to the level of immune competence. The status of metabolically active tissue is evaluated by creatinine height index analysis.

THE ANTHROPOMETRIC MEASUREMENTS

Anthropometric measurements are converted to percentages of standard. Anything less than 60% is classified as severe malnutrition. Moderate malnutrition is indicated when a measurement falls in the 60%-80% range.

339

Triceps skinfold

Measurement of the triceps skinfold provides an indication of available fat stores, which are a reflection of the body's caloric reserve. Fat stores are significantly diminished in marasmus (Table 15-1).

The midpoint of the upper portion of the patient's nondominant arm is identified. The skinfold at this point is measured over the triceps muscle with a skin-fold caliper. Three separate measurements are made, and the two closest results are averaged.

It should be remembered that body fat stores may remain normal, or may even be excessive, in the face of moderate to severe malnutrition. Therefore, the triceps skinfold measurement lacks sensitivitiy in the detection of malnutrition.

Mid–upper arm circumference (MUAC)

The mid–upper arm circumference provides an indication of the available fat and protein stores and facilitates an assessment of current nutri-

Table 15-1

Triceps skinfold measurements (mm), adults

| | | Percent of standard | | | |
	Standard	90	80	70	60
Male	12.5	11.3	10.0	8.8	7.5
Female	16.5	11.9	13.2	11.6	9.9

Table 15-2

Mid–upper arm circumferences (mm), adults

| | | Percent of standard | | | |
	Standard	90	80	70	60
Male	29.3	26.3	23.4	20.5	17.6
Female	28.5	25.7	22.8	20.0	17.1

Table 15-3

Arm muscle circumferences (mm), adults

| | | Percent of standard | | | |
	Standard	90	80	70	60
Male	25.3	22.8	20.2	17.7	15.2
Female	23.2	20.9	18.6	16.2	13.9

tional status in either kwashiorkor, a syndrome produced by severe protein deficiency, or marasmus, a condition characterized by generalized wasting and emaciation (Table 15-2).

The circumference at the midpoint of the upper portion of the nondominant arm is measured with the arm hanging freely.

Arm muscle circumference (AMC)

The arm muscle circumference provides an indication of the amount of muscle protein, which is usually diminished in kwashiorkor as opposed to pure marasmus (Table 15-3). The measurement is obtained by using the following formula:

Arm muscle circumference =
$$\text{arm circumference (cm)} - (0.314 \times \text{triceps skin fold [mm])}$$

A significant decrease in this measurement reflects a decrease in total muscle protein, and usually indicates kwashiorkor. If both total body fat and muscle protein are diminished, both kwashiorkor and marasmus should be suspected.

BIOCHEMICAL MEASUREMENTS

Serum albumin level

The serum albumin level provides an indication of visceral protein reserve; the albumin level is usually reduced when protein stores are lost. A serum albumin concentration of less than 3.4 gm/dl, in the absence of liver disease, indicates protein malnutrition.

Advantage

The serum albumin level correlates with changes in arm muscle circumference, and it is a reliable indicator of visceral protein activity.

Disadvantage

Because the half-life of albumin synthesis is long (16 to 18 days), serious protein and calorie depletion is already present by the time it is reflected in the serum albumin level, and early response to treatment is somewhat unpredictable. The half-life for albumin may be decreased in patients with infection, burns, severe injuries, and protein-losing enteropathies.

♦ Serum albumin levels and malnutrition

Mild: 3.0-3.5 gm/dl
Moderate: 2.1-3.0 gm/dl
Severe: <2.1 gm/dl

Serum transferrin level

Transferrin is a serum beta globulin that binds and transports iron. Therefore the transferrin level can be measured directly, or it can be estimated by multiplying the total iron-binding capacity by 0.8 and subtracting 43.

Advantage

Since transferrin has a shorter half-life than albumin, its level is reduced earlier, making it a more sensitive indicator of visceral secretory protein status.

Disadvantage

The transferrin level and the iron-binding capacity may be influenced by iron metabolism and low iron stores. Thus iron deficiency anemia can produce falsely elevated transferrin levels.

◆ Serum transferrin levels and malnutrition

Mild:	150-175 mg/dl
Moderate:	100-150 mg/dl
Severe:	<100 mg/dl

Levels of thyroxine-binding prealbumin and retinol-binding protein

These levels are probably better indicators of subclinical nutritional deficiency than of a substantial deficiency. Thyroxine-binding prealbumin has

Table 15-4

Ideal urinary creatinine values

Male		Female	
Height (cm)	Value (mg/24 hr)	Height (cm)	Value (mg/24 hr)
157.5	1288	147.3	830
160.0	1325	149.9	851
162.6	1359	152.4	875
165.1	1386	154.9	900
167.6	1426	157.5	925
167.6	1426	157.5	925
170.2	1467	160.0	949
172.7	1513	162.6	977
175.3	1555	165.1	1006
177.8	1596	167.6	1044
180.3	1642	170.2	1076
182.9	1691	172.7	1109
185.4	1739	175.3	1141
188.0	1785	177.8	1174
190.5	1831	180.3	1206
193.0	1891	182.9	1240

a half-life of only 2 days, and that of retinol-binding protein is only 12 hours. Both substances are sensitive to changes in protein and calories and respond rapidly to refeeding.

Creatinine-height index

Creatinine is a product of muscle metabolism; the 24-hour urinary excretion of creatinine is roughly proportional to the lean body mass or metabolically active tissue. A decrease in the 24-hour urinary output of creatinine reflects muscle protein depletion and a decrease in muscle mass.

The creatinine height index is obtained by multiplying the actual 24-hour urinary creatinine output by 100 and dividing by the ideal urinary creatinine output of a normal male or female of the same height as the person being tested. Table 15-4 lists the ideal 24-hour urinary creatinine outputs according to sex and height. To convert height in inches to height in centimeters, multiply the height in inches by 2.54. This index is a fairly accurate indicator of muscle protein depletion and decreases in muscle mass.

IMMUNOLOGIC TESTS

In malnutrition (both marasmus and kwashiorkor) there are apparently immunologic deficiencies, which disappear after malnutrition has been corrected. The following tests are usually performed.

Total lymphocyte count

Lymphocytes are sensitive to deficiencies in calories and precursor amino acids. Thus when protein malnutrition exists, the synthesis of lymphocytes is depressed, which in turn contributes to the impaired ability of the white cells to fight infection.

The total lymphocyte count is equal to the percentage of lymphocytes multiplied by the white blood cell count. This figure is then converted to a percentage of the standard, which is considered to be 1500/cu mm.

$$\text{Percentage of standard} = \frac{\text{total lymphocyte count} \times 100}{1500/\text{cu mm}}.$$

♦ Total lymphocyte count and malnutrition

Moderate: 800-1200/cu mm
Severe: <800/cu mm

Skin testing

An impaired ability of the white cells to fight infection, a situation that is linked to a decreased total lymphocyte count, can be recognized by means of skin testing. The usual antigens for skin testing are used, including streptokinase-streptodornase (SK-SD), mumps virus, *Candida* organisms, and purified protein derivative of tuberculin (PPD). The results are read in 24 to 48 hours. A normal response is positive, indicated by the appearance of a wheal 5 mm or more in diameter within 24 to 48 hours. An abnormal response is negative (anergy). Some clinicians try to quantitate the response, arguing that a wheal between 10 and 15 mm indicates mild deficiency, a wheal between 5 and 10 mm indicates moderate deficiency, and a wheal of less than 5 mm indicates severe immune deficiency and anergy. However, such a classification is not very accurate, and it is probably better simply to characterize the reaction as positive (indicating cellular immunity) or negative (indicating depressed cellular immunity).

Disadvantages

Anergy also occurs as a result of acute fevers, sepsis, steroid treatment, certain tumors, shock, and circulating inhibititors of lymphocyte function, making the results of skin testing less than completely reliable.

TESTS FOR DEFICIENCIES OF VITAMINS OR NUTRIENTS

Deficiencies of specific vitamins or nutrients can be identified by means of laboratory tests, as follows:

Vitamin A: deficiency evaluated by serum assay. A low serum vitamin A level plus a low serum carotene level strongly suggests a vitamin A deficiency, although serum carotene levels themselves reflect only the recent dietary intake.

Vitamin B_1 (thiamine): deficiency best identified by recognition of diminished erythrocyte transketolase activity, the test for which is not readily available

Vitamin B_2 (riboflavin): deficiency best assessed through the use of the glutathione reductase assay, not readily available

Vitamin B_6: deficiency detected by an enzymatic assay, not readily available

Vitamin B_{12}: assays readily available clinically

Vitamin D: serum 25-OH-D_3 assay, not routinely employed; serum alkaline phosphatase level, easily determinable but indirect measure; serum calcium and phosphorus levels, also easily available but indirect measures

Vitamin E: serum tocopherol measurement, not readily available. (Tocopherols are substances possessing vitamin E activity.)

Vitamin K: level indirectly measured by prothrombin time

Folic acid: serum levels readily available. The red cell folate level is more accurate in the diagnosis of chronic deficiency and depletion of tissue stores, and correlates well with the clinical syndromes associated with folic acid deficiency.

Iron and iron-binding capacity: serum assay readily available. However, the results can be variable, inaccurate, and sometimes misleading.

Ferritin: determination of serum ferritin level. Such a determination is fairly accurate, and the ferritin level is a good index of iron stores, correlating very well with a bone marrow iron stain level for the diagnosis of iron deficiency. One pitfall is that the ferritin level is elevated in acute inflammatory diseases, infections, and lymphomas; such an elevation thus does not reflect iron stores.

DIAGNOSIS OF SUBCLINICAL NUTRITIONAL DEFICIENCIES

Subclinical nutritional deficiency is not an established clinical entity. In the future it may or may not be considered clinically significant. However, we would like to alert you to the possibility that it may. For example, although clinical beriberi is very rare in the United States, the majority of alcoholics have red cell transketolase levels that are significantly diminished, indicating subclinical deficiencies of vitamin B_1, which respond to the administration of thiamine. It is difficult to establish the significance of such a decreased transketolase level in the clinical setting. However, one can say that in alcoholics, in view of the decreased transketolase level, there is subclinical B_1 deficiency.

The serum ferritin level is another example. A ferritin level of 10 mg/dl or less with microcytic anemia is diagnostic of iron deficiency anemia. However, in the absence of anemia and in the presence of apparent microcytosis, a ferritin level of 10 to 40 mg/dl is definitely associated with decreased bone marrow iron levels, as shown by bone marrow stains, and with decreased bone marrow stores. Before iron deficiency anemia sets in or before there is a decrease in hemoglobin level, or hematocrit, the levels of certain iron-dependent enzymes decrease. There is strong clinical evidence that these decreases contribute significantly to the symptoms of iron deficiency anemia, suggesting that a ferritin level between 10 and 40 mg/dl indicates a subclinical deficiency of iron. For example, in a patient who is complaining of fatigue and who has a ferritin level of 20 mg/dl without anemia, there is evidence to suggest that before frank anemia develops there is a definite decrease in the iron-dependent enzyme levels, and that this decrease is the cause of the symptoms.

These are just two examples to alert you to future developments in the area of subclinical nutritional deficiency.

SIXTEEN Miscellaneous diseases and laboratory tests

ALLERGY

Allergy in the true sense of the word means an adverse reaction to an antigen-antibody interaction, or, in some cases, an abnormal effect induced by an antigen in certain primed cells called T-lymphocytes. However, in general use the term has taken on a wider meaning. For example, patients with histories of rashes caused by ampicillin or sulfa drugs are told that they are "allergic" to those substances and never take them again. Such rashes, however, do not truly represent allergic reactions, because they have no immunologic basis. These rashes appear idiosyncratic in origin and absolutely unrelated to any antigen-antibody interaction. Several studies have shown that if a patient is rechallenged with a drug to which he is "allergic," there is no "allergy."

Allergic reactions may be divided into four types, only the first of which is discussed here:

1. Processes caused by interactions of antigens with IgE antibodies
2. Reactions resulting from antibodies that are directed toward membranes, as in an autoimmune hemolytic anemia
3. Pathologic damage caused by deposition of immune complexes, as in serum sickness
4. Adverse reactions resulting from cellular immunity, as in graft rejection

A type 1 (immediate hypersensitivity) allergic reaction occurs as follows: Immunoglobulin E, or IgE, is a circulating and tissue-fixed antibody that is present in extremely small amounts (10-200 ng/ml) in normal, nonatopic people but in excessive amounts in atopic individuals. This circulating antibody attaches itself to IgE receptors that are located mainly on circulating basophils and tissue-fixed mast cells. When all of the receptors on a cell are saturated with IgE, the cell becomes surrounded by molecules of excess IgE, all of which are extending their arms into the spaces between cells. When an antigen comes along, such as a drug, pollen, or grain, it can latch on to the free-floating arms of IgE, which is now attached to the cell. If two different IgE molecules are thereby brought together, a reaction in the cell is triggered through an extremely complex set of biochemical and biophysical interactions to ultimately allow calcium to enter the cell, which in turn triggers the release of endogenous substances. All of these substances, when released, can lead to an extremely noxious reaction that is manifested as allergic rhinitis (hay fever), allergic asthma, hives (urticaria), angioedema, or even frank anaphylaxis.

Intradermal skin tests

Intradermal skin tests are the most convenient, sensitive, highly reproducible, and economical means of finding out if a person has specific IgE antibodies mounted against common environmental antigens. Other ways include in vitro blood tests to evaluate the release of histamine by leukocytes in the presence of antigens.

In intradermal skin tests, small amounts of pollen and other allergens are injected into the superficial dermis, since there are large numbers of mast cells there. The reaction of these mast cells to the injected antigens triggers a release of histamine and leads to a wheal at the site of injection. This reaction occurs within 15 to 20 minutes.

Intradermal skin tests are an extremely fast and inexpensive way of detecting minutes amounts of IgE antibodies to particular antigens. If a skin test profile correlates well with a patient's history, it is fairly certain that there is an allergic phenomenon present, and desensitizing shots can be initiated.

PORPHYRIAS

Porphyrias are hereditary metabolic disorders of heme synthesis, the biochemical hallmark of which is overproduction of prophyrins and their precursors. Similar biochemical abnormalities are found in lead poisoning (both acute and chronic), which is a differential diagnosis. Several syndromes of porphyria have been described, two of which are mentioned here.

Erythropoietic porphyria is mainly characterized by skin lesions, photosensitivity, burning, and pruritus. Laboratory diagnosis is made on the basis of elevated uroporphyrin and coproporphyrin levels in the urine and in the red blood cells. In erythropoietic protoporphyria the erythrocyte protoprophyrin level is elevated.

Hepatic porphyria is characterized by acute intermittent abdominal pain and by neurologic abnormalities, neuropathies, and psychiatric disturbances. Laboratory diagnosis is made during an acute attack, on the basis of elevated urine levels of porphobilinogen (PBG) and δ-aminolevulinic acid (ALA). The RBC porphyrin level is normal.

Lead poisoning is also characterized by elevated urine levels of ALA and coproporphyrins and by high RBC levels of protoporphyrins. The elevated serum lead level, however, is diagnostic.

WILSON'S DISEASE (HEPATOLENTICULAR DEGENERATION)

Wilson's disease is an inherited abnormality in the hepatic excretion of copper; the disorder results in toxic levels of copper accumulating in various organs. Clinically, the disorder may manifest as a neurologic disease (athetoid chorea) and liver cirrhosis. Pathologically, there is abnormal deposition of copper in the brain, kidneys, cornea, and liver.

The diagnosis is suspected when the serum level of ceruloplasmin (a copper protein) is low, the urinary excretion of copper is greater than 150 μg/day, and biopsies of the kidney and the liver show increased deposition of copper.

◗ **Normal serum ceruloplasmin**

Varies depending on method of measurement

◗ **Normal serum copper**

100-180 μg/24 hr

◗ **Normal liver copper**

10-35 μg/g dry weight

◗ **Normal urine copper**

15-60 μg/24 hr

IRON STORAGE DISEASE (HEMOCHROMATOSIS)

Iron storage disease is characterized by increased deposition of iron in the liver, heart, and pancreas. Clinically the disorder presents as diabetes, liver cirrhosis, congestive heart failure, and arrhythmias.

Diagnosis is made on the basis of the serum iron level, which is elevated (usually greater than 200 μg/dl), and the serum iron-binding capacity, which is nearly at its maximum. The serum ferritin level is also elevated. The final diagnosis is made by liver and bone marrow biopsies, which show abnormal deposition of iron.

◗ **Normal serum iron**

Males: 70-170 μg/dl
Females: 65-170 μg/dl

◆ **Total iron-binding capacity**

250-390 μg/dl
Percent saturation: 20%-50%

◆ **Normal liver iron**

530-900 μg/gm dry weight

DIABETES MELLITUS

In general a *fasting blood glucose level* of 140 mg/dl or above found in two determinations is diagnostic, and no further testing is necessary. If the fasting blood glucose level is equivocal (110-130 mg/dl), a second step is necessary—a *2-hour postprandial test* following a high-carbohydrate meal. In diabetes mellitus this test shows the blood glucose level to be 180 mg/dl or above. If the results of both these tests are equivocal (fasting, 110 to 130 mg/dl; 2-hour postprandial, 140 to 180 mg/dl), the next step is an *oral glucose tolerance test*, for which there are several different regimens and criteria. The National Institutes of Health states that 2 hours after the administration of the glucose, the plasma glucose level should be greater than 200 mg/dl, which would be diagnostic. A level between 140 and 200 mg/dl is indicative of impaired glucose tolerance but is not necessarily diagnostic of diabetes mellitus.

In adults the major component hemoglobin is hemoglobin A (for "adult"). Among the remaining fractions are the glycohemoglobins, of which there are three types—a, b, and c. The levels of these minor hemoglobin components are all elevated in diabetes mellitus. However, it is the c fraction (Hb A_{Ic}) that is most abundant and whose level is easiest to measure. Some methods report all three levels together (Hb A_{Ia-c}), resulting in higher normal values. It is therefore important to know which method is being used.

The glycohemoglobins are synthesized from hemoglobin A through the addition of glucose to its structure, an irreversible reaction that progresses at a rate dependent upon the mean blood glucose level to which a red cell is exposed over its 120-day life span. Thus, in diabetics the level of Hb A_{Ic} reflects the degree of metabolic control of the diabetes and may be two to three times that of a normal individual.

◆ **Hemoglobin A_{Ic} levels (expressed as % of total hemoglobin)**

Normal:	3.5%-5.9%
Diabetics on diet therapy:	4.8%-11.5%
Diabetics taking oral hypoglycemic agents:	5.3%-16.5%
Diabetics using insulin:	6.1%-16.9%

AMYLOIDOSIS

In amyloidosis, a disorder of protein metabolism, fibrillar protein is deposited in the extracellular spaces, a situation that is manifested clinically by hepatomegaly, congestive heart failure, neuropathies, and malabsorption syndrome.

The best diagnostic test is a rectal mucosal biopsy, with staining being done for amyloid with Congo red.

BREAST TUMORS AND CANCER

Breast tumors are usually discovered either by means of self-palpation or by means of palpation performed by a physician. Several laboratory tests have been employed for diagnosis and/or management of breast tumors; the following are the ones most frequently used.

Xeromammography

Radiography brings into contrast the different tissues of the breast, differentiating the abnormal from the normal.

There is a recognized error of around 20%-40% in this procedure, and the oncogenic potential of the radiation limits its use as a routine screening test to postmenopausal women and to women in whom the risk of a breast tumor is high.

Cytologic examination

Cytologic examination of serosanguineous or serous discharges from the nipple and of fluid aspirated from cystic tumors may lead to a diagnosis. However, a negative result does not rule out carcinoma.

Biopsy

Biopsy is the only definitive means of making a cytologic diagnosis in a case of breast tumor. The biopsy specimen may be obtained by aspiration, excision, or incision, depending upon the clinical setting.

Estradiol and progesterone receptor assays

The major use of estradiol and progesterone assays is to predict whether a tumor will respond to endocrine manipulation or endocrine ablation. Usually, 1 gm of tumor tissue is used for the laboratory procedure. Initially, this procedure was only an estrogen receptor assay, and the results were reported as either estrogen receptor–positive or estrogen receptor–negative. Recently, however, a progesterone receptor assay has been added. The combined assays give more information and indicate more clearly whether a tumor will respond to endocrine manipulation.

♦ **Estrogen receptor assay**

Positive: >3 Fentomoles (FMOL)/mg
Negative: <3 Fentomoles/mg

♦ **Progesterone receptor assay**

Positive: >5 Fentomoles/mg
Negative: <5 Fentomoles/mg

• • •

Thermography, sonography, and CT scanning of the breast are still being evaluated for clinical use.

CANCER OF THE CERVIX AND UTERUS

All epithelia desquamate their surface cells; malignant epithelia do so more rapidly. The Papanicolaou (Pap) technique for staining provides a means of detecting such malignant cells before the clinical manifestation of cervical cancer.

The use of Pap smears of the vaginal mucosa and of exocervical and endo-cervical scrapings has an accuracy rate of 95% in the detection of carcinoma of the cervix, as does the examination of a Pap smear of aspirate from the endometrial cavity in the diagnosis of carcinoma of the uterus. Usually, two samples are taken at the same time, increasing the diagnostic yield. The results are reported as negative or as carcinoma of class I, II, III, or IV.

Although the Pap smear is useful for cytologic diagnosis, dilatation and curettage, with or without biopsy, is the most frequently employed technique for the diagnosis of uterine masses.

VAGINAL DISCHARGE

The usual cause of vaginal discharge is infection with *Candida* organisms, *Trichomonas vaginalis*, or *Hemophilus vaginalis*.

For candidiasis, a wet potassium hydroxide smear is the method of laboratory diagnosis. One can see the spores and filaments characteristic of this fungal infection.

For a *Trichomonas vaginalis* infection, a wet saline smear is the mode of diagnosis. The active motile organism is seen in most cases, and one seldom has to grow a culture.

Hemophilus vaginalis is the cause of nonspecific vaginitis; the presence of this organism is usually suspected because of the character of the discharge and the odor. After ruling out a *Trichomonas* infection and candidiasis, a clinician should use a wet saline smear to test for a *Hemophilus vagi-*

nalis infection. The appearance of the epithelial granular-looking cells called Clue cells suggests this diagnosis. The diagnosis can be confirmed by culturing the organism.

PREGNANCY TESTS

In the differential diagnosis of secondary amenorrhea in females of childbearing age, it is essential to rule out pregnancy. The diagnosis of pregnancy is based on the detection of *human chorionic gonadotropin (HCG)*, a placental hormone, in the maternal urine. A test may be positive as early as 4 days after the expected date of menstruation; it is more than 95% reliable by the tenth to fourteenth day.

The usual tests available detect the presence of the total HCG molecule, which has the same alpha subunits as luteinizing hormone, creating a problem of specificity, since there may be cross-reacting between the two hormones.

With the availability of a specific assay for the beta subunits of HCG, the pregnancy test has become more specific, making possible a diagnosis as early as 9 days after the estimated date of ovulation. The result of a beta subunit test is usually positive in tubal pregnancy, while the result of the routine HCG assay may be negative in up to 50% of tubal pregnancies.

For the following reasons, the *progesterone provocative test* should never be performed: (1) Failure to show withdrawal bleeding after administration of progesterone is not diagnostic of pregnancy. (2) Administration of progesterone during the early stages of pregnancy may cause fetal abnormalities.

CYTOGENETICS

Chromosome analysis and cytogenetics have become an important part of the laboratory diagnosis of certain disease entities. The following is a discussion of some of the most commonly encountered diseases in which the diagnosis is based on analysis of chromosomes.

Normally there are 46 chromosomes in human cells—44 somatic chromosomes and 2 sex chromosomes. The somatic chromosomes are numbered and the sex chromosomes are designated either X, for female, or Y, for male. Thus a normal female is designated 46XX, indicating 44 normal somatic chromosomes and 2 female sex chromosomes. A normal male is designated 46XY, indicating 44 somatic chromosomes, 1 male sex chromosome, and 1 female sex chromosome.

Chromosomal abnormalities can be hereditary, or they may occur at any time after fertilization of the ovum. An abnormality can involve either deletion of a chromosome or duplication of a chromosome. Abnormalities develop into specific clinical syndromes, which may be diagnosed definitively only by chromosomal analysis. Such analysis is usually performed on lymphocytes, amniotic fluid, or cells obtained from smears of the buccal mucosa.

Down's syndrome

Before identification of the exact chromosomal abnormality was possible, Down's syndrome (trisomy 21, mongolism) was diagnosed only by the clinical picture. The disease is characterized by mental retardation and can be associated with a host of skeletal, eye, and skin abnormalities, as well as cardiovascular abnormalities and a predisposition to infections and leukemia.

Trisomy D₁ syndrome

Trisomy D_1 syndrome, which is rarer than Down's syndrome, involves additional chromosomes in positions 13 through 15. When the additional chromosomes are in the 16-18 group (E group), the disorder is designated trisomy E.

The definitive diagnosis is made by cytologic chromosomal analysis (karyotyping) of either smears of buccal mucosa or, prenatally, amniotic fluid. The chromosomal count reveals 47 instead of 46 chromosomes, with the extra one being in the 21st position.

Klinefelter's syndrome (XXY syndrome)

Klinefelter's syndrome, which affects only males, is characterized by testicular hypoplasia, underdevelopment of secondary sex characteristics, gynecomastia, azoospermia, and a high incidence of mental retardation. The pubic hair may have the distribution characteristic of females.

The diagnosis is made by chromosomal analysis, in which an extra X chromosome is detected. The karyotype designation is 47XXY. The extra X chromosome interferes with the survival of germ cells. Variants of this syndrome (48XXXY and 49XXXXY) are rare, and their effects are more extreme.

Turner's syndrome

Affected patients are females. The disease is usually characterized by primary amenorrhea, sexual infantilism, short stature, and absence or agenesis of ovaries. There are also congenital musculoskeletal and cardiac abnormalities, along with some mental deficiency. In the classic form of the disorder, the second X chromosome is absent, resulting in the syndrome being designated 45XO.

Noonan's syndrome is similar clinically to Turner's syndrome; however, affected patients have normal chromosomes. Noonan's syndrome is thought to be endocrine.

Polysomy X (super female) syndrome

Polysomy X syndrome, which is relatively rare, is usually characterized by mental retardation and ovarian dysfunction.

The diagnosis is made by chromosomal analysis, in which one or more extra X chromosomes are found (47XXX, 48XXXX, 49XXXXX). As the number of extra chromosomes increases, so does the severity of the clinical picture.

XYY (super male) syndrome

The XYY syndrome is a relatively common abnormality of males, with an estimated frequency of 1 in 1000 male births. This abnormality has been associated with mental illness and criminal tendencies. Affected persons are often male pseudohermaphrodites with female phenotypes, individuals with intersexual genitalia (true hermaphrodites), or tall males with normal genitalia and behavioral abnormalities. Infertility is not associated with this syndrome, and offspring have been normal.

Laboratory diagnosis is made by chromosome analysis, which shows an additional Y chromosome (47XYY).

Appendices

Tables of normal values*

Values may vary with different techniques or in different laboratories. Although only the more common tests are discussed in the text, values for other tests are included here for completeness.

The SI conversion units are found on pp. 491-493.

Abbreviations used in tables

<	= less than	ImU	= international milliunit
>	= greater than	mOsm	= milliosmole
dl	= deciliter (100 ml)	mμ	= millimicron
gm	= gram	mU	= milliunit
IU	= international unit	ng	= nanogram
kg	= kilogram	pg	= picogram
L	= liter	μEq	= microequivalent
mEq	= milliequivalent	μg	= microgram
mg	= milligram	IμU	= international microunit
ml	= milliliter	μl	= microliter
mM	= millimole	μU	= microunit
mm Hg	= millimeters of mercury	U	= unit

---

*Adapted, with permission, from Davidsohn, I., and Henry, J.B., editors: Todd-Sanford clinical diagnosis by laboratory methods, ed. 15, Philadelphia, 1974, W.B. Saunders Co., and from Scully, R.E., editor: Case records of the Massachusetts General Hospital, N. Engl. J. Med. **298:** 34, 1978.

Table A-1

Whole blood, serum, and plasma (chemistry)

Test	Material	Normal value	Special instructions
Acetoacetic acid			
Qualitative	Serum	Negative	
Quantitative	Serum	0.2-1.0 mg/dl	
Acetone			
Qualitative	Serum	Negative	
Quantitative	Serum	0.3-2.0 mg/dl	
Adrenocorticotropic hormone (ACTH)	Plasma	15-70 pg/ml	Place specimen on ice and send promptly to lab
Albumin, quantitative	Serum	3.2-4.5 gm/dl (salt fractionation) 3.2-5.6 gm/dl by electrophoresis 3.8-5.0 gm/dl by dye binding	
Alcohol	Serum or whole blood	Negative	
Aldolase	Serum	Adults: 1.3-8.2 U/dl Children: approximately 2 times adult levels Newborns: approximately 4 times adult levels	
Alpha-amino acid nitrogen	Plasma Serum	3.0-5.5 mg/dl 0.01-0.03 mg/dl	
δ-Aminolevulinic acid	Blood	80-110 μg/dl	
Ammonia			Collect with sodium heparinate; specimen must be delivered packed in ice and analyzed immediately
Amylase	Serum	4-25 U/ml	
Argininosuccinic lyase	Serum	0-4 U/dl	
Arsenic	Whole blood	<3 μg/dl	
Ascorbic acid (vitamin C)	Plasma Whole blood	0.6-1.6 mg/dl 0.4-1.5 mg/dl	Analyze immediately
Barbiturates	Serum, plasma, or whole blood	Negative Coma level: phenobarbital, approximately 10 mg/dl; most other drugs, 1-3 mg/dl	
Base excess	Whole blood	Male: −3.3 to +1.2 Female: −2.4 to +2.3	
Base, total	Serum	145-160 mEq/L	
Bicarbonate	Plasma	21-28 mM/L	
Bile acids	Serum	0.3-3.0 mg/dl	
Bilirubin	Serum	Up to 0.4 mg/dl (direct or conjugated) Total: 0.7 mg/dl Newborns total: 1-12 mg/dl Indirect is total minus direct	

Table A-1—cont'd

Whole blood, serum, and plasma (chemistry)

Test	Material	Normal value	Special instructions
Blood gases			
pH		7.38-7.44 arterial	
		7.36-7.41 venous	
Pco₂		35-40 mm Hg arterial	
		40-45 mm Hg venous	
Po₂		95-100 mm Hg arterial	
Bromide	Serum	Toxic level: 17 mEq/L	
BSP (sulfobromo-phthalein) (5 mg/kg)	Serum	<5% retention after 45 min	
Calcitonin	Plasma	Undetectable in normals >100 pg/ml in medullary carcinoma	
Calcium	Serum	Ionized: 4.2-5.2 mg/dl 2.1-2.6 mEq/L or 50%-58% of total Total: 9.0-10.6 mg/dl 4.5-5.3 mEq/L Infants: 11-13 mg/dl	
Carbon dioxide			
CO₂ content	Whole blood, arterial	19-24 mM/L	
	Plasma or serum, arterial	24-30 mEq/L 20-26 mEq/L in infants (as HCO₃)	
	Whole blood, venous	22-26 mM/L	
	Plasma or serum, venous	24-30 mM/L	
CO₂ combining power	Plasma or serum, venous	24-30 mM/L	
CO₂ partial pressure (Pco₂)	Whole blood, arterial	35-40 mm Hg	
	Whole blood, venous	40-45 mm Hg	
Carbonic acid	Whole blood, arterial	1.05-1.45 mM/L	
	Whole blood, venous	1.15-1.50 mM/L	
	Plasma, venous	1.02-1.38 mM/L	
Carboxyhemoglobin (carbon monoxide hemoglobin)	Whole blood	Suburban nonsmokers: >1.5% saturation of hemoglobin Smokers: 1.5-5.0% saturation Heavy smokers: 5.0-9.0% saturation	
Carotene, beta	Serum	40-200 μg/dl	
Cephalin cholesterol flocculation	Serum	Negative to 1+ after 24 hr 2+ or less after 48 hr	
Ceruloplasmin	Serum	23-50 mg/dl	
Chloride	Serum	100-106 mEq/L	

Continued.

Table A-1—cont'd

Whole blood, serum, and plasma (chemistry)

Test	Material	Normal value	Special instructions
Cholesterol			
Total	Serum	150-250 mg/dl (varies with diet and age)	
Esters	Serum	65-75% of total cholesterol	
Cholinesterase	Erythrocytes	0.65-1.00 pH units	
Pseudocholinesterase	Plasma	0.5-1.3 pH units	
		8-18 IU/L at 37° C	
Citric acid	Serum or plasma	1.7-3.0 mg/dl	
Congo red test	Serum or plasma	>60% after 1 hour	Severe reactions may occur if dye is injected twice; check patient's record
Copper	Serum or plasma	100-200 μg/dl	
Cortisol	Plasma	8 A.M.: 5-25 μg/dl	
		8 P.M.: <10 μg/dl	
Creatine	Serum or plasma	0.6-1.5 mg/dl	
Creatine phosphokinase (CK)	Serum	Males: 5-55 mU/ml	See Chapter 4
		Females: 5-35 mU/ml	
Creatinine	Serum or plasma	0.6-1.2 mg/dl	
Creatinine clearance (endogenous)	Serum or plasma and urine	Male: 123 ± 16 ml/min	
		Female: 97 ± 10 ml/min	
Cryoglobulins	Serum	Negative	Keep specimen at 37° C
Doriden (Glutethimide)	Serum	0	
Electrophoresis, protein	Serum		

	percent	gm/dl
Albumin	52-65	3.2-5.6
Alpha 1	2.5-5.0	0.1-0.4
Alpha 2	7.0-13.0	0.4-1.2
Beta	8.0-14.0	0.5-1.1
Gamma	12.0-22.0	0.5-1.6

Test	Material	Normal value	Special instructions
Ethanol	Blood	0.3-0.4%, marked intoxication	Collect in oxalate and refrigerate
		0.4-0.5%, alcoholic stupor	
		0.5% or over, alcoholic coma	
Fats, neutral	Serum or plasma	0-200 mg/dl	
Fatty acids			
Total	Serum	9-15 mM/L	
Free	Plasma	300-480 μEq/L	
Fibrinogen	Plasma	200-400 mg/dl	
Fluoride	Whole blood	<0.05 mg/dl	
Folate	Serum	5-25 ng/ml (bioassay)	
	Erythrocytes	166-640 ng/ml (bioassay)	
Galactose	Whole blood	Adults: none	
		Children: <20 mg/dl	
Gammaglobulin	Serum	0.5-1.6 gm/dl	
Gastrin	Plasma	0-200 pg/ml	

Table A-1—cont'd

Whole blood, serum, and plasma (chemistry)

Test	Material	Normal value	Special instructions
Globulins, total	Serum	2.3-3.5 gm/dl	
Glucose, fasting	Serum or plasma	70-110 mg/dl	Collect with heparin-fluoride mixture
	Whole blood	60-100 mg/dl	
Glucose-6-phosphate dehydrogenase (G-6-PD)	Erythrocytes	250-500 units/10^9 cells 1200-2000 mIU/ml of packed erythrocytes	
Glucose tolerance Oral	Serum or plasma	Fasting: 70-110 mg/dl 30 min: 30-60 mg/dl above fasting 60 min: 20-50 mg/dl above fasting 120 min: 5-15 mg/dl above fasting 180 min: fasting level or below	Collect with heparin-fluoride mixture
Glucose tolerance IV	Serum or plasma	Fasting: 70-110 mg/dl 5 min: maximum of 250 mg/dl 60 min: significant decrease 120 min: below 120 mg/dl 180 min: fasting level	Collect with heparin-fluoride mixture
γ-Glutamyl transpeptidase	Serum	2-39 U/L	
Glutathione	Whole blood	24-37 mg/dl	
Growth hormone	Serum	<10 ng/ml	
Heptoglobin	Serum	100-200 mg/dl as hemoglobin binding capacity	
Hemoglobin	Serum or plasma	Qualitative: negative Quantitative: 0.5-5.0 mg/dl	
	Whole blood	Female: 12.0-16.0 gm/dl Male: 13.5-18.0 gm/dl	
Hemoglobin A_2	Whole blood	1.5-3.5% of total hemoglobin	
α-Hydroxybutyric dehydrogenase	Serum	140-350 U/ml	
17-Hydroxycorticosteroids	Plasma	Male: 7-17 μg/dl Female: 9-21 μg/dl After 25 USP units of ACTH IM: 35-55 μg/dl	Perform test immediately or freeze plasma
Immunoglobulins	Serum		
IgG		800-1600 mg/dl	
IgA		50-250 mg/dl	
IgM		40-120 mg/dl	
IgD		0.5-3.0 mg/dl	
IgE		0.01-0.04 mg/dl	
Insulin	Plasma	11-24 IμU/ml (bioassay) 4-24 μU/ml (radioimmunoassay)	

Continued.

Table A-1—cont'd

Whole blood, serum, and plasma (chemistry)

Test	Material	Normal value	Special instructions
Insulin tolerance	Serum	Fasting: glucose of 70-100 mg/dl 30 min: fall to 50% of fasting level 90 min: fasting level	Collect with heparin-fluoride mixture
Iodine			
Butanol extraction (BEI)	Serum	3.5-6.5 μg/dl	Test not reliable if iodine-containing drugs or radiographic contrast media were given prior to test
Protein bound (PBI)	Serum	4.0-8.0 μg/dl	
Iron			
Total	Serum	50-150 μg/dl	Hemolysis must be avoided
Iron-binding capacity	Serum	250-410 μg/dl	
Iron saturation, percent	Serum	20-55%	
Isocitric dehydrogenase	Serum	50-250 U/ml	
Ketone bodies	Serum	Negative	
17-Ketosteroids	Plasma	25-125 μg/dl	
Lactic acid	Blood	0.6-1.8 mEq/L	Draw without stasis
Lactic dehydrogenase (LDH)	Serum	80-120 Wacker units 150-450 Wroblewski units 71-207 IU/L	See Chapter 4
Lactic dehydrogenase (heat stable)	Serum	60-120 U/ml	
Lactic dehydrogenase isoenzymes	Serum	Anode: LDH_1 17-27% LDH_2 27-37% LDH_3 18-25% LDH_4 3-8% Cathode: LDH_5 0-5%	
Lactose tolerance	Serum	Serum glucose changes are similar to those seen in a glucose tolerance test	
Lead	Whole blood	0-50 μg/dl	
Leucine aminopeptidase (LAP)	Serum	Male: 80-200 Goldbarg-Rutenburg units/ml Female: 75-185 Goldbarg-Rutenburg units/ml	
Lipase	Serum	0-1.5 Cherry-Crandall units/ml 14-280 U/ml	
Lipids	Serum		
Total		450-1000 mg/dl	
Cholesterol		120-200 mg/dl	
Triglycerides		40-150 mg/dl	

Table A-1—cont'd

Whole blood, serum, and plasma (chemistry)

Test	Material	Normal value	Special instructions
Phospholipids		9-16 mg/dl as lipid phosphorus	
Fatty acids		190-420 mg/dl	
Neutral fat		0-200 mg/dl	
Lipoprotein electrophoresis		40-150 mg/dl	
Lithium	Serum	Toxic level: 2 mEq/L Therapeutic level: 0.5-1.5 mEq/L	
Long-acting thyroid-stimulating hormone (LATS)	Serum	None	
Luteinizing hormone (LH)	Plasma	Male: <11 lmU/ml Female: midcycle peak >3 times base line value Premenopausal: <25 lmU/ml Postmenopausal: >25 lmU/ml	
Macroglobulins, total	Serum	70-430 mg/dl	
Magnesium	Serum	1.5-2.5 mEq/L	
Methanol	Blood	0	Level as low as 115 mg/dl may be fatal; collect in oxalate
Methemoglobin	Whole blood	0-0.24 gm/dl 0.4-1.5% of total hemoglobin	
Mucoprotein	Serum	80-200 mg/dl	
Nonprotein nitrogen (NPN)	Serum or plasma Whole blood	20-35 mg/dl 25-50 mg/dl	
5' Nucleotidase	Serum	0.3-3.2 Bodansky units	
Ornithine carbamyl transferase (OCT)	Serum	8-20 lmU/ml	
Osmolality	Serum	280-295 mOsm/L	
Oxygen			
Partial pressure (Po₂)	Whole blood, arterial	95-100 mm Hg	
Content	Whole blood, arterial	15-23 vol %	
Saturation	Whole blood, arterial	96-100%	
Parathyroid hormone	Serum	255 pg/ml (±50) at serum calcium level of 9-11 mg/dl	By RIA
pH	Whole blood, arterial	7.35-7.45	
	Whole blood, venous	7.36-7.41	
	Serum or plasma, venous	7.35-7.45	

Continued.

Table A-1—cont'd

Whole blood, serum, and plasma (chemistry)

Test	Material	Normal values	Special instructions
Phenylalanine	Serum	Adults: 0-2.0 mg/dl Newborns (term): 1.2-3.5 mg/dl Male total: 0.13-0.63 sigma U/ml Female total: 0.01-0.56 sigma U/ml Prostatic: 0-0.7 Fishman-Lerner U/dl	
Phosphatase, acid, total	Serum	0-1.1 U/ml (Bodansky) 1-4 U/ml (King-Armstrong) 0.13-0.63 U/ml (Bessey-Lowry) 1.4-5.5 U/ml (Gutman-Gutman) 0-0.56 U/ml (Roy) 0-6.0 U/ml (Shinowara-Jones-Reinhart)	Hemolysis must be avoided; perform test without delay or freeze specimen
Phosphatase, alkaline,	Serum total	Adults: 1.5-4.5 U/dl (Bodansky) 4-13 U/dl (King-Armstrong) 0.8-2.3 U/ml (Bessey-Lowry) 15-35 U/ml (Shinowara-Jones/Reinhart) Children: 5.0-14.0 U/dl (Bodansky) 3.4-9.0 U/dl (Bessey-Lowry) 15-35 U/dl (King-Armstrong)	
Phospholipid phosphorus	Serum	8-11 mg/dl	
Phospholipids	Serum	150-380 mg/dl	
Phosphorus, inorganic	Serum	Adults: 1.8-2.6 mEq/L 3.0-4.5 mg/dl Children: 2.3-4.1 mEq/L 4.0-7.0 mg/dl	Separate cells from serum promptly
Potassium	Plasma	3.8-5.0 mEq/L	
Primidone (Mysoline)	Serum	Therapeutic level: 4-12 μg/dl	
Prolactin	Serum	2-15 ng/ml	A.M. sample
Proteins	Serum		
Total		6.0-8.4 gm/dl	
Albumin		3.5-5.0 gm/dl	
Globulin		2.3-3.5 gm/dl	
Protoporphyrin	Erythrocytes	15-50 μg/dl	
Pyruvate	Whole blood	0.3-0.9 mg/dl	
Renin activity	Plasma	Supine: 1.1 ± 0.8 ng/ml/hr	EDTA tubes on ice; normal diet
		Upright: 1.9 ± 1.7 ng/ml/hr	
		Supine: 2.7 ± 1.8 ng/ml/hr	Low-sodium diet
		Upright: 6.6 ± 2.5 ng/ml/hr	
		Diuretics: 10.0 ± 3.7 ng/nl/hr	Low-sodium diet

Table A-1—cont'd

Whole blood, serum, and plasma (chemistry)

Test	Material	Normal value		Special instructions
Salicylates	Serum	Negative Therapeutic level: 20-25 mg/dl		
Sodium	Plasma	136-142 mEq/L		
Sulfate, inorganic	Serum	0.5-1.5 mEq/L 0.9-6.0 mg/dl as SO_4		Hemolysis must be avoided
Sulfhemoglobin	Whole blood	Negative		
Sulfonamides	Serum or whole blood	Negative		
Testosterone	Serum or plasma	Male: 400-1200 ng/dl Female: 30-120 ng/dl		
Thiocyanate	Serum	Negative		
Thymol flocculation	Serum	Up to 1+ in 24 hr		
Thyroid hormone tests	Serum	*Expressed as thyroxine*	*Expressed as iodine*	
T$_4$ (by column)		5.0-11.0 μg/dl	3.2-7.2 μg/dl	
T$_4$ (by competitive binding Murphy-Pattee)		6.0-11.0 μg/dl	3.9-7.7 μg/dl	
Free T$_4$		0.9-2.3 ng/dl	0.6-1.5 ng/dl	
T$_4$ (resin uptake)		25-38 relative % uptake		
Thyroxine-binding globulin (TBG)		15-25 μg/dl (expressed as T$_4$ uptake)		
Thyroid-stimulating hormone (TSH)	Serum	0.5-3.5 μU/ml		
Transaminases				
GOT	Serum	10-40 U/ml		
GPT	Serum	1-36 U/ml		
Triglycerides	Serum	10-190 mg/dl		
Urea clearance	Serum and urine	Maximum clearance: 64-99 ml/min Standard clearance: 41-65 ml/min or more than 75% of normal clearance		
Urea nitrogen	Blood	8-25 mg/dl		
Uric acid	Serum	3.0-7.0 mg/dl		
Vitamin A	Serum	0.15-0.6 μg/ml		
Vitamin A tolerance	Serum	Fasting: 15-60 μg/dl 3 hr or 6 hr after 5000 units vitamin A/kg: 200-600 μg/dl 24 hr: fasting values or slightly above		Administer 5000 units vitamin A in oil per kg weight
Vitamin B$_{12}$	Serum	Male: 200-800 pg/ml Female: 100-650 pg/ml		
Unsaturated vitamin B$_{12}$ binding capacity	Serum	1000-2000 pg/ml		

Continued.

Table A-1—cont'd

Whole blood, serum, and plasma (chemistry)

Test	Material	Normal value	Special instructions
Vitamin C	Plasma	0.6-1.6 mg/dl	Collect with oxalate and analyze within 20 min
Xylose absorption	Serum	25-40 mg/dl between 1 and 2 hr; in malabsorption, maximum approximately 10 mg/dl Dose Adult: 25 gm D-xylose Children: 0.5 gm/kg D-xylose	For children administer 10 ml of a 5% solution of D-xylose per kg of body weight
Zinc	Serum	50-150 µg/dl	
Zinc sulfate turbidity	Serum	<12 units	

Table A-2

Urine

Test	Type of specimen	Normal vlaue	Special instructions
Acetoacetic acid	Random	Negative	
Acetone	Random	Negative	
Addis count	12-hr collection	WBC and epithelial cells: 1,800,000/12 hr RBC: 500,000/12 hr Hyaline casts: 0-5000/12 hr	Rinse bottle with some neutral formalin; discard excess
Albumin			
Qualitative	Random	Negative	
Quantitative	24 hr	10-100 mg/24 hr	
Aldosterone	24 hr	2-26 µg/24 hr	Keep refrigerated
Alkapton bodies	Random	Negative	
Alpha-amino acid nitrogen	24 hr	100-290 mg/24 hr	
δ-Aminolevulinic acid	Random	Adult: 0.1-0.6 mg/dl Children: <0.5 mg/dl	
	24 hr	1.5-7.5 mg/24 hr	
Ammonia nitrogen	24 hr	20-70 mEq/24 hr 500-1200 mg/24 hr	Keep refrigerated
Amylase	2 hr	35-260 Somogyi units per hour	
Arsenic	24 hr	<50 µg/L	
Ascorbic acid	Random	1-7 mg/dl	
	24 hr	>50 mg/24 hr	
Bence Jones protein	Random	Negative	
Beryllium	24 hr	<0.05 µg/24 hr	
Bilirubin, qualitative	Random	Negative	

Table A-2—cont'd

Urine

Test	Type of specimen	Normal value	Special instructions
Blood, occult	Random	Negative	
Borate	24 hr	<2 mg/L	
Calcium			
Qualitative (Sulko-witch)	Random	1 + turbidity	Compare with standard
Quantitative	24 hr	Average diet: 100-250 mg/24 hr	
		Low calcium diet: <150 mg/24 hr	
		High calcium diet: 250-300 mg/24 hr	
Catecholamines	Random	Epinephrine <20 μg/24 hr	
	24 hr	Norepinephrine <100 μg/24 hr	
Chloride	24 hr	110-250 mEq/24 hr	
Chorionic gonado-tropin	First morning voiding	0	Specific gravity should be at least 1.015
Concentration test (Fishberg)	Random after fluid restriction	Specific gravity: >1.025 Osmolality: >850 mOsm/L	
Copper	24 hr	0-100 μg/24 hr	
Coproporphyrin	Random	Adult: 50-250 μg/24 hr	Use fresh specimen and do not expose to direct light; preserve 24-hr urine with 5 gm Na_2CO_3
	24 hr	Children: 0-80 μg/24 hr	
Creatine	24 hr	Under 100 mg/24 hr or less than 6% of creatinine	
		Pregnancy: up to 12%	
		Children: up to 30% of creatinine	
Creatinine	24 hr	15-25 mg/kg of body weight/24 hr	
Cystine, qualitative	Random	Negative	
Cystine and cysteine	10 ml	0	
Diacetic acid	Random	Negative	
Epinephrine	24 hr	0-20 μg/24 hr	
Estrogens, total	24 hr	Male: 5-18 μg/24 hr	Keep refrigerated
		Female	
		Ovulation: 28-100 μg/24 hr	
		Luteal peak: 22-105 μg/24 hr	
		At menses: 4-25 μg/24 hr	
		Pregnancy: up to 45,000 μg/24 hr	
		Postmenopausal: 14-20 μg/24 hr	
Estrogens Fractionated	24 hr	Nonpregnant, mid-cycle	
Estrone (E1)		2-25 μg/24 hr	
Estradiol (E2)		0-10 μg/24 hr	
Estriol (E3)		2-30 μg/24 hr	
Fat, qualitative	Random	Negative	

Continued.

Table A-2—cont'd

Urine

Test	Type of specimen	Normal value			Special instructions
FIGLU (*N*-formi-minoglutamic acid)	24 hr	<3 mg/24 hr After 15 gm of L-histidine: 4 mg/8 hr			
Fluoride	24 hr	<1 mg/24 hr			
Follicle-stimulating hormone (FSH)	24 hr	Follicular phase 5-20 IU/24 hr Mid-cycle 15-60 IU/24 hr Luteal phase 5-15 IU/24 hr Menopausal 50-100 IU/24 hr Men 5-25 IU/24 hr			
Fructose	24 hr	30-65 mg/24 hr			
Glucose					
Qualitative	Random	Negative			
Quantitative	24 hr				
Copper-reducing substances		0.5-1.5 gm/24 hr			
Total sugars		Average: 250 mg/24 hr			
Glucose		Average: 130 mg/24 hr			
Gonadotropins, pituitary (FSH and LH)	24 hr	10-50 mouse uterine units/24 hr			
Hemoglobin	Random	Negative			
Homogentisic acid	Random	Negative			
Homovanillic acid (HVA)	24 hr	<15 mg/24 hr			
17-Hydroxycortico-steroids	24 hr	Male: 5.5-14.5 mg/24 hr Female: 4-9-12.9 mg/24 hr Lower in children After 25 USP units ACTH, IM: a 2- to 4-fold increase			Keep refrigerated
5-Hydroxyindole-acetic acid (5-HIAA)	24 hr	2-9 mg/24 hr (women lower than men)			Some muscle relaxants and tranquilizers interfere with test
5-Hydroxyindoleacetic acid, quantitative	24 hr	<9 mg/24 hr			
Indican	24 hr	10-20 mg/24 hr			
Ketone bodies	Random	Negative			Fresh, keep cool
17-Ketosteroids	24 hr	*Age* *Males* 10 1-4 mg 20 6-21 mg 30 8-26 mg 50 5-18 mg 70 2-10 mg	*Females* 1-4 mg 4-16 mg 4-14 mg 3-9 mg 1-7 mg		Keep refrigerated
Androsterone		Male: 2.0-5.0 mg/24 hr Female: 0.8-3.0 mg/24 hr			
Etiocholanolone		Male: 1.4-5.0 mg/24 hr Female: 0.8-4.0 mg/24 hr			
Dehydroepiandro-sterone		Male: 0.2-2.0 mg/24 hr Female: 0.2-1.8 mg/24 hr			

Table A-2—cont'd

Urine

Test	Type of specimen	Normal value	Special instructions
11-Ketoandro-sterone		Male: 0.2-1.0 mg/24 hr Female: 0.2-0.8 mg/24 hr	
11-ketoetio-cholanolone		Male: 0.2-1.0 mg/24 hr Female: 0.2-0.8 mg/24 hr	
11-Hydroxyandro-sterone		Male: 0.1-0.8 mg/24 hr Female: 0.0-0.5 mg/24 hr	
11-Hydroxyetiochol-anolone		Male: 0.2-0.6 mg/24 hr Female: 0.1-1.1 mg/24 hr	
Lactose	24 hr	12-40 mg/24 hr	
Lead	24 hr	<100 μg/24 hr	
Magnesium	24 hr	6.0-8.5 mEq/24 hr	
Melanin, qualitative	Random	Negative	
3-Methoxy-4-hydroxy-mandelic acid	24 hr	1.5-7.5 mg/24 hr (adults) 83 μg/24 hr (infants)	No coffee or fruit 2 days prior to test
Mucin	24 hr	100-150 mg/24 hr	
Myoglobin			
Qualitative	Random	Negative	
Quanitative	24 hr	<1.5 mg/L	
Osmolality	Random	500-800 mOsm/L	May be lower or higher, depending on state of hydration
Pentoses	24 hr	2-5 mg/kg/24 hr	
pH	Random	4.6-8.0	
Phenosulfonphthalein (PSP)	Urine, timed after 6 mg PSP IV		
	15 min	20-50% dye excreted	
	30 min	16-24% dye excreted	
	60 min	9-17% dye excreted	
	120 min	3-10% dye excreted	
Phenylpyruvic acid, qualitative	Random	Negative	
Phosphorus	Random	0.9-1.3 mg/24 hr	Varies with intake
Porphobilinogen			
Qualitative	Random	Negative	
Quantitative	24 hr	0-2.0 mg/24 hr	
Potassium	24 hr	40-80 mEq/24 hr	Varies with diet
Pregnancy tests	Concentrated morning specimen	Positive in normal pregnancies or with tumors producing chorionic gonadotropin	
Pregnanediol	24 hr	Male: 0-1 mg/24 hr Female: 1-8 mg/24 hr Peak: 1 week after ovulation Pregnancy: 60-100 mg/24 hr Children: Negative	Keep refrigerated
Pregnanetriol	24 hr	Male: 1.0-2.0 mg/24 hr Female: 0.5-2.0 mg/24 hr Children: <0.5 mg/24 hr	Keep refrigerated

Continued.

Table A-2—cont'd

Urine

Test	Type of specimen	Normal value	Special instructions
Protein			
Qualitative	Random	Negative	
Quantitative	24 hr	10-100 mg/24 hr	
Reducing substances, total	24 hr	0.5-1.5 mg/24 hr	
Sodium	24 hr	80-180 mEq/24 hr	Varies with dietary ingestion of salt
Solids, total	24 hr	55-70 mg/24 hr Decreases with age to 30 mg/24 hr	
Specific gravity	Random	1.016-1.022 (normal fluid intake) 1.001-1.035 (range)	
Sugars (excluding glucose)	Random	Negative	
Titratable acidity	24 hr	20-50 mEq/24 hr	Collect with toluene
Urea nitrogen	24 hr	6-17 mg/24 hr	
Uric acid	24 hr	250-750 mg/24 hr	Varies with diet
Urobilinogen	2 hr	0.3-1.0 Ehrlich units	
	24 hr	0.05-2.5 mg/24 hr or 0.5-4.0 Ehrlich units/24 hr	
Uropepsin	Random	15-45 units/hr	
	24 hr	1500-5000 units/24 hr	
Uroporphyrins			
Qualitative	Random	Negative	
Quantitative	24 hr	10-30 μg/24 hr	
Vanillylmandelic acid (VMA)	24 hr	Up to 9 mg/24 hr	
Volume, total	24 hr	600-1600 ml/24 hr	
Zinc	24 hr	0.15-1.2 mg/24 hr	

Table A-3

Gastric fluid

Test	Normal value
Fasting residual volume	20-100 ml
pH	<2.0
Basal acid output (BAO)	0-6 mEq/hr
Maximal acid output (MAO) after histamine stimulation	5-40 mEq/hr
BAO/MAO ratio	<0.4

Table A-4

Hematology

Test	Normal value
Blood volume	Male: 69 ml/kg
	Female: 65 ml/kg
Coagulation factors	
Factor I (fibrinogen)	0.15-0.35 gm/dl
Factor II (prothrombin)	60-140%
Factor V (accelerator globulin)	60-140%
Factor VII-X (proconvertin-Stuart)	70-130%
Factor X (Stuart factor)	70-130%
Factor VIII (antihemophilic globulin)	50-200%
Factor IX (plasma thromboplastic cofactor)	60-140%
Factor XI (plasma thromboplastic ante-cedent	60-140%
Factor XII (Hageman factor)	60-140%
Coagulation tests	
Bleeding time (Ivy)	1-6 min
Bleeding time (Duke)	1-3 min
Clot retraction	½ the original mass in 2 hr
Dilute blood clot lysis time	Clot lyses between 6 and 10 hr at 37° C
Euglobin clot lysis time	Clot lyses between 2 and 6 hr at 37° C
Partial thromboplastin time (PTT)	60-70 sec
Kaolin activated	25-37 sec
Prothrombin time	12-14 sec
Venous clotting time	
3 tubes	5-15 min
2 tubes	5-8 min
Whole blood clot lysis time	None in 24 hr
Complete blood count (CBC)	
Hematocrit	Male: 40-54%
	Female: 38-47%
Hemoglobin	Male: 13.5-18.0 gm/dl
	Female: 12.0-16.0 mg/dl
Red cell count	Male: 4.6-6.2 $\times$ 10^6/μl
	Female: 4.2-5.4 $\times$ 10^6/μl
White cell count	4500-11,000/μl
Erythrocyte indices	
Mean corpuscular volume (MCV)	82-98 cu microns (fentoliters)
Mean corpuscular hemoglobin (MCH)	27-31 pg
Mean corpuscular hemoglobin concentration (MCHC)	32-36%
Haptoglobin	100-300 mg/dl
Hemoglobin A$_2$	1.5-3.5%
Hemoglobin F	<2%

Continued.

Table A-4—cont'd

Hematology

Test	Normal value		
Osmotic fragility			*% Lysis (after 24-hr incubation at 37° C)*
	% Na Cl	*% Lysis (fresh)*	
	0.20	97-100	95-100
	0.30	90-99	85-100
	0.35	50-95	75-100
	0.40	5-45	65-100
	0.45	0-6	55 95
	0.50	0	40-85
	0.55		15-70
	0.60		0-40
	0.65		0-10
	0.70		0-5
	0.75		0
Plasma volume	Male: 39 ml/kg		
	Female: 40 ml/kg		
Platelet count	200,000-350,000/mm		
Platelet function tests:			
Clot retraction	50-100% at 2 hr		
Platelet aggregation	Full response to ADP, 1-epinephrine, and collagen		
Platelet factor 3	35-57 sec		
Reticulocyte count	0.5-1.5%		
Sedimentation rate (ESR)	Men under 50 yr: <15 mm/hr		
(Westergren)	Men over 50 yr: <20 mm/hr		
	Women under 50 yr: <20 mm/hr		
	Women over 50 yr: <30 mm/hr		
Viscosity	1.4-1.8 times water		
White blood cell differential (adult)		*Mean percent*	*Range of absolute counts*
Segmented neutrophils		56%	1800-7000/μl
Bands		3%	0-7000/μl
Eosinophils		2.7%	0-450/μl
Basophils		0.3%	0-200/μl
Lymphocytes		34%	1000-4800/μl
Monocytes		4%	0-800/μl

Table A-5

Miscellaneous

Test	Specimen	Normal value
Bile, qualitative	Random stool	Negative in adults; positive in children
Carcinoembryonic antigen (CEA)	Plasma	0-2.5 ng/ml, 97% healthy nonsmokers
Chloride	Sweat	4-60 mEq/L
Clearances	Serum and timed urine	
Creatinine, endogenous		115 ± 20 ml/min
Iodopyracet (Diodrast)		600-720 ml/min
Inulin		100-150 ml/min
PAH		600-750 ml/min
Diagnex blue (tubeless gastric analysis)	Urine	Free acid present
Fat	Stool, 72 hr	Total fat: <5 gm/24 hr and 10-25% of dry matter or <4% of measured fat intake in 3 days
		Neutral fat: 1-5% of dry matter
		Free fatty acids: 5-13% of dry matter
		Combined fatty acids: 5-15% of dry matter
Immunoglobulins		
IgG	Blood	1140 mg/dl
		Range 540-1663
IgA		214 mg/dl
		Range 66-344
IgM		168 mg/dl
		Range 39-290
Immunologic tests		
Alpha-fetoglobulin	Blood	Abnormal if present
Alpha 1 antitrypsin	Blood	200-400 mg/dl
Antinuclear antibodies	Blood	Positive if detected with serum diluted 1:10
Anti-DNA antibodies	Blood	<15 units/ml
Bence Jones protein	Urine	Abnormal if present
Complement, total hemolytic	Blood	150-250 U/ml
C3	Blood	55-120 mg/dl
C4		20-50 mg/dl
Nitrogen, total	Stool, 24 hr	10% of intake or 1-2 gm/24 hr
Sodium	Sweat	10-80 mEq/L
Synovial fluid		
Glucose		Not less than 20 mg/dl lower than simultaneously drawn blood sugar
Mucin		Type 1 or 2
Thyroid ^{131}I uptake		7.5-25% in 6 hr
Trypsin activity	Random, fresh stool	Positive (2+ to 4+)
Urobilinogen		
Qualitative	Random stool	Positive
Quantitative	Stool, 24 hr	40-200 mg/24 hr
		30-280 Ehrlich units/24 hr

Table A-6

Serology

Test	Normal value
Antibovine milk antibodies	Negative
Antideoxyribonuclease (ADNAase)	<1:20
Antinuclear antibodies (ANA)	<1:10
Antistreptococcal hyaluronidase (ASH)	<1:256
Antistreptolysin-O (ASO)	<160 Todd units
Australia antigen	See hepatitis-associated antigen
Brucella agglutinins	<1:80
Coccidioidomycosis antibodies	Negative
Cold agglutinins	<1:32
Complement, C'3	100-170 mg/dl
C-reactive protein (CRP)	0
Fluorescent treponemal antibodies (FTA)	Nonreactive
Hepatitis-associated antigen (HAA or HBAg)	Negative
Heterophile antibodies	<1:56
Histoplasma agglutinins	<1:8
Latex fixation	Negative
Leptospira agglutinins	Negative
Ox cell hemolysin	<1:480
Rheumatoid factor	
Sensitized sheep cell	<1:160
Latex fixation	<1:80
Bentonite particles	<1:32
Streptococcal MG agglutinins	<1:20
Thyroid antibodies	
Antithyroglobulin	<1:32
Antithyroid microsomal	<1:56
Toxoplasma antibodies	<1:4
Trichina agglutinins	0
Tularemia agglutinins	<1:80
Typhoid agglutinins	
O	<1:80
H	<1:80
VDRL	Nonreactive
Weil-Felix (Proteus OX-2, OX-K, and OX-19 agglutinins)	Fourfold rise in titer between acute and convalescent sera

Table A-7

Cerebrospinal fluid

Test or constituent	Normal value	Special instructions
Albumin	10-30 mg/dl	
Albumin/globulin ratio	1.6-2.2	
Calcium	2.1-2.9 mEq/L	
Cell count	0-8 cells/μl	
Chloride	Adult: 118-132 mEq/L	These values are invalidated
	Children: 120-128 mEq/L	by admixture of blood
Colloidal gold curve	0001111000	
Globulins		
Qualitative (Pandy)	Negative	
Quantitative	6-16 mg/dl	
Glucose	45-75 mg/dl	
Lactic dehydrogenase (LDH)	Approximately $\frac{1}{10}$ of serum level	
Protein		
Total CSF	15-45 mg/dl	
Ventricular fluid	8-15 mg/dl	
Protein electrophoresis		
Prealbumin	4.1 ± 1.2%	
Albumin	62.4 ± 5.6%	
Alpha 1 globulin	5.3 ± 1.2%	
Alpha 2 globulin	8.2 ± 2.0%	
Beta globulin	12.8 ± 2.0%	
Gamma globulin	7.2 ± 1.1%	
Xanthochromia	Negative	

APPENDIX B

Normal values
for echocardiographic
examinations*

The following tables represent normal values for echocardiographic examinations. The adult subjects were examined between January 1971 and May 1975 by Mrs. Sonia Chang.

The children whose normal values are listed in Tables B-3 and B-4 were examined between January 1972 and June 1972 by Dr. Lee Konecke. All children were examined in the supine position. The values are arranged by both body weight and body surface area. The grouping of the data according to age did not prove to be useful.

Notes on tables: Right ventricular dimension (RVD) is the distance between the echoes of the anterior right ventricular wall and the right side of the interventricular septum at the R wave of the electrocardiogram. The left ventricular internal dimension (LVID) is between the left side of the septum and the posterior endocardium at the R wave of the electrocardiogram. Posterior left ventricular wall thickness is the distance between the posterior left ventricular endocardium and epicardium at the R wave of the electrocardiogram. Posterior left ventricular wall amplitude is the maximum amplitude of the posterior left ventricular endocardial echo. Interventricular septal (IVS) wall thickness is the distance between the left and right septal echoes at the R wave of the electrocardiogram. Mid interventricular septal (IVS) amplitude is the systolic amplitude of motion of the left septal echo with the ultrasonic beam traversing the mid portion of the left ventricle. Apical interventricular septal (IVS) amplitude is the systolic amplitude of motion of the left septal echo with the ultrasonic beam directed toward the

*Reproduced with permission from Feigenbaum, H.: Echocardiography, ed. 3, Philadelphia, 1981, Lea & Febiger.

apex in the vicinity of the papillary muscles. Left atrial dimension is the distance between the posterior surface of the posterior aortic wall echo and the anterior surface of the posterior left atrial wall echo at the level of the aortic valve at end-systole. Aortic root dimension is the distance between the anterior and posterior aortic echoes at the R wave of the electrocardiogram. Aortic cusps' separation is the distance between the anterior and posterior aortic valve leaflets in early systole.

Table B-1
Adult normal values

	Range (cm)	Mean (cm)	Number of subjects
Age (years)	13-54	26	134
Body surface area (m²)	1.45-2.22	1.8	130
RVD-flat	0.7-2.3	1.5	84
RVD-left lateral	0.9-2.6	1.7	83
LVID-flat	3.7-5.6	4.7	82
LVID-left lateral	3.5-5.7	4.7	81
Posterior LV wall thickness	0.6-1.1	0.9	137
Posterior LV wall amplitude	0.9-1.4	1.2	48
IVS wall thickness	0.6-1.1	0.9	137
Mid IVS amplitude	0.3-0.8	0.5	10
Aplical IVS amplitude	0.5-1.2	0.7	38
Left atrial dimension	1.9-4.0	2.9	133
Aortic root dimension	2.0-3.7	2.7	121
Aortic cusps' separation	1.5-2.6	1.9	93
Mean rate of circumferential shortening (Vcf)	1.02-1.94 circ/sec	1.3 circ/sec	38

Table B-2
Adult normal values, corrected for body surface area

	Range (cm)	Mean (cm)	Number of subjects
RVD/m²—flat	0.4-1.4	0.9	76
RVD/m²—left lateral	0.4-1.4	0.9	79
LVID/m²—flat	2.1-3.2	2.6	77
LVID/m²—left lateral	1.9-3.2	2.6	81
LAD/m²	1.2-2.2	1.6	127
Aortic root/m²	1.2-2.2	1.5	115

Table B-3

Normal values for children, arranged by weight

	Weight (lbs)	Mean (cm)	Range (cm)	Number of subjects
RVD	0-25	0.9	0.3-1.5	26
	26-50	1.0	0.4-1.5	26
	51-75	1.1	0.7-1.8	20
	76-100	1.2	0.7-1.6	15
	101-125	1.3	0.8-1.7	11
	126-200	1.3	1.2-1.7	5
LVID	0-25	2.4	1.3-3.2	26
	26-50	3.4	2.4-3.8	26
	51-75	3.8	3.3-4.5	20
	76-100	4.1	3.5-4.7	15
	101-125	4.3	3.7-4.9	11
	126-200	4.9	4.4-5.2	5
LV and IV septal wall thickness	0-25	0.5	0.4-0.6	26
	26-50	0.6	0.5-0.7	26
	51-75	0.7	0.6-0.7	20
	76-100	0.7	0.7-0.8	15
	101-125	0.7	0.7-0.8	11
	126-200	0.8	0.7-0.8	5
LA dimension	0-25	1.7	0.7-2.3	26
	26-50	2.2	1.7-2.7	26
	51-75	2.3	1.9-2.8	20
	76-100	2.4	2.0-3.0	15
	101-125	2.7	2.1-3.0	11
	126-200	2.8	2.1-3.7	5
Aortic root	0-25	1.3	0.7-1.7	26
	26-50	1.7	1.3-2.2	26
	51-75	2.0	1.7-2.3	20
	76-100	2.2	1.9-2.7	15
	101-125	2.3	1.7-2.7	11
	126-200	2.4	2.2-2.8	5
Aortic valve opening	0-25	0.9	0.5-1.2	26
	26-50	1.2	0.9-1.6	26
	51-75	1.4	1.2-1.7	20
	76-100	1.6	1.3-1.9	15
	101-125	1.7	1.4-2.0	11
	126-200	1.8	1.6-2.0	5

Table B-4

Normal values for children, arranged by body surface area

	BSA (m²)	Mean (cm)	Range (cm)	Number of subjects
RVD	0.5 or less	0.8	0.3-1.3	24
	0.6 to 1.0	1.0	0.4-1.8	39
	1.1 to 1.5	1.2	0.7-1.7	29
	over 1.5	1.3	0.8-1.7	11
LVID	0.5 or less	2.4	1.3-3.2	24
	0.6 to 1.0	3.4	2.4-4.2	39
	1.1 to 1.5	4.0	3.3-4.7	29
	over 1.5	4.7	4.2-5.2	11
LV and IV septal wall thickness	0.5 or less	0.5	0.4-0.6	24
	0.6 to 1.0	0.6	0.5-0.7	39
	1.1 to 1.5	0.7	0.6-0.8	29
	over 1.5	0.8	0.7-0.8	11
LA dimension	0.5 or less	1.7	0.7-2.4	24
	0.6 to 1.0	2.1	1.8-2.8	39
	1.1 to 1.5	2.4	2.0-3.0	29
	over 1.5	2.8	2.1-3.7	11
Aortic root	0.5 or less	1.2	0.7-1.5	24
	0.6 to 1.0	1.8	1.4-2.2	39
	1.1 to 1.5	2.2	1.7-2.7	29
	over 1.5	2.4	2.0-2.8	11
Aortic valve opening	0.5 or less	0.8	0.5-1.0	24
	0.6 to 1.0	1.3	0.9-1.6	39
	1.1 to 1.5	1.6	1.3-1.9	29
	over 1.5	1.8	1.5-2.0	11

Normal values for cardiac catheterization

Table C-1

Normal values for pressures (at rest) in the cardiac chambers and vessels (mm Hg)

Location	Mean	Range
Right atrium		
Mean	2.8	1-5
a wave	5.6	2.5-7
z point	2.9	1-5.5
c wave	3.8	1.5-6
x' wave	1.7	0-5
v wave	4.6	2-7.5
y wave	2.4	0-6
Right ventricle		
Peak systolic	25	17-32
End-diastolic	4	1-7
Pulmonary artery		
Mean	15	9-19
Peak systolic	25	17-32
End-diastolic	9	4-13
Pulmonary artery wedge		
Mean	9	4-13
Left atrium		
Mean	7.9	2-12
a wave	10.4	4-16
z point	7.6	1-13
v wave	12.8	6-21
Left ventricle		
Peak systolic	130	90-140
End-diastolic	8.7	5-12
Brachial artery		
Mean	85	70-105
Peak systolic	130	90-140
End-diastolic	70	60-90

Table C-2

Normal values for cardiac output and related measurements

Measurements	Units	±SD
O_2 uptake	143/ml/min/m²	14.3
Arteriovenous O_2 difference	4.1 vol %	0.6
Cardiac index	3.5 L/min/m²	0.7
Stroke index	46 ml/beat/m²	8.1

Table C-3

Oxygen content and saturation

Location	O_2 content (vol %)	O_2 saturation
Superior vena cava (SVC)	14 (±1)	70%
Inferior vena cava (IVC)	16 (±1)	80%
Right atrium (RA)	15 (±1)	75%
Pulmonary artery (PA)	15.2 (±1)	75%
Right ventricle (RV)	15.2 (±1)	75%
Brachial artery (BA)	19.0 (±1)	95%

Table C-4

Other measurements obtained during cardiac catheterization

$$\text{Pulmonary arteriolar resistance} = \frac{\text{Mean PA pressure} - \text{Mean PAW pressure (mm Hg)}}{\text{Pulmonary blood flow (L/min)}}$$

where: PA = Pulmonary artery
PAW = Pulmonary artery wedge
Normal values for PAR = Less than 2.0 resistance units (less than 160 dynes sec cm^5)

$$\text{Total pulmonary resistance (TPR)} = \frac{\text{Mean PA pressure} - \text{LV mean diastolic pressure (mm Hg)}}{\text{Pulmonary blood flow (L/min)}}$$

where: PA = Pulmonary artery
LV = Left ventricle
Normal values for TRP = Less than 3.5 resistance units (less than 280 dynes sec cm^5)

$$\text{Mitral valve area (cm}^2) = \frac{\text{Mitral valve flow (ml/sec)}}{31\sqrt{\text{Diastolic gradient across the mitral valve}}}$$

where: $\text{Mitral valve flow} = \dfrac{\text{Cardiac output (ml/min)}}{\text{Diastolic filling period (sec/min)}}$

Diastolic filling period (sec/min) = Diastolic period per beat (sec/beat) × Heart rate (beats/min)
Diastolic gradient across the mitral valve (mm Hg) = Left atrial mean pressure (mm Hg) − Left ventricular mean diastolic pressure (mm Hg)
31 = Empirical constant

$$\text{Aortic valve area (cm}^2) = \frac{\text{Aortic valve flow (ml/sec)}}{44.5\sqrt{\text{Systolic pressure gradient across the aortic valve}}}$$

where: $\text{Aortic valve flow (ml/sec)} = \dfrac{\text{Cardiac output (ml/min)}}{\text{Systolic ejection period (sec/min)}}$

Systolic ejection period (sec/min) = Systolic ejection period per beat (sec/beat) × Heart rate (beats/min)
Systolic pressure gradient across the aortic valve (mm Hg) = Left ventricular mean systolic pressure (mm Hg) − Aortic mean systolic pressure (mm Hg)
44.5 = Gravity acceleration factor

$$\text{Cardiac output (L/min)} = \frac{1}{Ct} \times 60$$

where: I = Amount of indicator injected
C = Mean concentration of indicator for the first circulation (mg/L)
t = Time for the first circulation of indicator (seconds)

$$\text{Cardiac output (ml/min)} = \frac{\text{Oxygen consumption (ml/min)}}{\text{Arterial O}_2 \text{ content} - \text{Mixed venous O}_2 \text{ content}} \times 100$$
$$\text{(vol \%)} \qquad\qquad \text{(vol \%)}$$

APPENDIX D

Common drugs affecting clinical laboratory tests*

Table D-1

Drugs affecting thyroid function tests

Drug	Free thyroxine index	^{131}I uptake	T$_3$ uptake	T$_4$ (Murphy-Pattee)
Ampicillin		−		
Aspirin	−†	−	+	−
Barium		−		
Bromides		−		
Cascara		−		
Chlordiazepoxide		−	−	
Corticosteroids	−	−	+	
Coumarin			+	
Dicumarol			+	
Digitalis		−		
Digitoxin		−		
Heparin			+	−
Levodopa				+
Oral contraceptives	+		−	−
Penicillin		−	+	−
Pentobarbital		−		
Phenylbutazone	−	−	+	
Phenytoin sodium	−		+	+
(Pregnancy)			−	−
Propylthiouracil		−	−	−
Quinidine		−		
Secobarbital		−		
Sulfonamides		−	+	
Thiazides		−		
Thyroid		−	+	

*Sources for the material in these tables are as follows: Davies, D.M., editor: Textbook of adverse drug reactions, New York, 1977, Oxford University Press, Inc.; Wallach, J.: Interpretation of diagnostic tests, ed. 3, Boston, 1978, Little, Brown & Co.; Young, D.S., Pestaner, L.C., and Gibberman, V.: Effects of drugs on clinical laboratory tests, Clin. Chem. **21**(5):240D-399D, 1975.

†+, increased value; −, decreased value; blank, no effect.

DRUGS AFFECTING PROTHROMBIN TIME

Drugs such as salicylates, phenylbutazone, oxyphenbutazone, indometh-acin, and some sulfonamides can displace the anticoagulants from the plas-ma protein to which they are bound. This will make more anticoagulants available, thus increasing the prothrombin time.

Other drugs, such as barbiturates, griseofulvin, and glutethimide, induce the formation of enzymes by the liver that metabolize coumarin and phen-indione derivatives, thus decreasing the prothrombin time. If any of these drugs is withdrawn from a patient who has been stabilized on an anticoagu-lant plus the drug, a critical fall in prothrombin level may result.

Additionally, vitamin K may be suppressed by broad-spectrum anti-biotics and some oral sulfonamides that change the intestinal flora and in-hibit the microorganisms responsible for vitamin K production, thus increas-ing the prothrombin time. By the same token, the patient who is taking vitamin K or daily mineral oil (which enhances vitamin K absorption) may have prothrombin time decreased.

The commonly used drugs affecting prothrombin time are listed in Table D-2.

Table D-2

Most common drugs affecting prothrombin time

Increased time	Comment	Increased time	Comment
Acenocoumarol		Indomethacin	Displaces anticoagu-
Acetaminophen			lants from binding
Allopurinol	Patients on coumarin		proteins
Aminosalicylic acid	Suppresses pro-	Mefenamic acid	Displaces coumarin
	thrombin for-		from albumin
	mation	Mercaptopurine	
Anabolic steroids		Methyldopa	
Aspirin	In large doses	Methylphenidate	Inhibits metabolism
Cathartics			of coumarin
Chloral hydrate	Displaces anticoagu-	Monoamide oxidase	
	lants from albumin	(MAO) inhibitors	
Chloramphenicol	May lower prothrom-	Nalidixic acid	Displaces coumarin
	bin		from albumin
Chlorthalidone	Patients on coumarin	Neomycin	
Clofibrate		Oxyphenbutazone	Displaces anticoagu-
Diazoxide	Displaces anticoagu-		lants from albumin
	lants from albumin	Phenylbutazone	
Dicumarol		Phenyramidol	
Disulfiram	Patients on coumarin	Propylthiouracil	
Diuretics	May prolong action	Quinidine	
	of anticoagulants	Quinine	
Erythromycin		Streptomycin	May decrease vita-
Ethacrynic acid	Patients on coumarin		min K synthesis
Glucagon	Patients on coumarin	Sulfinpyrazone	
Guanethidine		Sulfonamides	
Heparin		Thyroid	
		Tolbutamide	

Decreased time	Comment	Decreased time	Comment
Anabolic steroids		Diuretics	Patients on anticoag-
Antacids	May shorten anti-		ulant
	coagulant action	Ethchlorvynol	Patients on coumarin
Antihistamines	Anticoagulant metab-	Glutethimide	Patients on coumarin
	olism accelerated	Griseofulvin	
Ascorbic acid	Anticoagulant action	Heptabarbital	Anticoagulants me-
	may shorten		tabolized by liver
Aspirin	In small doses	Oral contraceptives	
Barbiturates	Patients on coumarin	Phenobarbital	
Chloral hydrate	Patients on coumarin	Secobarbital	Patients on coumarin
Colchicine	Patients on coumarin	Tetracycline	May partially counter-
Corticosteroids	Anticoagulant metab-		act action of
	olism accelerated		heparin
Cortisone	Patients on coumarin	Vitamin K	

Table D-3

Drugs affecting urinalysis

Test	Increased value	Decreased value
Creatine	Caffeine Methyltestosterone PSP	Anabolic steroids Androgens Thiazides
Creatinine	Ascorbic acid* Corticosteroids Levodopa* Methyldopa* Nitrofurans* PSP*	Anabolic steroids Androgens Thiazides
Diagnex blue excretion	Aluminum salts Barium salts Calcium salts Iron salts Kaolin Magnesium salts Methylene blue* Nicotinic acid Quinacrine* Quinidine* Quinine* Riboflavin* Sodium salts* Vitamin B*	Caffeine benzoate

Glucose	Aminosalicylic acid
	Aspirin
	Corticosteroids
	Ephedrine
	Furosemide
	Phenytoin sodium
		With glucose-oxidase method
		  Ascorbic acid*
		  Aspirin*
		  Levodopa*
		  Mercurial diuretics*
		  Tetracycline*

Hematuria or hemoglobinuria	Acetanilid Acetophenetidin Acetylsalicylic acid Amphotericin B Bacitracin Coumarin Indomethacin Phenylbutazone	
17-Hydroxycorticosteroids	Acetazolamide Chloral hydrate Chlordiazepoxide Chlorpromazine Colchicine Erythromycin Etryptamine Meprobamate	Estrogens Oral contraceptives Phenothiazines Reserpine

*Method-affected.

Table D-3—cont'd
Drugs affecting urinalysis

Test	Increased value	Decreased value
	Oleandomycin Paraldehyde Quinidine Quinine Spironolactone	
17-Ketosteroids	Chloramphenicol Chlorpromazine Cloxacillin Dexamethasone Erythromycin Ethinamate Meprobamate Nalidixic acid Oleandomycin Penicillin Phenaglycodol Phenazopyridine Phenothiazines Quinidine Secobarbital Spironolactone	Chlordiazepoxide Estrogens Meprobamate Metyrapone Probenecid Promazine Reserpine
pH	Aldosterone Parathyroid extract Prolactin Sodium bicarbonate	
Porphyrins (fluorometric method)	Acriflavine Antipyretics Barbiturates Ethoxazene Phenazopyridine Phenylhydrazine Sulfamethoxazole Sulfonamides Tetracycline	
Pregnancy test (DAP test)	False positive Chlorpromazine (frog, rab- bit; immunologic) Phenothiazines (frog, rab- rib; immunologic) Promethazine (Gravindex)	False negative Promethazine
Protein	Drugs causing nephrotoxicity, such as: Aminosalicylic acid Ampicillin Aspirin	

Continued.

Table D-3—cont'd

Drugs affecting urinalysis

Test	Increased value	Decreased value
Protein—cont'd	Bacitracin	
	Cephaloridine	
	Corticosteroids	
	Insecticides	
	Mercurial diuretics	
	Neomycin	
	Penicillin (large doses)	
	Phenylbutazone	
	Radiographic agents (post-aortography)	
	Streptomycin	
	Sulfonamides	
	Turbidimetric procedures*	
	(false positive)	
	Aminosalicylic acid	
	Cephaloridine	
	Chlorpromazine	
	Penicillin (large doses)	
	Promazine	
	Sulfisoxazole	
	Thymol	
Specific gravity	Dextran*	
	(Diurnal variation)	
	Radiographic agents	
	Sucrose*	
Vanillylmandelic acid (VMA)	Aminosalicylic acid*	Clofibrate*
	Aspirin*	Guanethidine analogs
	Bromsulphalein (BSP)	Imipramine
	Glyceryl guaiacolate*	Methyldopa
	Mephenesin*	Monoamine oxidase (MAO) inhibitor
	Nalidixic acid*	
	Oxytetracycline*	
	Penicillin*	
	Phenazopyridine*	
	PSP*	
	Sulfa drugs*	

Table D-4

Drugs affecting blood tests

Test	Increased value	Decreased value
Amylase	Cholinergics Codeine Drugs inducing acute pancreatitis Ethanol Meperidine Methacholine Morphine Oral contraceptives	
Bilirubin	Ajmaline Antimalarials Aspirin Cholinergics Coumarin Ethoxazene Morphine Oral contraceptives Penicillin Phenylbutazone Primaquine Procainamide Quinidine Quinine Radiographic agents Rifampin Streptomycin Sulfa drugs Tetracycline Thiazides	Barbiturates Corticosteroids Phenobarbital Sulfonamides Thioridazine
Calcium	Anabolic steroids Antacids (Ca containing) Calcium gluconate (newborns) Estrogens Hydralazine Oral contraceptives Secretin Thiazides	Corticosteroids Diuretics (mercurial) Gastrin Insulin Laxatives (excess) Mestranol Oral contraceptives Phenytoin sodium (chronic use) Sulfates
Chloride	Chlorothiazide (prolonged therapy) Corticosteroids Guanethidine Marijuana Phenylbutazone	Aldosterone Bicarbonates Corticosteroids Corticotropin Cortisone Diuretics Laxatives (chronic abuse) Prednisolone

Continued.

Table D-4—cont'd

Drugs affecting blood tests

Test	Increased value	Decreased value
Cholesterol	Anabolic steroids	Allopurinol
	Cinchophen	Azathioprine
	Cortisone	Clofibrate
	Epinephrine	Clomiphene
	Heparin (after cessation)	Corticotropin
	Oral contraceptives	Erythromycin
	Phenytoin sodium	Garlic
	(Pregnancy)	Isoniazid
	Promazine	Kanamycin
	Sulfadiazine	MAO inhibitors
	Sulfonamides	Neomycin
	Thiazides	Tetracycline
	Thiouracil	Thiouracil
CO_2 content	Aldosterone	Acetazolamide
	Bicarbonates	Dimercaprol
	Ethacrynic acid	Dimethadione
	Hydrocortisone	Methicillin
	Laxatives (chronic abuse)	Nitrofurantoin
	Metolazone	Phenformin
	Prednisone	Tetracycline
	Thiazides	Triamterene
	Tromethamine	
	Viomycin	
Coombs' test	Positive	
	Chlorpromazine	
	Chlorpropamide	
	Dipyrone	
	Ethosuximide	
	Hydralazine	
	Isoniazid	
	Levodopa	
	Mefenamic acid	
	Melphalan	
	Oxyphenisatin	
	Phenylbutazone	
	Phenytoin sodium	
	Procainamide	
	Quinidine	
	Quinine	
	Streptomycin	
	Sulfonamides	
	Tetracycline	
Creatinine	Clofibrate	
	Clonidine	
	Colistimethate	
	Colistin	
	Doxycycline	

Table D-4—cont'd

Drugs affecting blood tests

Test	Increased value	Decreased value
	Drugs causing nephrotoxicity, such as: Amphotericin B Capreomycin Carbutamide Cephaloridine Chlorthalidone	
Erythrocyte sedimentation rate (ESR)	Dextrans Methyldopa Methysergide Penicillamine Theophylline Trifluperidol Vitamin A	Quinine Salicylates Steroids
Glucose	Aminosalicylic acid Aspirin Caffeine Chlorpromazine Chlorthalidone Coffee Corticosteroids Cortisone Dopamine Ephedrine Epinephrine Estrogens Ethacrynic acid Furosemide Hydralazine Levodopa Phenylbutazone Phenytoin Prednisolone Reserpine Secretin Thiazides Thyroid	Dicumarol Erythromycin Ethacrynic acid Guanethidine Insulin Sulfaphenazole Sulfonamides Sulfonylureas
Lactic dehydrogenase (LDH)	Anesthetic agents Codeine Dicumarol Morphine (Muscular exercise)	
Leucine aminopeptidase	Estrogens Morphine Oral contraceptives (Pregnancy) Thorium dioxide	

Continued.

Table D-4—cont'd

Drugs affecting blood tests

Test	Increased value	Decreased value
Lipase	Cholinergics Codeine Heparin (10 min postinjection) Meperidine Methacholine Morphine Narcotics	Protamine Saline (at molar concentrations)
Phosphate	Anabolic steroids Methicillin Phosphates Phospho-Soda	Alkaline antacids Anticonvulsants Calcitonin Epinephrine Insulin (Menstruation) Oral contraceptives Phenobarbital
Potassium	Amphotericin B Epinephrine Heparin Histamine (IV) Marijuana Methicillin Spironolactone Tetracycline	Aldosterone Amphotericin B Aspirin Bicarbonates Corticosteroids Cortisone Diuretics Ethacrynic acid Furosemide Gentamicin Insulin Licorice Polythiazide Sodium bicarbonate Thiazides
Protein	Anabolic steroids Androgens Corticosteroids Corticotropin Digitalis Epinephrine Insulin Thyroid	Estrogens Oral contraceptives
SGOT/SGPT	Ascorbic acid Cholinergics Codeine Guanethidine Hydralazine Isoniazid Meperidine Morphine Tolbutamide	

Table D-4—cont'd

Drugs affecting blood tests

Test	Increased value	Decreased value
Sodium	Anabolic steroids Bicarbonate Clonidine Corticosteroids Cortisone Estrogens Guanethidine Marijuana Methoxyflurane Oral contraceptives Phenylbutazone Prolactin (IM) Tetracycline	Ammonium chloride Cathartics (excessive) Chlorpropamide Ethacrynic acid Furosemide Mannitol Metolazone Spironolactone Thiazides Triamterene
Triglycerides	Birth control pills Cholestyramine Estrogens	Ascorbic acid Asparaginase Clofibrate Metformin Phenformin
Urea nitrogen (BUN)	Drugs causing nephrotoxicity, and also the following: Anabolic steroids Androgens Arginine Bacitracin Calcium salts Clonidine Dextran Guanethidine Licorice Marijuana Mephenesin Methoxyflurane Methsuximide Metolazone Minocycline	Glucose (Muscular exercise) Paramethasone (Pregnancy)
Uric acid	Acetazolamide Aspirin Ethacrynic acid Furosemide Hydralazine Propylthiouracil Thiazides	Allopurinol Chlorpromazine Cinchophen Clofibrate Corticosteroids Corticotropin Cortisone Coumarin Dicumarol Phenylbutazone Probenecid Radiographic agents

Recommended procedure for necessary contrast studies in patients with history of reaction to contrast material

PREMEDICATION

Items 1 and 2 are recommended for *all patients;* items 3 and 4 are recommended as additional premedication for patients considered to be high risk.*

1. Prednisone (or equivalent steroid) 150 mg/day, in divided doses ($\times$ 24 hr, before the study; $\times$ 12 hr, after the study)
2. Benadryl 25-50 mg slow IVP just before the procedure or 50 mg PO or IM 1 hr before the procedure
3. Methylprednisolone 1 gm IV 1 hr before the study
4. Cimetidine (Tagamet) 300 mg IVPB over 15 min, 30 min before the study (limited experience with this agent)

---

*With combined use of premedications 1, 2, 3, and 4, risk of severe reactions should be substantially less than 1%.

GENERAL PRECAUTIONS

1. Secure IV line.
2. Have airway and bag/valve available for respiratory support.
3. Have anesthesiologist available (in the hospital).
4. Have crash cart available.
5. Observe patient closely for 1 hour *after* the procedure.
6. Obtain informed consent (indicating the need for the study and the fact that the patient is aware of the risks).
7. Skin testing and small graded doses of contrast material are of no diagnostic or predictive value.

ASSESSMENT OF RISK

If patient has history of reaction, and no premedication is given: 15%-30% chance of acute allergic reaction

If patient has history of reaction and premedications 1 and 2 are given: 5%-10% chance of mild reaction; <1% chance of severe reaction

Critical limits (panic values) for laboratory tests and drug levels

The following laboratory values indicate potentially life-threatening situations. When such values are encountered and confirmed, the nurse and the physician responsible for the patient's care should be notified immediately. Sometimes these values are called "panic values." It should be clearly understood, however, that the patient's overall condition and clinical status ultimately determine the significance of these extreme laboratory variations.

In addition to the values listed here, results of all laboratory studies ordered "stat," as well as all positive blood, acid-fast, and cerebrospinal fluid cultures, should be reported immediately to the responsible nurse and physician.

LABORATORY TEST RESULTS

Hemoglobin	<5 gm/dl
Hematocrit	<15%
Platelet count	<30,000/cu mm
Prothrombin time	<10%

Any atypical antibodies detected during cross-matching

Serum sodium	<120 mEq/L or >160 mEq/L
Serum potassium	<3.0 mEq/L or >6.5 mEq/L
Serum glucose	<40 mg/dl or >400 mg/dl
Serum calcium	<6.0 mg/dl or >14.0 mg/dl
Serum magnesium	<1.0 mEq/L or >5.0 mEq/L
Serum lithium	>2.5 mEq/L

DRUG LEVELS

Digoxin	>4.0 ng/ml
Procainamide	>15 μg/ml
Dilantin	>25 μg/ml
Quinidine	>10 μg/ml
Lidocaine	>8 μg/ml
Theophylline	>21 μg/ml
Digitoxin	>40 ng/ml
Disopyramide (Norpace)	>70 μg/ml

BLOOD GAS LEVELS

PO_2	<50 mm Hg
PCO_2	>60 mm Hg
pH	<7.20

References

Anthony, C.P., and Thibodeau, G.A.: Textbook of anatomy and physiology, ed. 10, St. Louis, 1979, The C.V. Mosby Co.

Barrocas, A., and Giardina, M.A.: Nutritional assessment in the community hospital, South. Med. J. **73**(1):55, 1980.

The bio-science handbook, California, 1979, Bio-Science Laboratories.

Blackburn, G.L., and Thornton, P.A.: Nutritional assessment of the hospitalized patient, Med. Clin. North Am. **63**(5):1103, Sept., 1979.

Bordow, R.A., Stool, E.W., and Moser, K.M.: Manual of clinical problems in pulmonary medicine, Boston, 1980, Little, Brown & Co.

Braunwald, E., editor: Heart disease, Philadelphia, 1980, W.B. Saunders Co.

Chang, S.: M-mode echocardiographic techniques and pattern recognition, Philadelphia, 1976, Lea & Febiger.

Conn, H.F., and Conn, R.B., Jr.: Current diagnosis, Philadelphia, 1980, W.B. Saunders Co.

Costello, D., and Glover, M.: Two-dimensional echocardiography, West. J. Med. **135**:112, 1981.

Ennis, C.E., and Andrassy, R.J.: Nutritional management of the surgical patient, AORN J. **31:** 1217, 1980.

Feingenbaum, H.: Echocardiography, ed. 3, Philadelphia, 1981, Lea & Febiger.

Felson, B.: Fundamentals of chest roentgenology, Philadelphia, 1973, W.B. Saunders Co.

Forse, R.A., and Shizgal, H.M.: The assessment of malnutrition, Surgery **88**:17, 1980.

Frankel, S., Reitman, S., and Sonnenwirth, A.C., editors: Gradwohl's clinical laboratory methods and diagnosis: a textbook on laboratory procedures and their interpretation, vols. 1 and 2, ed. 7, St. Louis, 1970, The C.V. Mosby Co.

Guyton, A.C.: Textbook of medical physiology, ed. 5, Philadelphia, 1976, W.B. Saunders Co.

Halsted, J.A., editor: The laboratory in clinical medicine: interpretation and application, Philadelphia, 1976, W.B. Saunders Co.

Harper, H.A.: Review of physiological chemistry, ed. 16, Los Altos, Calif., 1977, Lange Medical Publications.

Henry, J.B., editor: Todd-Sanford and Davidson clinical diagnosis by laboratory methods, ed. 16, Philadelphia, 1979, W.B. Saunders Co.

Hume, M., and Fremont-Smith, P.: Role of noninvasive techniques in diagnosing leg thrombosis, Hosp. Pract. **10**(12):57, 1975.

Hurst, J.W., editor: The heart, ed. 4, New York, 1978, McGraw-Hill Book Co.

Mendel, D.: Practice of cardiac catheterization, ed. 2, Oxford, 1974, Blackwell Scientific Publications, Inc.

Michel, L., Serrano, A., and Malt, R.A.: Nutritional support of hospitalized patients. In Medical intelligence: current concepts, N. Engl. J. Med. **304**:1147, 1981.

Pugatch, R.D., and Faling, L.J.: Computed tomography of the thorax: a status report, Chest **80**(5):618, 1981.

Ravel, R.: Clinical laboratory medicine: application of laboratory data, ed. 2, Chicago, 1973, Year Book Medical Publishers, Inc.

Salmond, S.W.: How to assess the nutritional status of acutely ill patients, Am. J. Nurs. (5): 922, May 1980.

Schottelius, B.A., and Schottelius, D.D.: Textbook of physiology, ed. 18, St. Louis, 1978, The C.V. Mosby Co.

Schwartz, A.R., and Lyons, H.: Acid base and electrolyte balance: normal regulation and clinical disorder, New York, 1977, Grune & Stratton, Inc.

Scully, R.E., editor: Case records of the Massachusetts General Hospital, New Engl. J. Med. **298:**34, Jan. 5, 1978.

Skydell, B., and Crowder, A.S.: Diagnostic procedures: a reference for health practitioners and a guide for patient counseling, Boston, 1975, Little, Brown & Co.

Slisenger, M.H., and Fordtran, J.S.: Gastrointestinal disease, pathophysiology, diagnosis, management, Philadelphia, 1973, W.B. Saunders Co.

Stollerman, G.H., editor: Advances in internal medicine, vols. 18 and 19, Chicago, 1972, Year Book Medical Publishers, Inc.

Strandness, D.E.: Noninvasive evaluation of carotid artery disease, J. Cardiovasc. Med. **5:**841, September, 1980.

Tavell, M.E.: Clinical phonocardiography and external pulse recording, ed. 2, Chicago, 1972, Year Book Medical Publishers, Inc.

Thorn, G.W., and others, editors: Harrison's principles of internal medicine, ed. 7, New York, 1977, McGraw-Hill Book Co.

Usdin, G., and Hawkins, D.R.: The office guide to sleep disorders, New York, 1980, KPR Infor/media Corp.

Weisler, A.M.: Noninvasive cardiology, New York, 1974, Grune & Stratton, Inc.

West, J.B.: Respiratory physiology, ed. 2, Baltimore, 1980, The Williams & Wilkins Co.

Wright, R.A.: Nutritional assessment, J.A.M.A. **244:**559, 1980.

Index

Boldface page numbers indicate main discussion.

Copper—cont'd
  urinary, 348, 367
Coproporphyrins, urinary, 347, 367
  lead poisoning and, 348
Cor pulmonale, 146
Cord compression, 299
Cordarone; *see* Amiodarone
Corgard; *see* Nadolol
Cornea, copper in, 348
Coronary angioplasty, transluminal, **116**
Coronary artery disease
  arteriography in, **116**, 118
  blood lipids and, **94-96**
  blood tests in, 97, 99
  cardiac catheterization and, 116, 117
  echocardiography in, 106
  electrocardiogram and, **69-71**, 72, 74
    exercise, 81, 82
  esophagitis and, 193
  fluoroscopy and, 87
  glucose tolerance test and, 96
  hypercholesterolemia and, 7
  hyperuricemia in, 29
  obstructive
    exercise electrocardiography in infarcts
      with, 82
    myocardial perfusion studies in, 112
  silent, bundle-branch block in, 75
Coronary artery spasm
  arteriography and, 116
  S-T elevations in, 70
Coronary recanalization, transluminal, **116**
Corpus luteum
  luteinizing hormone and, 253
  regressing, 223
Cortex
  adrenal; *see* Adrenal cortex
  renal, **166,** 167
Corticosteroids; *see also* Steroids
  blood tests and, 389, 391, 392, 393
  neutrophils and, 36, 58
  prothrombin time and, 385
  thyroid function tests and, 383
  thyrotropin-releasing hormone and, 230
  urinalysis and, 386
Corticosterone, 238
Corticotropine, 390, 392, 393
Corticotropine-releasing factor, 239, 250
Cortisol, **238**
  in Addison's disease, 248
  adrenal insufficiency and, 242
  and adrenocorticotropic hormone stimula-
    tion, 239, 244, 245
  Cushing's syndrome and, 246

Cortisol—cont'd
  free, 238
    urinary assay of, **241**
  growth hormone deficiency and, 252
  pituitary adenomas and, 251
  plasma, 238, **240-241,** 360
    in Addison's disease, 248
    in adrenocorticotropic hormone stimula-
      tion test, 244
    dexamethasone suppression test and, 244
    diurnal variation of, 240-241
    hypothalamus and, 239
  as regulator
    of adrenocorticotropic hormone, 239
    of corticotropic-releasing hormone, 239
  renal function and, **169,** 241
  sleep and, 333
  test for production of, 243
Cortisone
  adrenocorticotropic hormone and, 222
  blood tests and, 389, 390, 391, 392, 393
  eosinophils and, 59
  leukopenia and, 34
  prothrombin time and, 385
Cosyntropin, 244; *see also* Adrenocorticotropic
    hormone
Cough
  bronchitis and, 161
  restrictive lung disease and, 163
Coulter panel, **38**
Coumadin, 179
Coumarins, 179
  blood tests and, 389, 391, 393
  prothrombin time and, 98, 265
    drugs and, 384
  thyroid function tests and, 383
  urinalysis and, 386
Cow's milk, 26
Coxsackie A and B viruses, 325
CPA, **107-109, 126;** *see also* Carotid arteries
Cramps, abdominal, 205
Creat; *see* Creatinine
Creatine, 360
  hyperuricemia with, 29
  urinary, 367
    drugs and, 386
Creatine kinase, **91-93**
Creatine phosphokinase, serum, 360
  Duchenne dystrophy and, 299
  muscle disease and, 305, 308
Creatinine, 53
  clearance of; *see* Creatinine clearance
  electrolytes and, 9
  glomerular disease and, 26

Conversion factors to SI units for some biochemical components of blood*

Component	Normal range in units as customarily reported	Conversion factor	Normal range in SI units, molecular units, international units, or decimal fractions
Acetoacetic acid (S)	0.2-1.0 mg/dL	98	19.6-98.0 μmol/L
Acetone (S)	0.3-2.0 mg/dL	172	51.6-344.0 μmol/L
Albumin (S)	3.2-4.5 g/dL	10	32-45 g/L
Ammonia (P)	20-120 μg/dL	0.588	11.7-70.5 μmol/L
Amylase (S)	60-160 Somogyi units/dL	1.85	111-296 U/L
Base, total (S)	145-160 mEq/L	1	145-160 mmol/L
Bicarbonate (P)	21-28 mEq/L	1	21-28 mmol/L
Bile acids (S)	0.3-3.0 mg/dL	10	3-30 mg/L
		2.547	0.8-7.6 μmol/L
Bilirubin, direct (S)	Up to 0.3 mg/dL	17.1	Up to 5.1 μmol/L
Bilirubin, indirect (S)	0.1-1.0 mg/dL	17.1	1.7-17.1 μmol/L
Blood gases (B)			
P_{CO_2} arterial	35-40 mm Hg	0.133	4.66-5.32 kPa
P_{O_2} arterial	95-100 mm Hg	0.133	12.64-13.30 kPa
Calcium (S)	8.5-10.5 mg/dL	0.25	2.1-2.6 mmol/L
Chloride (S)	95-103 mEq/L	1	95-103 mmol/L
Creatine (S)	0.1-0.4 mg/dL	76.3	7.6-30.5 μmol/L
Creatinine (S)	0.6-1.2 mg/dL	88.4	53-106 μmol/L
Creatinine clearance (P)	107-139 mL/min	0.0167	1.78-2.32 mL/s
Fatty acids (total) (S)	8-20 mg/dL	0.01	0.08-2.00 mg/L
Fibrinogen (P)	200-400 mg/dL	0.01	2.00-4.00 g/L
Gamma globulin (S)	0.5-1.6 g/dL	10	5-16 g/L
Globulins (total) (S)	2.3-3.5 g/dL	10	23-35 g/L
Glucose (fasting) (S)	70-110 mg/dL	0.055	3.85-6.05 mmol/L
Insulin (radioimmuno-	4-24 μIU/mL	0.0417	0.17-1.00 μg/L
assay) (P)	0.20-0.84 μg/L	172.2	35-145 pmol/L
Iodine, BEI (S)	3.5-6.5 μg/dL	0.079	0.28-0.51 μmol/L
Iodine, PBI (S)	4.0-8.0 μg/dL	0.079	0.32-0.63 μmol/L
Iron, total (S)	60-150 μg/dL	0.179	11-27 μmol/L
Iron-binding capacity (S)	300-360 μg/dL	0.179	54-64 μmol/L
17-Ketosteroids (P)	25-125 μg/dL	0.01	0.25-1.25 mg/L
Lactic dehydrogenase (S)	80-120 units at 30 °C	0.48	38-62 U/L at 30 °C
	Lactate → pyruvate		
	100-190 U/L at 37 °C	1	100-190 U/L at 37 °C
Lipase (S)	0-1.5 U/mL	278	0-417 U/L
	(Cherry-Crandall)		
Lipids (total) (S)	400-800 mg/dL	0.01	4.00-8.00 g/L
Cholesterol	150-250 mg/dL	0.026	3.9-6.5 mmol/L
Triglycerides	75-165 mg/dL	0.0114	0.85-1.89 mmol/L
Phospholipids	150-380 mg/dL	0.01	1.50-380 g/L
Free fatty acids	9.0-15.0 mM/L	1	9.0-15.0 mmol/L

*This is a selected (not a complete) list of biochemical components. The ranges listed may differ from those accepted in some laboratories and are shown to illustrate the conversion factor and the method of expression in SI molecular units. For a more complete listing, see Henry, J.B., editor: Todd-Sanford-Davidsohn clinical diagnosis and management by laboratory methods, ed. 16, Philadelphia, W.B. Saunders Co.

Continued.

491

Conversion factors to SI units for some biochemical components of blood—cont'd

Component	Normal range in units as customarily reported	Conversion factor	Normal range in SI units, molecular units, international units, or decimal fractions
Nonprotein nitrogen (S)	20-35 mg/dL	0.714	14.3-25.0 mmol/L
Phosphatase (P)			
Acid (units/dL)	Cherry-Crandall	2.77	0-5.5 U/L
	King-Armstrong	1.77	0-5.5 U/L
	Bodansky	5.37	0-5.5 U/L
Alkaline (units/dL)	King-Armstrong	1.77	30-120 U/L
	Bodansky	5.37	30-120 U/L
	Bessey-Lowry-Brock	16.67	30-120 U/L
Phosphorus, inorganic (S)	3.0-4.5 mg/dL	0.323	0.97-1.45 mmol/L
Potassium (P)	3.8-5.0 mEq/L	1	3.8-5.0 mmol/L
Proteins, total (S)	6.0-7.8 g/dL	10	60-78 g/L
Albumin	3.2-4.5 g/dL	10	32-45 g/L
Globulin	2.3-3.5 g/dL	10	23-35 g/L
Sodium (P)	136-142 mEq/L	1	136-142 mmol/L
Testosterone: Male (S)	300-1,200 ng/dL	0.035	10.5-42.0 nmol/L
Female	30-95 ng/dL	0.035	1.0-3.3 nmol/L
Thyroid tests (S)			
Thyroxine (T_4)	4-11 μg/dL	12.87	51-142 nmol/L
T_4 expressed as iodine	3.2-7.2 μg/dL	79.0	253-569 nmol/L
T_3 resin uptake	25%-38% relative uptake	0.01	0.25%-0.38% relative uptake
TSH (S)	10 μU/mL	1	$<10^{-3}$ IU/L
Urea nitrogen (S)	8-23 mg/dL	0.357	2.9-8.2 mmol/L
Uric acid (S)	2-6 mg/dL	59.5	0.120-0.360 mmol/L
Vitamin B_{12} (S)	160-950 pg/mL	0.74	118-703 pmol/L

Some hematology values*

Component	Normal range in units as customarily reported	Conversion factor	Normal range in SI units, molecular units, international units, or decimal fractions
Red cell volume (male)	25-35 mL/kg body weight	0.001	0.025-0.035 L/kg body weight
Hematocrit	40%-50%	0.01	0.40-0.50
Hemoglobin	13.5-18.0 g/dL	10	135-180 g/L
Hemoglobin	13.5-18.0 g/dL	0.155	2.09-2.79 mmol/L
RBC count	4.5-6 × 10^6/μL	1	4.6-6 × 10^{12}/L
WBC count	4.5-10 × 10^3/μL	1	4.5-10 × 10^9/L
Mean corpuscular volume	80-96 μm^3	1	80-96 fL

*The International Committee for Standardization in Hematology recommends that the numbers remain the same but that the units change, so that hemoglobin is expressed as grams per deciliter (g/dL) even though other measurements are expressed as units per liter (U/L).

Equivalent values of kPa and mm Hg units*

kPa	0.1	0.2	0.3	0.4	0.5	0.6	0.7	0.8	0.9
mm Hg	0.750	1.50	2.25	3.00	3.75	4.50	5.25	6.00	6.75

kPa	mm Hg	kPa	mm Hg
1	7.50	21	158
2	15.0	22	165
3	22.5	23	172
4	30.0	24	180
5	37.5	25	188
6	45.0	26	195
7	52.5	27	202
8	60.0	29	210
9	67.5	29	218
10	75.0	30	225
11	82.5	31	232
12	90.0	32	240
13	97.5	33	248
14	105	34	255
15	112	35	262
16	120	36	270
17	128	37	278
18	135	38	285
19	142	39	292
20	150	40	300

*From World Health Organization: The SI for the health professions, Geneva, 1977, The Organization, p. 40.